Critical Skills and Procedures in Emergency Medicine

Editors

JORGE L. FALCON-CHEVERE
JOSE G. CABANAS

EMERGENCY MEDICINE
CLINICS OF NORTH AMERICA

www.emed.theclinics.com

Consulting Editor
AMAL MATTU

February 2013 • Volume 31 • Number 1

ELSEVIER

1600 John F. Kennedy Boulevard • Suite 1800 • Philadelphia, Pennsylvania 19103-2899

http://www.theclinics.com

EMERGENCY MEDICINE CLINICS OF NORTH AMERICA Volume 31, Number 1
February 2013 ISSN 0733-8627, ISBN-13: 978-1-4557-4938-6

Editor: Patrick Manley
Developmental Editor: Donald Mumford

Emergency Medicine Clinics of North America (ISSN 0733-8627) is published quarterly by Elsevier Inc., 360 Park Avenue South, New York, NY, 10010-1710. Months of issue are February, May, August, and November. Business and Editorial Offices: 1600 John F. Kennedy Boulevard, Suite 1800, Philadelphia, PA 19103-2899. Customer Service Office: 6277 Sea Harbor Drive, Orlando, FL 32887-4800. Periodicals postage paid at New York, NY, and additional mailing offices. Subscription prices are $142.00 per year (US students), $281.00 per year (US individuals), $478.00 per year (US institutions), $201.00 per year (international students), $404.00 per year (international individuals), $576.00 per year (international institutions), $201.00 per year (Canadian students), $347.00 per year (Canadian individuals), and $576.00 per year (Canadian institutions). International air speed delivery is included in all *Clinics'* subscription prices. All prices are subject to change without notice. **POSTMASTER:** Send address changes to *Emergency Medicine Clinics of North America*, Elsevier Periodicals Customer Service, 11830 Westline Industrial Drive, St. Louis, MO 63146. Customer Service (orders, claims, online, change of address): Elsevier Periodicals Customer Service, 11830 Westline Industrial Drive, St. Louis, MO 63146. Tel: 1-800-654-2452 (U.S. and Canada); 314-453-7041 (outside U.S. and Canada). Fax: 314-453-5170. E-mail: journalscustomerservice-usa@elsevier.com (for print support); journalsonline support-usa@elsevier.com (for online support).

Reprints. For copies of 100 or more of articles in this publication, please contact the Commercial Reprints Department, Elsevier Inc., 360 Park Avenue South, New York, NY 10010-1710. Tel.: 212-633-3812; Fax: 212-462-1935; E-mail: reprints@elsevier.com.

Emergency Medicine Clinics of North America is covered in *MEDLINE/PubMed (Index Medicus)*, *Current Contents/Clinical Medicine*, *EMBASE/Excerpta Medica*, *BIOSIS*, *SciSearch*, *CINAHL*, *ISI/BIOMED*, and *Research Alert*.

Printed and bound by CPI Group (UK) Ltd, Croydon, CR0 4YY

Transferred to digital print 2012

Contributors

CONSULTING EDITOR

AMAL MATTU, MD
Professor and Vice Chair, Department of Emergency Medicine, University of Maryland School of Medicine, Baltimore, Maryland

GUEST EDITORS

JORGE L. FALCON-CHEVERE, MD, FAAEM, FACEP
Program Director and Assistant Professor, Emergency Medicine Department, University of Puerto Rico School of Medicine, San Juan, Carolina, Puerto Rico

JOSE G. CABANAS, MD, FACEP
Assistant Professor, Emergency Medicine Residency, University Medical Center Brackenridge, UT Southwestern at Austin; Deputy Medical Director, Austin, Texas

AUTHORS

ANGELISSE ALMODOVAR, MD
Senior Resident, Department of Emergency Medicine, Hospital UPR Dr Federico Trilla, University of Puerto Rico School of Medicine, Carolina, Puerto Rico

STUART E. BOSS, MD
Resident, Department of Emergency Medicine, The University of Texas Medical School at Houston, Houston, Texas

ISABEL BREA, MD
Clinical Instructor and Emergency Medical Services Fellow, Department of Emergency Medicine, Life Lion and Critical Care Transport, Penn State Hershey Medical Center, College of Medicine, Hershey, Pennsylvania

PAV BRECKON, MD
Chief Resident, Emergency Medicine Residency, Florida Hospital, Orlando, Florida

JANE H. BRICE, MD, MPH
Department of Emergency Medicine, University of North Carolina, Chapel Hill, North Carolina

KRIS CHILES, MD
Department of Emergency Medicine, Florida Hospital-East Orlando, Orlando, Florida

STEPHANIE A. CRAPO, MD
Resident Physician, Department of Emergency Medicine, University of North Carolina, Chapel Hill, North Carolina

JORGE L. FALCON-CHEVERE, MD, FAAEM, FACEP
Program Director and Assistant Professor, Department of Emergency Medicine, University of Puerto Rico School of Medicine, Carolina, Puerto Rico

LAUREANO GIRALDEZ, MD
Chief Resident, Department of Otolaringology, University of Puerto Rico School of Medicine, San Juan, Puerto Rico

ERIC HAWKINS, MD, MPH
Department of Emergency Medicine, Carolinas Medical Center, Charlotte, North Carolina

HEATHER HEATON, MD
Department of Emergency Medicine, University of North Carolina Hospitals, Chapel Hill, North Carolina

CHARLOTTE HENNINGSEN, MS
Adjunct Faculty, Sonography Department, Florida Hospital College; Adjunct Faculty, Immediate Past President SDMS, EM Residency Program, FL Hospital, Orlando, Florida

CALVIN HUANG, MD, MPH
Ultrasound Fellow, Research Fellow, Massachusetts General Hospital, Boston, Massachusetts

ANITA J. L'ITALIEN, MD
Attending Physician, Department of Emergency Medicine, Wake Emergency Physicians, PA, Raleigh; Associate Professor, Department of Emergency Medicine, University of North Carolina, Chapel Hill, North Carolina

GEMMA C. LEWIS, MD
Resident Physician, Department of Emergency Medicine, University of North Carolina, Chapel Hill, North Carolina

RESA E. LEWISS, MD
Director of Emergency Ultrasound Division, Department of Emergency Medicine, St. Luke's Roosevelt Hospital Center, New York, New York

SAMUEL D. LUBER, MD, MPH, FACEP
Assistant Professor, Department of Emergency Medicine, The University of Texas Medical School at Houston, Houston, Texas

CHARLES MADDOW, MD, FACEP
Associate Professor, Department of Emergency Medicine, The University of Texas Medical School at Houston, Houston, Texas

JENNIFER A. MARTIN, MD
Emergency Ultrasound Fellow, Department of Emergency Medicine, St. Luke's Roosevelt Hospital Center, New York, New York

DANA MATHEW, MD
Staff Emergency Physician, Wake Emergency Physicians, WakeMed Health & Hospitals, Raleigh; Adjunct Clinical Professor, Emergency Medicine, University of North Carolina, Chapel Hill, North Carolina

ROBERTO MEDERO-COLON, MD
Department of Emergency Medicine, University of Puerto Rico School of Medicine, Carolina, Puerto Rico

AMIT M. MEHTA, MD
Resident, Department of Emergency Medicine, The University of Texas Medical School at Houston, Houston, Texas

BRIAN MENDEZ, MD
Department of Emergency Medicine, University of Puerto Rico, San Juan, Puerto Rico

LORRAINE MENDEZ-CARRENO, MD
Department of Emergency Medicine, University of Puerto Rico School of Medicine, Carolina, Puerto Rico

JOANNA MERCADO, MD, MSc
Assistant Professor and Research Section Director, Department of Emergency Medicine, University of Puerto Rico, San Juan, Puerto Rico

ALISON MURPHY, MD
Department of Pediatric Emergency Medicine, Wolfson Children's Hospital, Jacksonville, Florida

HAWNWAN PHILIP MOY, MD
Department of Emergency Department, Barnes Jewish Hospital, Washington University School of Medicine, Saint Louis, Missouri

MICHAEL C. MURPHY, MD
Clinical Instructor and Director of Emergency Ultrasound, Department of Emergency Medicine, Mount Auburn Hospital, Harvard Medical School, Cambridge, Massachusetts

ARUN NAGDEV, MD
Director of Emergency Ultrasound and Assistant Clinical Professor of Emergency Medicine, Ultrasound Fellowship Director, Department of Emergency Medicine, Highland General Hospital, University of California, Oakland, California

VICKI E. NOBLE, MD
Chief and Associate Professor, Emergency Ultrasound Division, Department of Emergency Medicine, Massachusetts General Hospital, Harvard University, Boston, Massachusetts

HILSA QUINONES, MD
Department of Emergency Medicine, University of Puerto Rico, San Juan, Puerto Rico

MARIA R. RAMOS-FERNANDEZ, MD, FACEP
Assistant Professor and Assistant Program Director, Department of Emergency Medicine, University of Puerto Rico School of Medicine, Carolina, Puerto Rico

EVAN RICHARDS, MS-IV
2nd Lt, USAF, Uniformed Services University, San Antonio, Texas

JOSE O. RIVERA-RIVERA, MD
Chief Resident, Department of Emergency Medicine, University of Puerto Rico School of Medicine, Carolina, Puerto Rico

DAVID RODRIGUEZ, MD
Department of Emergency Medicine, University of Puerto Rico, San Juan, Puerto Rico

FERNANDO SOTO, MD
Assistant Professor in Emergency Medicine and Emergency Medicine Clerkship Director, Pediatric Emergency Medicine Section, University of Puerto Rico School of Medicine, San Juan, Puerto Rico

ADAM SIVITZ, MD
Director of Pediatric Emergency Medicine Education, Newark Beth Israel Medical Center, The Children's Hospital of New Jersey, New Jersey

TITO SUERO-SALVADOR, MD
Senior Resident, Department of Emergency Medicine, University of Puerto Rico School of Medicine, Carolina, Puerto Rico

ALFREDO TIRADO, MD
Assistant Medical Director, EM US Director for Florida Emergency Physicians, EM Residency Program, FL Hospital, Orlando, Florida

MARIA UZCATEGUI-CORDER, MD
Chief Resident, Department of Emergency Medicine, Hospital UPR Dr Federico Trilla, University of Puerto Rico School of Medicine, Carolina, Puerto Rico

JEFFERSON G. WILLIAMS, MD, MPH
Clinical Assistant Professor, Department of Emergency Medicine, University of North Carolina, Chapel Hill; Associate Medical Director, Wake County Emergency Medical Services; Associate Director of Medical Services, North Carolina State Highway Patrol, Raleigh, North Carolina

TERESA WU, MD
Director, EM Ultrasound Program and Fellowship, Co-Director, Simulation Program and Fellowship, Associate Program Director, EM Residency Program, Department of Emergency Medicine, Maricopa Medical Center, College of Medicine, University of Arizona, Phoenix, Arizona

Contents

Foreword: Critical Skills and Procedures xiii

Amal Mattu

Preface xv

Jorge L. Falcon-Chevere and Jose G. Cabanas

Critical Airway Skills and Procedures 1

Eric Hawkins, Hawnwan Philip Moy, and Jane H. Brice

> Airway management is a critical procedure and essential skill necessary for all physicians working in the emergency department. Optimal resuscitative treatment of medical and trauma patients often revolves around timely and effective airway interventions that can be challenging in the acute setting, especially in critical patients. Time-honored airway techniques and procedures combined with recent advances in rapid sequence intubation, video laryngoscopy, and further advanced airway techniques now offer emergency clinicians a wide range of exciting new options for improving this crucial component of acute care and management.

Critical ENT Skills and Procedures in the Emergency Department 29

Jorge L. Falcon-Chevere, Laureano Giraldez, Jose O. Rivera-Rivera, and Tito Suero-Salvador

> Injuries and illness to the ears, nose, and throat are frequently seen in the emergency department. The emergency medicine physician must be proficient in recognizing these injuries and their associated complications and be able to provide appropriate management. This article discusses the most common otorrhinolaringologic procedures in which emergency physicians must be proficient for rapid intervention to preserve function and avoid complications. A description of each procedure is discussed, as well as the indications, contraindications, equipment, technique and potential complications.

Critical Skills and Procedures in Emergency Medicine: Vascular Access Skills and Procedures 59

Gemma C. Lewis, Stephanie A. Crapo, and Jefferson G. Williams

> The venous and/or arterial vasculature may be accessed for fluid resuscitation, testing and monitoring, administration of blood product or medication, or procedural reasons, such as the implantation of cardiac pacemaker wires. Accessing the vascular system is a common and often critically important step in emergency patient care. This article reviews methods for peripheral, central venous, and arterial access and discusses adjunct skills for vascular access such as the use of ultrasound guidance, and other forms of vascular access such as intraosseus and umbilical cannulation, and peripheral venous cut-down. Mastery of these skills is critical for the emergency medicine provider.

Ultrasound-Guided Procedures in the Emergency Department—Needle Guidance and Localization   87

Alfredo Tirado, Arun Nagdev, Charlotte Henningsen, Pav Breckon, and Kris Chiles

Ultrasound has rapidly become an essential tool in the emergency department, specifically in procedural guidance. Its use has been demonstrated to improve the success rate of procedures, while decreasing complications. In this article, we explore some of these specific procedures involving needle guidance and structure localization with ultrasound.

Ultrasound-Guided Procedures in the Emergency Department—Diagnostic and Therapeutic Asset   117

Alfredo Tirado, Teresa Wu, Vicki E. Noble, Calvin Huang, Resa E. Lewiss, Jennifer A. Martin, Michael C. Murphy, and Adam Sivitz

Bedside ultrasound is an extremely valuable and rapidly accessible diagnostic and therapeutic modality in potentially life- and limb-threatening situations in the emergency department. In this report, the authors discuss the role of ultrasound in quick assessment of pathologic conditions and its use to aid in diagnostic and therapeutic interventions.

Critical Cardiovascular Skills and Procedures in the Emergency Department   151

Anita J. L'Italien

The management of cardiovascular emergencies is a fundamental component of the practice of an emergency practitioner. Delays in the evaluations and management can lead to significant morbidity or mortality. It is of vital importance to be familiar with procedures such as pericardiocentesis, cardioversion, defibrillation, temporary pacing, and options for the management of tachyarrhythmias. This article discusses the most common cardiovascular procedures encountered in an emergency setting, including the indications, contraindications, equipment, technique, and complications for each procedure.

Critical Obstetric and Gynecologic Procedures in the Emergency Department   207

Joanna Mercado, Isabel Brea, Brian Mendez, Hilsa Quinones, and David Rodriguez

Obstetric and gynecologic emergencies are common reasons for emergency department visits. Therefore, emergency physicians must be proficient in the management and treatment of these emergencies. This article reviews critical procedures and provides an overview of each procedure and the indications, contraindications, technique, and potential complications.

Critical Urologic Skills and Procedures in the Emergency Department   237

Maria R. Ramos-Fernandez, Roberto Medero-Colon, and Lorraine Mendez-Carreno

The evaluation and management of genitourinary emergencies is a fundamental component of the training and practice of emergency physicians. Urologic procedures are common in the emergency room. Emergency physicians play a vital role in the initial evaluation and treatment because delays in management can lead to permanent damage. This article discusses the most common urologic procedures in which emergency physicians must be proficient for rapid intervention to preserve function and avoid complications. An overview of each procedure is discussed as well as indications, contraindications, equipment, technique, and potential complications.

Critical Orthopedic Skills and Procedures 261

Stuart E. Boss, Amit Mehta, Charles Maddow, and Samuel D. Luber

Musculoskeletal injury and diseases are common presentations in the Emergency Department. Emergency physicians must be versed in the critical procedural skills necessary to diagnose joint infection, manage fractures and dislocations, and assess for compartment syndrome. Arthrocentesis, splinting, dislocation reduction, and the evaluation of limb compartment syndrome are reviewed.

Critical Trauma Skills and Procedures in the Emergency Department 291

Jorge L. Falcon-Chevere, Joanna Mercado, Dana Mathew, Maria Uzcategui-Corder, Angelisse Almodovar, and Evan Richards

Injuries and illness associated with major trauma that require lifesaving procedures, such as surgical airway, chest tube thoracotomy, emergency department thoracotomy, early recognition and treatment of compartment syndrome, and venous cutdown, are seen in the emergency department. The emergency medicine physician must be proficient in recognizing these injuries and their associated complications and be able to provide appropriate management. This article discusses the most common trauma-related procedures in which emergency physicians must be proficient. A description of each procedure is discussed as well as the indications, contraindications, equipment, technique, and potential complications.

Critical Procedures in Pediatric Emergency Medicine 335

Fernando Soto, Alison Murphy, and Heather Heaton

Children comprise approximately one-quarter of all visits to most emergency departments. Children are generally healthier than adults, yet there are similar priorities in assessment and management of pediatric patients. The initial approach to airway, breathing, and circulation still applies and is first and foremost in the evaluation of young infants and children. There are certain anatomic, physiologic, developmental, and social considerations that are unique to this population and must be taken into account during their evaluation and treatment. In this review, we present and discuss an evidence-based approach to high-yield procedures necessary for all emergency physicians taking care of children.

Index 377

Critical Skills and Procedures in Emergency Medicine

EMERGENCY MEDICINE CLINICS OF NORTH AMERICA

FORTHCOMING ISSUES

May 2013
Head, Ears, Eyes, Nose, and Throat Emergencies
Alisa Gibson, MD, and Kip Benko, MD, *Guest Editors*

August 2013
Pediatric Emergency Medicine
Mimi Lu, MD, Dale Woolridge, MD, PhD, and Ann Dietrich, MD, *Guest Editors*

November 2013
Dangerous Fever in the Emergency Department
Emilie Calvello MD and Christian Theodosis MD, *Guest Editors*

RECENT ISSUES

November 2012
OB/GYN Emergencies
Kathleen Wittels, MD, and Sarah Sommerkamp, MD, *Guest Editors*

August 2012
Acute Ischemic Stroke
Lauren M. Nentwich, MD, Brendan G. Magauran Jr, MD, and Joseph H. Kahn, MD, *Guest Editors*

May 2012
Thoracic Emergencies
Joel Turner, MD, *Guest Editor*

PROGRAM OBJECTIVE:
The goal of *Emergency Medicine Clinics of North America* is to keep practicing emergency medicine physicians and emergency medicine residents up to date with current clinical practice in emergency medicine by providing timely articles reviewing the state of the art in patient care.

TARGET AUDIENCE
All practicing physicians and healthcare professionals who provide patient care utilizing findings from *Emergency Medicine Clinics of North America*.

ACCREDITATION
The Elsevier Office of Continuing Medical Education (EOCME) is accredited by the Accreditation Council for Continuing Medical Education (ACCME) to provide continuing medical education for physicians.

The EOCME designates this journal-based CME activity for a maximum of 11 *AMA PRA Category 1 Credit*(s)™. Physicians should claim only the credit commensurate with the extent of their participation in the activity.

All other health care professionals completing continuing education credit for this activity will be issued a certificate of participation.

DISCLOSURE OF CONFLICTS OF INTEREST
The EOCME assesses conflict of interest with its instructors, faculty, planners, and other individuals who are in a position to control the content of CME activities. All relevant conflicts of interest that are identified are thoroughly vetted by EOCME for fair balance, scientific objectivity, and patient care recommendations. EOCME is committed to providing its learners with CME activities that promote improvements or quality in healthcare and not a specific proprietary business or a commercial interest.

The planning committee, staff, authors and editors listed below have identified no financial relationships or relationships to products or devices they or their spouse/life partner have with commercial interest related to the content of this CME activity:
Angelisse Almodovar, MD; Stuart E. Boss, MD; Isabel Brea, MD; Pav Breckon, MD; Jane H. Brice, MD, MPH; Jose G. Cabanas, MD, FACEP; Kris Chiles, MD; Stephanie A. Crapo, MD; Jorge L. Falcon-Chevere, MD; Jeannette Forcina; Laureano Giraldez, MD; Eric Hawkins, MD, MPH; Heather Heaton, MD; Charlotte Henningsen, MS; Calvin Huang, MD, MPH; Anita J. L'Italien, MD; Gemma C. Lewis, MD; Resa E. Lewiss, MD; Samuel D. Luber, MD, MPH; Charles Maddow, MD; Jennifer A. Martin, MD; Dana Mathew, MD; Amal Mattu, MD; Jill McNair; Roberto Medero-Colon, MD; Amit Mehta, MD; Brian Mendez, MD; Lorraine Mendez-Carreno, MD; Joanna Mercado, MD, MSc; Hawnwan Philip Moy, MD; Alison Murphy, MD; Michael C. Murphy, MD; Arun Nagdev, MD; Vicki E. Noble, MD; Nagaraj Paramasivam; Hilsa Quinones, MD; Maria R. Ramos-Fernandez, MD; Evan Richards, MS-IV; Jose O. Rivera-Rivera, MD; David Rodriguez, MD; Adam Sivitz, MD; Fernando Soto, MD; Katelynn Steck; Tito Suero-Salvador, MD; Alfredo Tirado, MD; Maria Uzcategui-Corder, MD; Jefferson G. Williams, MD, MPH; and Teresa Wu, MD.

UNAPPROVED/OFF-LABEL USE DISCLOSURE
The EOCME requires CME faculty to disclose to the participants:

1. When products or procedures being discussed are off-label, unlabelled, experimental, and/or investigational (not US Food and Drug Administration (FDA) approved; and
2. Any limitations on the information presented, such as data that are preliminary or that represent ongoing research, interim analyses, and/or unsupported opinions. Faculty may discuss information about pharmaceutical agents that is outside of DA-approved labelling. This information is intended solely for CME and is not intended to promote off-label use of these medications. If you have any questions, contact the medical affairs department of the manufacturer for the most recent prescribing information.

TO ENROLL
To enroll in the *Emergency Medicine Clinics* Continuing Medical Education program, call customer service at 1-800-654-2452 or sign up online at http://www.theclinics.com/home/cme. The CME program is available to subscribers for an additional annual fee of $212.

METHOD OF PARTICIPATION
In order to claim credit, participants must complete the following:

1. Complete enrolment as indicated above.
2. Read the activity.
3. Complete the CME Test and Evaluation. Participants must achieve a score of 70% on the test. All CME Tests and Evaluations must be completed online.

CME INQUIRIES/SPECIAL NEEDS
For all CME inquiries or special needs, please contact elsevierCME@elsevier.com.

Foreword

Critical Skills and Procedures

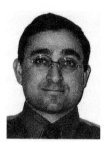

Amal Mattu, MD
Consulting Editor

Any practicing emergency physician will attest that emergency medicine is a procedure-oriented specialty. Although there is a great deal of internal medicine and pediatric medicine that makes up the routine practice of this specialty, emergency medicine is often considered the primary interface between these more cerebral specialties and the very hands-on surgical specialties. On any given day, an emergency physician may perform basic and advanced forms of vascular access, endotracheal intubation, placement of a transvenous pacemaker, joint dislocation reductions, tube thoracostomy, or thoracotomy. In fact, as our specialty has evolved, the scope of procedures that we "own" and train our residents to perform has increased remarkably. A notable difference between emergency medicine practice in the United States versus emergency medicine practice in countries that are still struggling to develop the specialty lies in the extent of procedural competency of the practitioners. Procedural competency is critical to the development of our specialty.

Not surprisingly, emergency medicine residency programs in the United States are required to closely track procedures performed among the trainees, and a major portion of the emergency medicine Core Curriculum is focused on procedural competency. Cadaver-based and simulation-based procedure courses are common in residencies as well as in continuing medical education courses around the country. These courses target the more experienced practitioners who seek to update their skills and knowledge regarding procedures. Several textbooks and journals in emergency medicine now provide online video training in procedures as well. The numerous venues for learning procedures reflect the importance of procedural competency in our specialty. A well-trained emergency physician must be competent at performing a multitude of emergency procedures. A poorly trained emergency physician, on the other hand, is forced to repeatedly consult other services to perform procedures, resulting in delays in patient care and potential adverse outcomes.

Fortunately for those seeking to increase their knowledge in emergency medicine procedures, guest editors Drs Cabanas and Falcon-Chevere have assembled an

Emerg Med Clin N Am 31 (2013) xiii–xiv
http://dx.doi.org/10.1016/j.emc.2012.09.012
emed.theclinics.com

outstanding group of emergency care providers to bring you the latest regarding the critical procedural skills that emergency physicians must have for optimal practice in today's emergency departments. Articles discuss procedures that experienced clinicians would consider "bread and butter," such as vascular access, basic trauma and obstetric/gynecological skills, ear-nose-throat procedures, and orthopedic reductions. But other articles are also devoted to more challenging and advanced topics, such as advanced vascular access; cardiovascular procedures; and more challenging trauma, obstetric, and pediatric airway skills. These are often the procedures that create anxiety in even the most experienced practitioners. Two additional articles are provided that focus on the use of bedside ultrasound as a diagnostic test and to assist in other procedures in order to decrease complications. The frequent use of charts, boxes, and tables within the text makes for easy and quick reading so that the issue can be used in real-time, even in a busy Emergency Department.

This issue of *Emergency Medicine Clinics of North America* represents an important addition to the emergency medicine literature. Drs Cabanas, Falcon-Chevere, and their colleagues have provided an important and practical resource for either quick use or for more in-depth reference when caring for patients in a busy Emergency Department. Emergency care providers in every type of practice setting will find this issue immensely useful. Kudos to the contributors for an outstanding issue!

Amal Mattu, MD
Department of Emergency Medicine
University of Maryland School of Medicine
110 South Paca Street, Sixth Floor, Suite 200
Baltimore, MD 21201, USA

E-mail address:
AMattu@smail.umaryland.edu

Preface

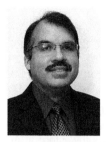 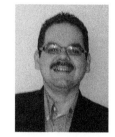

Jorge L. Falcon-Chevere, MD, Jose G. Cabanas, MD, FACEP
      FAAEM, FACEP

Guest Editors

This edition of *Emergency Medicine Clinics of North America* is focused on critical skills and procedures emergency medicine physicians must master while providing care to ill or injured patients. Emergency physicians are sometimes faced with difficult clinical challenges, which require immediate procedural intervention in order to preserve life, which, added to the sometimes limited access to specialties and subspecialty consultants in the emergency department, makes this issue a most valuable one.

Our goal was to focus on critical procedures performed by emergency clinicians during the evaluation and treatment of common and challenging conditions that present to the emergency department. A comprehensive emergency procedures curriculum was assembled. It includes important topics such as difficult airway, ultrasound-guided procedures, and trauma-related procedures, among others. Emphasis was given on the practical application of techniques, indications, contraindications, and complications.

We hope this edition of the *Emergency Medicine Clinics of North America* is a valuable reference for emergency medicine physicians that practice in different clinical settings and this reference serves as a useful tool for clinicians, educators, and emergency medicine residents.

We would like to thank all the authors who contributed to this project, for their dedication and commitment while spending numerous hours reviewing the literature and

Emerg Med Clin N Am 31 (2013) xv–xvi
http://dx.doi.org/10.1016/j.emc.2012.10.003
0733-8627/13/$ – see front matter © 2013 Elsevier Inc. All rights reserved.

writing their articles. We would also like to thank our families for their unconditional support throughout our careers.

Jorge L. Falcon-Chevere, MD, FAAEM, FACEP
Emergency Medicine Department
University of Puerto Rico School of Medicine
PO Box 29207
65th Infantry Station
San Juan, PR 00929

Jose G. Cabanas, MD, FACEP
Emergency Medicine Residency
UT Southwestern at Austin
University Medical Center Brackenridge
1400 North IH-35
CEC 2.230
Austin, TX 78701

E-mail addresses:
jfalconc@gmail.com (J.L. Falcon-Chevere)
jgcabanas@me.com (J.G. Cabanas)

Critical Airway Skills and Procedures

Eric Hawkins, MD, MPH[a], Hawnwan Philip Moy, MD[b],
Jane H. Brice, MD, MPH[b],*

KEYWORDS

- Airway • Airway adjuncts • Endotracheal intubation

KEY POINTS

- Airway management is a critical skill for emergency physicians.
- Careful airway assessment and preplanning are essential in determining which patients require invasive airway management and what equipment will be required to successfully manage the patients' airway.
- Airway management is a team-based procedure, and the emergency physician must be receptive and responsive to team input to maximize the safety of the procedure.

Airway management is a critical procedure and essential skill necessary for all physicians working in the emergency department. Optimal resuscitative treatment of medical and trauma patients often revolves around timely and effective airway interventions that can be challenging in the acute setting, especially in critical patients. Time-honored airway techniques and procedures combined with recent advances in rapid sequence intubation (RSI), video laryngoscopy, and further advanced airway techniques now offer emergency clinicians a wide range of exciting new options for improving this crucial component of acute care and management.

AIRWAY MANAGEMENT DECISION MAKING AND BASIC MANAGEMENT

Initial patient assessment forms the cornerstone of further advanced airway management, and the primary evaluation should focus on the quick identification of those who may need respiratory support. This evaluation includes assessment for the patency of

Disclosures: (1) Dr Hawkins has nothing to disclose. (2) Dr Moy has nothing to disclose. (3) Dr Brice is the recipient of grant funding from the Emergency Medical Services for Children and the National Highway Traffic Safety Administration.
^a Department of Emergency Medicine, Carolinas Medical Center, Medical Education Building, Third Floor, 1000 Blythe Boulevard, Charlotte, NC 28203, USA; ^b Department of Emergency Medicine, University of North Carolina, CB# 7594, Chapel Hill, NC 27599-7594, USA
* Corresponding author.
E-mail address: brice@med.unc.edu

the airway and adequacy of ventilatory effort, potential hypoxia, or presence of illness or injury that could result in further deterioration of the patients' respiratory status. These initial efforts should then guide proper management techniques and interventions to improve the patients' overall condition and optimize both oxygenation and ventilation.

In general, patients with airway management issues may be divided into those who need an immediate definitive intervention versus those who are more stable or less urgent. The first category is generally identified as a *crash airway* and must be managed without delay.[1] The second group may be assessed in a more systematic fashion in an effort to determine the next best step in treatment and to identify factors that could make airway management difficult.

Primary efforts should focus on airway patency, and any potential obstruction should be immediately treated. Simple airway repositioning may improve occlusion from the tongue and may include varied techniques, such as the jaw thrust or chin lift method. Inspection may also demonstrate airway occlusion from blood, vomit, or other foreign bodies that should be quickly removed. Patients with altered levels of consciousness may not protect their airway and may require insertion of an oropharyngeal airway or a nasopharyngeal airway in an effort to overcome posterior tongue displacement or loss of pharyngeal muscle tone.

In cases of potential respiratory compromise, it is also wise to identify early those patients who may have difficulty with airway management and include this as a component of the initial assessment. The commonly used mnemonic MOANS (**Table 1**) can help identify those who may be difficult to provide ventilatory support via a bag valve mask (BVM), and its individual components have been validated in multiple studies.[2–4] Similarly, the mnemonic LEMON (**Table 2**) may be used to identify potential difficulties with endotracheal (ET) intubation.[5,6]

The initial evaluation using pulse oximetry to identify hypoxia is now almost universal in prehospital and emergency triage vital signs and provides a useful initial screen for those with potential respiratory issues and complaints.[7] Pulse oximetry also gives useful feedback on the effects of supplemental oxygen and assessment of further treatment, delivering easily obtainable and noninvasive real-time information for providers. In more critical patients, continuous pulse oximetry is essential for the process of RSI and for further management of patients on noninvasive positive pressure ventilation or mechanical ventilation (MV). As with all technology, there are limitations, including factors like motion artifact and cardiac arrhythmias, and physical barriers, like nail polish that may cause false readings.[8,9] Pulse oximetry also provides

Table 1	
MOANS: a mnemonic for identifying patients at risk for poor bag-valve-mask seal	
MOANS[2]	**Criteria**
Mask seal	Beards, facial injury
Obesity/obstruction	BMI >26, airway obstruction, obstetric patients
Age	Aged older than 55 years
No teeth	
Stiffness	Increased airway resistance (asthma, COPD), stiff lungs (pulmonary edema, CHF, pneumonia)

Abbreviations: BMI, body mass index; CHF, congestive heart failure; COPD, chronic obstructive pulmonary disease.

Table 2
LEMON: a mnemonic for identifying patients at risk for difficult endotracheal intubation

LEMON[4]	Criteria
Look	A quick external examination of the patient for potential signs of airway management problems.
Evaluate the 3-3-2 Rule	Examine the airway for structural and anatomic factors that may make intubation difficult. Normal findings should show a mouth opening that accommodates 3 of the patient's fingers, a mandible measuring 3 fingers from the mentum to the hyoid bone, and a distance of 2 fingers from the hyoid bone to the thyroid notch. When present, these factors predict sufficient spatial relationships between the mouth, the mandible, temporamandibular joint mobility, and the larynx to allow for successful direct laryngoscopy and eventual endotracheal intubation.
Mallampati Score	Assessment of the posterior oropharyngeal structures visualized when the mouth is open and the tongue is fully protruded.
Obstruction	Upper airway obstruction from foreign bodies, edema, stridor, or soft tissue masses.
Neck Mobility	Assessment of difficulty of potential neck positioning to assure optimum angles for visualization of the glottis. Examples include potential cervical spine injuries, rheumatoid arthritis, or degenerative arthritis.

information solely on oxygenation and gives no information on ventilatory status, carbon dioxide levels, or acid base status.[7]

An additional useful noninvasive measurement of respiratory status and ventilation is the use of capnography. This technology measures the partial pressure of carbon dioxide (CO_2) during ventilation and provides a useful proxy measurement of arterial CO_2. This measurement may occur as a one-time measurement, as in the use of a colorimetric end-tidal CO_2 detector, or as an ongoing measurement of exhaled CO_2 displayed as a continuous capnogram. At present, these measurements are most useful in confirming and assessing ET tube placement, for procedural sedation, and for monitoring patients with obstructive lung disease, like chronic obstructive pulmonary disease (COPD) or asthma, that may result in CO_2 retention and potential subsequent acidosis.[10]

Patients who are found to have inadequate ventilation may require assistance with a BVM to deliver positive pressure ventilation in addition to supplemental oxygen. This technique relies on an experienced operator who can ensure a tight mask seal and works well in conjunction with an oropharyngeal or nasopharyngeal device (**Fig. 1**). During the initial evaluation, patients who may be difficult candidates for adequate BVM should be identified by the use of the mnemonic MOANS, as described earlier, or by the identification of any factor that may make the seal of the mask inadequate. The major drawbacks to BVM revolve around issues of lack of protection from pulmonary aspiration and gastric inflation, both of which may occur with increased airway pressures necessary for adequate ventilation.

BRIDGING ADJUNCTS

Although advanced airway procedures are often required to manage patients with impending respiratory failure, there are a few alternatives to consider before

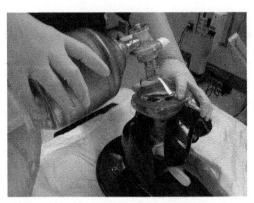

Fig. 1. Correct hand placement and technique for bag-valve mask ventilation.

proceeding to ET intubation or other invasive airway interventions. ET intubation is not without risk. Commonly reported adverse events surrounding intubation include trauma to the upper airway structures, ET tube–induced tissue necrosis, loss of protective anatomic barriers to infection and the resulting nosocomial pneumonias, patient discomfort and agitation, as well as increased intensive care use and associated costs.[11–13]

Noninvasive ventilation (NIV) is delivered via positive pressure applied through either a face mask or nose mask to spontaneously breathing patients. For optimal use, patients must have sufficient respiratory effort to be able to effectively use the device. NIV has been acknowledged as a viable airway management strategy since biblical times when bellows and other positive pressure devices were used to maintain respiration during resuscitation.[14] In more modern times, NIV was used during the polio epidemics of the 1950s to sustain the ventilation of patients with polio using devices, such as the chest shell and the iron lung.[15] In today's emergency department, 2 noninvasive adjuncts should be at the fingertips of an emergency physician: continuous positive airway pressure (CPAP) and bilevel positive airway pressure (BiPAP).

CPAP is a critical airway procedure that requires patients to breathe against a continuous and constant positive pressure that is delivered through a tight-fitting face mask. Breathing against a continuous positive pressure encourages the recruitment on atelectatic lungs, reduces the work of breathing, improves pulmonary compliance, and may decrease the need for intubation.[16] The typical settings are 10.0 to 12.5 cm H_2O.

BiPAP ventilation cycles between 2 modes of positive airway pressure. During inspiration, BiPAP ventilation provides high-flow inspiratory positive airway pressure. Sensing the patient's native flow rate, the BiPAP ventilator responds with high-flow pressure for either a fixed time period or until the gas flow rate decreases less than a preset threshold, usually 25% of the expiratory volume. At the conclusion of inspiration, the device switches to the expiratory positive airway pressure, delivering a lower positive pressure to splint open alveoli and to maintain a fixed alveolar pressure. Common starting settings are 10 cm of inspiratory pressure and 5 cm of expiratory pressure.

Five conditions warrant consideration of noninvasive ventilation, and only 3 of which apply directly to the emergency department setting.[17] The use of NIV in COPD is strongly supported by the medical literature.[18–22] Both CPAP and BiPAP have demonstrated decreased intubation rates for patients with acute cardiogenic pulmonary edema and should be considered the first-line therapy for appropriate patients (**Table 3**).[23–27] An emerging use of NIV, which is not typically considered in the

Table 3 Indications and contraindications of use of NIV	
Indications	Contraindications
Alert and cooperative patient	Decreased mental status (GCS <10)
Severe dyspnea at rest	Uncooperative patient
Use of accessory muscles of respiration	Poor respiratory effort
Respiratory rates >30 bpm	Aspiration risk
Hypercarbic respiratory failure	Inability to clear secretions
Acute respiratory acidosis (pH <7.30)	Hemodynamic instability
	Face trauma, surgery, or deformity
	Upper gastrointestinal bleeding
	Cardiac or respiratory arrest

Abbreviation: GCS, Glasgow Coma Scale.

emergency setting, is the application of NIV for patients who are immunocompromised.[28,29] ET intubation and MV are associated with significant morbidity, particularly nosocomial pneumonias. Avoidance of ET intubation in this patient population may come with resulting decreases in mortality and intensive care length of stays.[28] NIV ventilation may also be particularly useful for patients with hematological malignancies, patients who have elected a do-not-intubate status, and for relief of severe dyspnea in patients with cancer.[29] Nonemergency department indications include the use of NIV in extubation failure among patients with COPD and use in postoperative patients.[30–33] Although promising, controversy exists regarding the use of NIV in patients with asthma.[34,35]

Two hours is considered an adequate trial if NIV is to be implemented.[36,37] Improvements in acidosis and carbon dioxide retention should be demonstrated within this time window. Failure to demonstrate improvement should lead the clinician to proceed to intubation and MV. Of course, any worsening of these parameters during the trial should prompt the clinician to more aggressively manage the patients' ventilation. Other criteria for failed NIV trial are worsening mental status or agitation, worsening oxygenation, hemodynamic instability, or inability to tolerate the mask.[7] There are few complications associated with use of NIV. The most common complication is skin breakdown or necrosis secondary to the tight-fitting masks. Some patients may experience retention of secretions or gastric distention. Others may find the mask itself intolerable and the NIV trial may fail because of patient anxiety or inability to tolerate the tight-fitting mask.

ET INTUBATION

ET intubation is a key procedure for emergency physicians and is taught in every emergency medicine residency in the United States. Often, clinicians are quick to jump to ET intubation in patients who might be better managed using skills we have already discussed, such as simple airway positioning maneuvers; nasal or oral airways; or bridging adjuncts, such as BiPAP. The physical skill of ET intubation is relatively easy to master with enough practice, but applying the appropriate assessment skills and knowledge to know when to intubate is often very complex.

Indications

Indications for ET intubation fall into 2 categories: reflexive and relative. The most obvious reflexive indication is for those patients who are not breathing. Patients with severe facial injuries or those who are so obtunded that they can no longer protect their airway also require ET intubation. It has been traditionally taught that the absence of a gag reflex signals the need to intubate; however, Davies and colleagues[38] demonstrated that approximately 37% of the general population have an absent gag reflex. It may be more prudent to assess patients' ability to swallow spontaneously and handle their secretions. These reflexive indications require rapid patient assessment and intervention to prevent fatal outcomes.

Relative indications allow the emergency clinician a bit more time to prepare and assess patients using the assessment techniques, such as LEMON, mentioned earlier in the article. Patients failing bridging adjuncts, such as BiPAP, or those who present in extremis from COPD, asthma, or other respiratory emergency will also ultimately require intubation. In addition, patients with a clinical condition, such as facial trauma, abscess, or burns, may also require intubation as a more elective procedure should their condition suggest eventual deterioration and airway compromise.

Preplanning

In an airway emergency, the only critical failure is a failure to ventilate. Failing to successfully intubate patients is not a critical failure. Beginning with the end in mind will improve airway management success rates and will improve patient outcomes. Inability to ventilate patients is a true emergency and requires the emergency clinician to move rapidly to place an ET tube or proceed to surgical airway.

Perhaps the most important airway procedure occurs months in advance of the particular need to intubate an individual. Preplanning for airway emergencies will make the emergency intubation not only more efficient and successful but also safer for patients. Emergency physician practice groups should consider either developing or adopting an emergency airway checklist. Evidence from our intensive care and anesthesia colleagues has demonstrated the utility of checklists in decreasing complications and adverse outcomes.[39–42] Emergency physicians should plan well in advance for airway emergencies by assembling all essential airway equipment and supplies, including rescue devices and surgical equipment, in an airway cart or similar depot that can be easily moved to the patients' bedside; this should be a standard emergency department policy. While the airway cart is being moved to the patients' bedside, the clinician should assess the patients' anatomy and airway while keeping in mind which rescue devices might be most appropriate should intubation prove difficult. Patients should be preoxygenated, and the intubator should conduct a brief time-out to ensure that every team member understands their role in the procedure and that all the required equipment, personnel, and supplies are in the room.

Equipment

The required equipment for ET intubation is listed in **Table 4**. It should be standard practice to monitor patients with a cardiac monitor, pulse oximetry, blood pressure measurements, and capnography. All of these are essential to adequately evaluate patients during an airway emergency.

The BVM device should come with a variety of facial mask sizes to accommodate large adults as well as children. Suction must be available at the bedside with an attached yankauer suction tip. Oropharyngeal or nasopharyngeal airways will improve the ability of the person bagging the patients to ventilate the patients and should always be available within short reach.[43] Oropharyngeal airways are measured from the corner of the mouth to the angle of the jaw. They should only be used in unresponsive patients with an absent gag reflex so as not to stimulate vomiting and subsequently increase the risk of aspiration.[43] Nasopharyngeal airways are measured

Table 4	
Equipment for ET intubation	
ET Intubation Equipment	**Backup Devices**
BVM	Bougie
Suction	Laryngeal mask airway
Airways (oropharyngeal and nasopharyngeal)	King airway
ET tubes of appropriate sizes	Flexible fiberoptic endoscope
Stylet	Cricothyroidotomy
Laryngoscope	
Laryngoscope blades (both curved and straight)	
Magill forceps	
10-mL syringe	
Stethoscope	

from the nares to the tragus of the ear and are inserted using a lubricant into the nares at an angle perpendicular to the face.[43] These devices should not be used in patients with facial trauma or basilar skull fractures and should be used with caution in anticoagulated patients or those with nasal deformities.[43]

ET tubes are usually made of polyvinyl chloride and are available in a variety of sizes (2.0–10.5 mm of internal diameter) (**Fig. 2**). For most adults, ET tubes between 7.5 mm and 8.5 mm will provide an acceptable first pass rate as well as an adequate ventilation capacity.[44] It is useful to have a full range of sizes readily at hand to accommodate unexpected airway sizes. For children, the Broselow Pediatric Emergency Tape (Armstrong Medical Industries, Lincolnshire, IL, USA)[45] will provide guidance for the appropriate ET tube size based on patient size. Adult tubes are usually cuffed, whereas pediatric tubes come in both cuffed and uncuffed varieties. An intubating stylet is a useful aid, which lends rigidity to the ET tube and provides the intubator with the ability to form the stylet and ET tube to the patients' specific anatomy (see **Fig. 2**). Although many advocate a stylet as an adjunct for difficult airways, it may be a useful tool in every intubation.

The laryngoscope is simply a viewing device to bring the airway anatomy into view under lighted conditions to facilitate the correct placement of the ET tube. The traditional laryngoscope is a left-handed instrument consisting of a handle housing

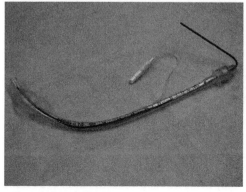

Fig. 2. Endotracheal tube with stylet in place.

batteries that power a light on the end of a blade inserted into the handle. More recently, emergency physicians have begun to use video laryngoscopes that use a digital video camera that projects the airway anatomy onto a video monitor (**Fig. 3**). This device allows the intubator a larger image of the airway and facilitates both increased first pass success rates and decreased intubation time.[46] The lighted blade attached to the laryngoscope handle comes essentially in 2 varieties: curved and straight (**Fig. 4**). Each variety is available in sizes ranging from 0 for infants to 4 for large adults. There are many blades on the market, each differing slightly in construction with a flange here and an extra ridge there, but essentially it all boils down to intubator preference and the specific anatomy of the patient being intubated. Emergency physicians may have a preference for curved versus straight blades but should be facile with both types.

Other standard equipment for intubation should include Magill forceps,[47] which may be useful in guiding the ET tube into the larynx when an anterior airway is encountered, as well as a 10-mL syringe to inflate the cuff once the ET tube is placed successfully and a stethoscope as one adjunct to confirm tube placement.

Technique

The technical aspects of intubation are simple to write but hard to perform without focused mentored practice. Intubation is a core skill acquired in an emergency medicine residency, but it is not enough to learn the skill during residency because skills deteriorate without practice.[48] Most emergency physicians intubate frequently enough to maintain skills, but difficult airway algorithms and skills are more difficult to retain because these instances occur so infrequently. Many are currently advocating the use of simulators for skill practice and retention; but community emergency

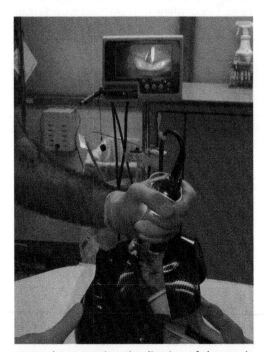

Fig. 3. Video laryngoscopy demonstrating visualization of the vocal cords in a manequin model.

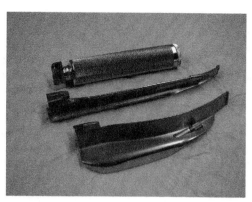

Fig. 4. Laryngoscope handle and two blades.

physicians may not have access to simulators, which are more commonly located in large academic medical centers.[49,50] Other options for skill retention include operating room skill performance through collegial relationships with anesthesia or mannequin practice. It is incumbent on the emergency physician to maintain skill performance.

Once the emergency physician has conducted a brief time-out to ensure that every team member understands their role in the procedure; that all the required equipment, personnel, and supplies are in the room; and that the equipment is functional, the next step should be to position the patient. Taking time to properly position the patient can spell the difference between success and failure. The stretcher should be at about the height of the intubator's midchest.[51] Except in the setting of suspected cervical spine injury, the patient should be placed into a sniffing position. The sniffing position allows for an optimal view of the glottic opening by aligning the oral, pharyngeal, and laryngeal axes.[52] This position may be accomplished be flexing the neck and extending the head. Recent evidence suggests that simply extending the head as a single maneuver may be as effective as the combined maneuver of neck flexion and head extension.[53] Suspected cervical spine injury mandates immobilization of the neck, thus, preventing the intubator from using the sniffing position and care must be taken to assign a team member to maintain cervical spine immobilization during the procedure. The patient should be preoxygenated with 100% O_2 using a non-rebreather mask if the patient has an adequate ventilatory effort or using the BVM technique if there is inadequate effort. During the procedure, a team member should be appointed to apply the Sellick maneuver. Consisting of firm pressure over the thyroid cartilage, the intended outcome of the maneuver is primarily to minimize the risk of gastric aspiration. The maneuver should be initiated at the beginning of positive pressure ventilation and continued until the ET tube cuff is inflated in the trachea. Some have questioned this maneuver's effectiveness, but it remains a recommended part of the intubation process.[54]

From this point forward, it is assumed that the patient is awake and spontaneously breathing. For those patients who are not breathing, the sedation and paralytic steps can be skipped as part of a *crash airway* algorithm. The patient should be properly sedated before proceeding. Once sedated, the patient's mouth is opened using a scissoring motion with a crossed right forefinger and thumb. The forefinger is placed on the patient's upper teeth and the thumb on the lower teeth to use a scissoring motion to open the mouth. After assuring adequate preoxygenation and the ability to ventilate the patient using the BVM technique, the patient may be chemically paralyzed using RSI techniques detailed later in this article.

The laryngoscope handle is held in the intubator's left hand, and the blade is inserted into the right side of the mouth to sweep the tongue into the left side of the mouth. The laryngoscope is then advanced into the airway slowly taking note of the airway anatomy with a goal of visualizing the epiglottis (**Fig. 5**).[52] If a curved blade is being used, then the blade is placed into the vallecula and forward pressure is applied to lift the epiglottis and bring the vocal cords into view.[52] If a straight blade is being used, the blade is placed beneath the epiglottis.[52] Using an upward and slightly forward motion, the vocal cords are brought into view. Care must be taken to never use the teeth as leverage. Once the vocal cords are visualized, the ET tube is taken in the right hand and advanced into the airway until the cuff passes through the cords. The laryngoscope can now be removed from the mouth and the stylet removed from the ET tube. ET intubation attempts should be limited to no longer than 30 seconds, although shorter limits may be required based on patient oxygen saturation and heart rate.[55] If the intubator is unable to place the tube within the time limit, then the attempt should be aborted, the patient ventilated, and preparations made for another attempt.

A failed attempt at intubation provides an opportunity to remediate or correct problems in positioning, equipment, or procedure. The intubator may want to consider placing a rolled towel beneath the patient's shoulder to optimize positioning.[52] A change in laryngoscope blade may be warranted or suction may be required. The BURP maneuver may also be a useful addition to the procedure: firm backward (B), upward (U), rightward (R) pressure (P) is applied to the patient's thyroid cartilage to bring the vocal cords into better view.[56,57] Although some have questioned the utility of this maneuver, it may be a useful adjunctive maneuver in a difficult intubation situation.[58]

Even when done correctly by the most skilled clinician, intubation can occasionally have complications.[59] These complications include airway trauma, such as dental

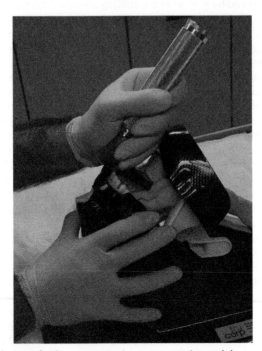

Fig. 5. Correct technique for laryngoscopy in a mannequin model.

injury and bruising or laceration of the lip, tongue, or mucosa. Many patients complain of sore throat after intubation. Other reported complications of emergency intubation are glottic injury, aspiration, retropharyngeal bruising, or rarely perforation.[60]

Postintubation Procedures

Once the ET tube has been placed through the vocal cords, the cuff should be inflated with 10 cm^3 of air. After tube confirmation is assured, the cuff inflation pressure should be measured and the least amount of air necessary to create a seal during ventilation should be used. There are many methods for confirming tube placement; but unfortunately no one method has proven to be 100% reliable, and relying on any single confirmation method is suboptimal.[61,62] Suggested methods are noted in **Box 1**. Li[61] published a meta-analysis of capnographic clinical trials in 2001. Using a sample of 2192 intubations, he reported a 93% sensitivity (95% confidence interval [CI] 92%–94%) and a 97% specificity (CI 93%–99%) for ET tube placement confirmation using capnography. He also reported the false-negative failure rate (tube in trachea but capnography reports esophagus) to be 7% and the false-positive rate (tube in esophagus but capnography reports trachea) to be 3%. Most usefully, he translates this information into a number needed to harm using capnography as a sole confirmation procedure. For every 10 patients in whom ET intubation is confirmed with capnography alone, one will be harmed (number needed to harm: 14 for false negative, 33 for false positive, and 10 for both).[61] Although waveform capnography is not perfect, it is the best among the recommended confirmation methods.[63] There is evidence, though, that waveform capnography is not widely available in emergency departments in the United States.[64]

Recently, several studies have examined the usefulness of ultrasonography to evaluate the placement of an ET tube.[65–68] Ultrasound can be used in 2 different ways to confirm placement. First, the application of the transducer to the neck can visualize the placement of the tube during the procedure of intubation. Secondly, using the sliding lung sign during bag ventilation, ET tube placement can be confirmed.

BACKUP DEVICES

Not every intubation procedure goes as planned, and emergency physicians must always have a backup plan in mind. During the initial assessment of the patient's

---

Box 1
Methods of ET tube placement confirmation

Waveform capnography

Colorimetric end-tidal carbon dioxide detector

Auscultation of breath sounds

Ultrasonography

Direct visualization of the tube between the cords

Self-inflating esophageal bulb

Fogging of the ET tube

Rise and fall of the chest

Pulse oximetry readings

Improvement in the patients' condition (color, heart rate)

airway anatomy, the emergency physician should have made some decisions about which backup devices might be most appropriate for that specific patient. Once it is clear that the intubation procedure is difficult, the emergency physician should move quickly to a backup device or procedure.

The bougie is an intubation aid that many clinicians find useful in patients with anterior airway anatomy or poor visualization of the vocal cords such as occurs in trauma patients with cervical spine immobilization.[69,70] The bougie is a semirigid, straight rod with a hockey-stick bend at one end and can be inserted into the airway to locate the trachea and then to serve as an introducer over which the ET tube can be placed. Typically, the bougie is used under direct laryngoscopy but may be used to facilitate nasotracheal intubation,[71,72] retrograde intubation,[73] or cricothyrotomy.[74]

The bougie is inserted into the airway under direct visualization using a laryngoscope. Passing the bougie tip beneath the epiglottis and into the trachea, vibrations or clicks are palpated through the bougie shaft as the tip of the bougie passes against the rigid tracheal rings. The inability to advance the bougie past 40 cm in an adult also indicatives tracheal placement because the bougie will be stopped at the carina or by the small lumen of the bronchus.[75] If it was in the esophagus, there would be no impediment to its advancement. Kidd and colleagues[76] studied the reliability of these two signs for predicting placement of the bougie in the trachea. They reported 89.7% accuracy for tracheal clicks and 100% accuracy for "tracheal hold up." Once tracheal placement is confirmed, the ET tube can be advanced over the bougie. Advancement past the vocal cords can occasionally require gentle pressure and 90°counterclockwise tube rotation.[77]

Extraglottic devices can also provide the clinician with an airway alternative allowing for oxygenation and ventilation without the requirement to thread an ET tube through the vocal cords. Useful in both difficult and failed airways, extraglottic devices are commonly used in the operating room, the emergency department, and in prehospital environments. There are many such devices on the market but this discussion is confined to the most common devices: the Laryngeal Mask Airway (LMA International N.V. Willemstad, Curacao), the Combitube (Kendall-Sheridan, Mansfield, MA, USA), and the King Airway (King Systems, Noblesville, IN, USA).

The LMA is a large-bore stem with a flexible cuffed mask on the end designed to fit over the tracheal inlet (**Fig. 6**). It is a blind insertion device often used in anesthesia when ET intubation is unnecessary or in emergency situations when intubation fails.[78] Once inserted and seated, the cuff is inflated to create a low-pressure seal around the

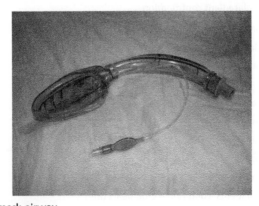

Fig. 6. Laryngeal mask airway.

tracheal inlet. Several investigators report the utility of this device in the hands of less experienced clinicians as a first-line device as well as a rescue device for failed airways in any setting.[79–81]

The LMA is available in a variety of adult and pediatric sizes as well as several different models with differing functions. Notably, an intubating version of the LMA (I-LMA. Laryngeal Mask Airway. LMA International N.V. Willemstad, Curacao) exists and allows for the passage of an ET tube through the mask and into the trachea. The I-LMA is placed blindly using a metal handle, and an enlarged stem lumen allows for the passage of an ET tube through the stem and into the trachea through the mask. The I-LMA uses a proprietary nonkinking ET tube. Many investigators report up to a 95% success rate for intubation of the trachea using an I-LMA.[82–88] It should be noted that none of the LMA devices protect the trachea from aspiration in patients with full stomachs or copious secretions. Some investigators advocate the use of the bougie through an LMA as a tracheal placeholder and then passage of an ET tube over the bougie.[89]

The Combitube device has been used extensively in the prehospital environment as a rescue device with success rates of up to 93%.[90] The Combitube is a blind insertion, dual-lumen airway designed to be placed in the esophagus but can also be used when inserted into the trachea. The Combitube has a large cuff that, when correctly positioned, will lie in the posterior pharynx above the glottis. The distal end of the tube has a smaller cuff that, when placed in the esophagus, occludes that passage to force air into the tracheal inlet. The Combitube is gradually losing favor to the newer and easier-to-use King Airway.[91]

The King Laryngeal Tube (LT) Airway (King Systems, Noblesville, IN, USA) is a blind insertion, single-lumen tube that is shorter, easier to manipulate, and easier to position than the Combitube (**Fig. 7**). Additionally, it only has a single cuff inflation port, which inflates both cuffs at the same time. When properly positioned, the proximal cuff seals the hypopharynx and the distal cuff seals the esophagus, allowing for ventilation through the port positioned between the cuffs and at the laryngeal inlet. Russi and colleagues[92] demonstrated the ease and speed with which a King LT can be placed in a difficult airway simulator, whereas Guyette and colleagues[93] have demonstrated its successful use in the actual rescue of difficult and failed intubations. The King LT ventilating tube is large enough to allow for the passage of a flexible endoscope, a tracheal tube introducer, or a bougie. The use of these adjunct devices, along with the King LT, may allow for the subsequent passage of an ET tube, although complications, such as perforation of the trachea, have been reported.[94–96]

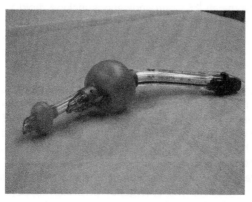

Fig. 7. King airway.

BACKUP PROCEDURES

In addition to backup devices, the emergency physician must also be facile with backup procedures. Two alternative airway procedures are discussed: nasal intubation and flexible fiberoptic intubation. Cricothyrotomy is discussed in the next section.

Nasal intubation can be performed for a variety of reasons and in a variety of situations. For example, it may be preferred as an awake intubation technique along with fiberoptic visualization in the setting of oral airway obstruction, such as severe lingual edema or trauma.[97,98] Nasal intubation may also be used in the setting of breathing patients in whom oral intubation has failed. Three techniques are possible in accomplishing nasal intubation. In the blind insertion technique, the lubricated ET tube is introduced into a nare and advanced over the floor of the nasopharynx into the hypopharynx while the intubator listens at the tube end for breath sounds. As the patient inhales, the tube is advanced in the direction of air movement into the laryngeal inlet and through the vocal cords. Devices, such as directional tipped ET tubes or the Beck airway airflow monitor may increase success rates in blind nasal intubation attempts.[99] Alternatively, in situations when nasal intubation can be accomplished using direct laryngoscopy, the ET tube is advanced along that nasal floor through the nasal pharynx until visualized in the posterior pharynx and then guided through the vocal cords under direct visualization. Severe midface trauma is a relative contraindication for nasal intubation.[100,101]

Fiberoptic intubation allows for indirect visualization of the laryngeal inlet and vocal cords to facilitate the correct placement of the ET tube via either an oral or nasal route.[102] Using a flexible fiberoptic endoscope over which an ET tube has been threaded, the intubator directs the flexible endoscope into the hypopharynx visualizing landmarks and anatomy as the tube progresses. The tube is passed through the vocal cords, and the ET tube is threaded off of the bronchoscope and into position in the trachea.[102] Preparation for fiberoptic intubation requires time and patient cooperation. Patients should be awake, breathing spontaneously, and adequately oxygenated. The technique requires physician experience and practice with the device well in advance of the immediate need to intubate. Additionally, the device and associated equipment is expensive and not maintained in many emergency departments.

Fiberoptic intubation is particularly useful for patients in whom the initial airway assessment has suggested a difficult airway and in whom chemical paralysis would be dangerous.[102] Examples of patients for whom fiberoptic intubation could be considered include those with limited mouth opening, facial trauma, lingual edema or trauma, oral obstructions from infection or tumor, or unusual upper airway anatomy (whether congenital or postsurgical).[102] Contraindications include rapid airway compromise; extensive secretions, such as emesis or bleeding; hypoventilation; or poor patient cooperation.[102]

RSI

RSI is often chosen in emergency settings because it rapidly induces unconsciousness and chemical paralysis of previously awake and breathing patients in a controlled manner. It is critical to remember that emergency patients have often not fasted and are at much higher risk of aspiration of secretions or emesis.[103] A decision to use RSI also requires that the emergency physician has made a thorough assessment of the patient's airway and has planned for the difficult airway scenario.

RSI requires a sequential series of steps to be safely and efficiently completed.[104] The first step is preparation. The emergency physician must prepare 3 elements: the equipment, the patient, and the team. The authors have previously discussed appropriate intubation equipment to have at the bedside and readily available. This equipment should include backup devices and equipment. Patients should be informed and preferably consented to the procedure if time and circumstances allow. Patients should also be preoxygenated with high-flow oxygen through a non-rebreather mask for up to 5 minutes before proceeding. Emergency airway management and the patients' condition may not allow for this ideal preoxygenation interval. Preoxygenation allows for supersaturation of the alveoli through nitrogen washout. Baraka and colleagues[105] have demonstrated that 3 minutes of tidal volume breathing is sufficient to preoxygenate patients. In ideal models, investigators suggest that preoxygenation can buy the clinician about 8 minutes before the oxygen saturation levels drop less than 90%; however, both Famery and Mort have shown that this ideal desaturation curve is not reliable or valid in the critically ill patients that most emergency physicians will be intubating using RSI.[106–108] The final preparatory element is the team. RSI requires a team of personnel, each of whom understands their role in the event and each of whom is alert to possible safety concerns or possible human error.[109] The team leader should ensure that team members know each other, that they understand their role, and that they acknowledge the need to speak up when they are concerned about the evolution of the procedure.

Once the preparatory phase is complete, the second step is medication, which has 2 phases. The emergency physician may consider pretreatment with medications, such as lidocaine, an analgesic, atropine, and a defasciculating agent, although the evidence for these pretreatments is unconvincing and conflicting. Typically administered 2 to 3 minutes before induction and paralysis, these medications are proposed as blunting the physiologic response to intubation. It has been suggested that lidocaine (1.5 mg/kg intravenously) as a pretreatment medication may blunt the increases in intracranial pressure, heart rate, and mean arterial pressure during intubation. These findings have not been consistently demonstrated; although it is advocated for use in patients with head injuries or bleeding or intracranial tumors, its use is left to the judgment of the clinician.[110–112] Analgesic administration also carries no convincing evidence to suggest routine use as a pretreatment.[113,114] Although atropine may decrease the incidence of bradydysrhythmias in children during intubation, these dysrhythmias are usually self-limited and of little consequence. Atropine should at least be available during the intubation of young children.[115,116] Defasciculating doses on nondepolarizing agents may decrease the intensity and duration of muscle fasciculation after the administration of succinylcholine.

Induction agents should be administered after pretreatment medication (if any). Producing a rapid loss of consciousness, induction medications allow for control of patients and prevent psychological harm during the administration of paralytic agents. One of 4 induction agents is typically used in the emergency department: etomidate, propofol, ketamine, or midazolam.

Etomidate is one of the most commonly used agents in the United States for RSI induction.[117] This anesthetic agent has a short half-life and rapid onset of action. Additionally, it is very useful in patients with hemodynamic instability because it is less likely than other agents to cause decreases in blood pressure and very useful in patients with suspected head injury because it reportedly decreases intracranial pressure while maintaining normal arterial pressure.[118–120] Propofol also has a rapid onset of action, short duration, and is cerebroprotective; however, it is not useful in patients with hemodynamic instability because of its myocardial depressive profile.

Ketamine has regained popularity in the adult emergency department for use in RSI.[121] An N-methyl-d-aspartate receptor antagonist, ketamine carries both analgesic properties and the ability to create a dissociative state in patients. Once thought to cause increases in intracranial pressure, new research suggests that ketamine may improve cerebral perfusion and may have neuroprotective properties.[122–125] Midazolam is a benzodiazepine with relatively slower onset of action and longer duration of action that limits its effectiveness in RSI.[118] Additionally, midazolam often causes hypotension, making it not useful in the setting of hemodynamic instability.[118]

The final phase of the medication step is the administration of paralytics. The purpose of paralytic agents is to obliterate the patient's protective reflexes to facilitate efficient placement of the ET tube. It is important to remember that paralytic agents only paralyze; they do not provide sedation, amnesia, or analgesia and the clinician must remember to maintain adequate levels of appropriate medications to also meet these important needs. The clinician must choose between depolarizing agents, such as succinylcholine, and nondepolarizing agents, such as rocuronium, for paralysis. Succinylcholine has a very rapid onset requiring the clinician to be ready to manage the patient's airway as soon as the medication is delivered and a short duration of action. Succinylcholine is associated with the release of intracellular potassium and should be used with caution in patients who are known or suspected to be hyperkalemic.[126] Nondepolarizing agents, such as rocuronium, have both longer onset and duration of action. Potassium release is not associated with nondepolarizing agents, making these drugs useful in patients who are hyperkalemic; however, the use of nondepolarizing agents in patients with suspected difficult airways is not recommended to avoid the *cannot ventilate, cannot intubate* scenario. Having now completed the preparation phase and the medication phase, the final phase is the actual procedure of intubation. The procedure itself is no different from that described previously.

DIFFICULT AIRWAYS

One of the most important decisions an emergency physician can make when managing an airway is identifying a difficult airway. A difficult airway exists in patients when basic facemask ventilation is problematic or tracheal intubation is difficult. When a physician finds himself or herself in such a situation, this should immediately prompt the use of a difficult airway algorithm that includes the use of difficult airway adjuncts.[2,5,127] One should have experience with one or all of the following adjuncts before a difficult airway were to present itself.

In addition to the difficult airway adjuncts that have been mentioned previously, the lighted stylet presents a viable option in the setting of excessive secretions, blood, or trismus. The lighted stylet requires transillumination of the anterior neck and can be hindered by obesity or excessive ambient light.[128] One should consider dimming the lights when using this technique. The lighted stylet is a semirigid stylet with a light on the end and an ET tube preloaded on the stylet.[129] With the patient in the sniffing position, the lighted stylet is advanced blindly into the posterior pharynx. While advancing, one should look for evidence of a single light shining through the skin. On reaching the trachea, a distinct light will shine through the thin tracheal membranes and skin. Once visualized in this manner, the ET tube can be advanced and verified using standard technique. Visualizing a diffuse glow as opposed to a distinct point of light can identify an esophageal intubation.

The fiberoptic stylet (FOS) is another difficult airway adjunct.[130] The FOS is extremely useful in anterior airways and significantly cheaper than a video laryngoscope. However, if there is an abundance of secretions or blood, visualization is limited, making intubation that much more difficult. The FOS contains a fiberoptic device at the distal end of the stylet, allowing the physician to obtain a direct view of the posterior pharynx. Like the lighted stylet, the FOS is placed blindly into the posterior pharynx with the ET tube preloaded; but unlike the lighted stylet, the FOS can be advanced toward the trachea with direct visualization seen through an eyepiece at the proximal end of the stylet. Once the vocal cords are visualized, the stylet is advanced into the trachea and, subsequently, so too is the ET tube. Confirmation is obtained using the standard technique.

Another adjunct often forgotten is the retrograde wire intubation (RWI).[131] Because 2 operators are often required (one at the neck and one at the mouth), it is invasive, and can be complicated by upper airway obstruction or poor direct visualization, RWI is typically the very last option in rescuing a difficult airway. However, RWI can be rapidly attempted before a surgical airway is decided on and has less morbidity than a surgical airway.[131]

The neck should be prepped with povidone-iodine followed by the identification of the cricothyroid membrane. Subsequently, an 18-gauge needle should be placed through the cricothyroid membrane with immediate aspiration of air, thus, confirming placement of the needle in the airway. Once the needle is repositioned cephalad, a guidewire can be advanced through the needle. As the guidewire is advanced far enough into the oropharynx, one can use a McGill or alligator forceps to firmly grasp the distal tip of the wire. Immediately extract the wire out of the mouth. Once secured, the ET tube can be advanced over the wire using a Seldingerlike technique.[131] Placement can then be confirmed using the standard measures.

FAILED AIRWAYS

When intubation has failed and oxygenation cannot be adequately obtained a *failed airway* has occurred. The 2 traditional approaches, surgical open cricothyroidotomy and needle cricothyroidotomy, are the 2 solutions for a failed airway. When anticipating a failed airway, the LMA, Combitube, and King Airway previously mentioned may provide oxygenation while preparing for a surgical airway. Nonetheless, when a clinician is forced down this path, preparation is the key and includes a firm understanding of the involved anatomy as well as the complications of each technique.

The cricothyroid membrane is easily palpated between the thyroid and cricoid cartilages.[132,133] However, in patients with abnormal anatomy, the cricothyroid membrane can be found approximately one-third of the distance midline from the manubrium to the chin. The thyroid cartilage is the largest cartilage on the neck and often referred to as the *Adam's apple*.[134] The beginning of the cricothyroid membrane is inferior to the thyroid cartilage. Vasculature includes the cricothyroid artery and vein located at the superior border of the cricothyroid membrane and the inferior portion of the thyroid cartilage. Typically, there is no vasculature near the superior aspect of the cricoid cartilage, although there is a small percentage of patients who have an inferior thyroid artery variant called a *thyroid IMA* artery, which arises from the aortic arch or, in some cases, the subclavian artery and passing over the inferior portion of the membrane.[135]

There are 2 techniques for the surgical cricothyroidotomy: open cricothyroidotomy and Seldinger cricothyroidotomy (**Boxes 2** and **3**).[136] The Seldinger technique has been shown to be quicker as well as has fewer complications.[137,138] Typically, cricothyroidotomy kits come already prepared, with the Melker kit (Cook Critical Care, Bloomington, IN, USA) being the most popular because it allows for both an open and Seldinger technique. However, if your institution does not have a commercially available kit, a kit should be prepared ahead of time, being mindful that the inner diameter of the tube should NOT exceed 6.0 mm. A 6.0- or 5.0-mm internal diameter cuffed ET tube should be used if a cuffed emergency cricothyroidotomy catheter is not

Box 2
Procedure for open cricothyroidotomy approach

The clinician should stand on one side of the patient. A right-handed clinician should stand on the right and a left-handed clinician should stand on the left.

Feel for the thyroid prominence at the midline of the thyroid cartilage and then roll the index finger caudally by 1 to 2 cm until a small hollow is felt. This is the cricothyroid membrane.

Use the thumb and middle finger of the nondominant hand to stabilize the 2 cartilages.

A vertical skin incision is then made in the midline of the region between the thyroid cartilage and cricoid cartilage. (A vertical incision is made to avoid vasculature and can be extended if it is too high or too low.)

Once the cricothyroid membrane is exposed, turn the scalpel horizontally and perforate at the midline inferior portion of the membrane using a horizontal stabbing motion approximately 1 cm deep to avoid complications. A horizontal incision is made so as not to cut the cricoid cartilage as one might with a vertical incision.

Insert the back handle of the scalpel into the cricothyroid membrane and rotate it 90° to widen the opening.

Place the ET tube in the opening and inflate the balloon as in a traditional intubation. Connect the ET tube to the BVM and confirm placement with standard protocol.

Secure the ET tube with adhesive tape.

Obtain a chest radiograph to verify placement.

Data from Farcy DA, Chiu MC, Flaxman A, et al. Critical care emergency medicine. New York: McGraw Hill Professional; 2011.

Box 3
Procedure for Seldinger cricothyroidotomy approach

Open the kit and insert the dilator with the wire into the airway catheter.

Locate the cricothyroid membrane as stated before.

Attach the sheath to the needle and fill the syringe with a small amount of water. Insert the needle into the cricothyroid membrane pointing toward the feet at a 45 to 50° angle. Gently puncture until air bubbles appear in the syringe.

As soon as air bubbles appear, advance the sheath at a 45° angle, knowing that an overzealous advancement may get the sheath stuck on the posterior aspect of the cricoid cartilage.

Withdraw the syringe and advance the guidewire through the sheath. Then remove the sheath when the guidewire is advanced far enough.

Take the 15-blade scalpel; create a 0.5-cm vertical skin incision on both sides of the wire.

Insert the external end of the wire into the dilator (which you had already placed into the airway catheter in step 1) and insert them as a unit through the cricothyroid membrane, following the curvature of the dilator. Advance until the catheter is flush against the skin.

Once in place, remove the dilator and inflate the cuff.

Secure the cricothyroidotomy airway catheter with the provided wrap.

Data from Farcy DA, Chiu MC, Flaxman A, et al. Critical care emergency medicine. New York: McGraw Hill Professional; 2011.

available. Be aware that if an ET tube is being used, it is difficult to secure and may end up with a right main stem bronchus intubation. It is often prudent to be aware of the cricothyrotomy kit in your emergency department as well as its equipment before a failed airway has presented itself.

MECHANICAL VENTILATION

With the increasing demand on emergency departments and prolonged boarding times of ICU patients in the emergency department, the management of mechanical ventilation (MV) is becoming an ever more crucial skills for an emergency physician. It is critical that an emergency physician understand the basics of MV for varying disease processes, with the special consideration that every patient is different.

To date, there are no fixed indications for MV; but generally patients are intubated for respiratory failure, protection of the airway from potential aspiration of various causes, and predicted clinical course of facilitating either a workup or a definitive treatment. Placement of the ET tube has now removed all protective functions of the upper airway: warming of air, air filtration, prevention of aspiration, and removal of secretions. Additionally, MV is providing paradoxic breathing in which positive pressure is being forced into sensitive lung tissues allowing for possible ventilator-induced lung injury, acute lung injury, and barotrauma/volutrauma.[139] Nonetheless, with a general understanding of MV, one can navigate through the hazards of critically ill intubated patients.

The most crucial iatrogenic injury associated with MV is ventilator-induced lung injury.[139] In lung diseases that require MV, the underlying disease is usually not distributed uniformly throughout the lungs. Thus, inflation volumes are preferentially shunted toward normal lungs, which may cause hyperinflation, producing stress fractures at the alveolar-capillary interface. This condition may be a result of excessive alveolar pressures (barotrauma) or excessive alveolar volumes (volutrauma).[139] In turn, the fractures may cause increased inflammation in the normal lung volumes leading to an acute respiratory distress syndrome (ARDS)–like picture.

As a result, a large study published in the *New England Journal of Medicine* demonstrated in more than 800 patients that ventilation with low tidal volumes was associated with a 9% absolute reduction in mortality when the end-inspiratory plateau pressure was more than 30 cm H_2O.[140] In essence, low volume (6 mL/kg) is now recommended for all patients with ARDS and is now considered a beneficial strategy in all patients with acute respiratory failure.[141] Additionally, low lung volumes cause repeated opening and closing of the alveoli at the end of expiration resulting in possible acute lung injury. To ameliorate this, adding positive end-expiratory pressure (PEEP) stents opens the airways and prevents further injury. A sample protocol designed to reduce ventilator-induced lung injury is described in **Box 4**.[142,143]

POSTINTUBATION SEDATION

Once patients are intubated and MV management has begun, it is important to minimize discomfort. Despite the tradition of a long-term paralytic followed by a benzodiazepine for postintubation management, there is now a push to move toward a pain-first paradigm.[144] The goal is to optimize analgesia and then add in sedative agents.

Typically, after intubation or during rapid sequence intubation, providing a fentanyl or morphine bolus will address pain issues and perhaps keep you ahead of the game. Once analgesia has been initiated, the clinician has to decide what sedative/analgesic combination to provide. This depends on the type of pathologic condition patients have on intubation. Sedation choices are provided in **Table 5**.

Box 4
Protocol for lung protective ventilation

1. Select assist-control mode and fraction of inspired oxygen (FIO_2) = 100%

2. Set initial tidal volume (Vt) at 8 mL/kg using the patient's predicted body weight (PBW)

    a. Men: PBW = 50 + (2.3 × [height in inches − 60])

    b. Women: PBW = 45.5 + (2.3 × [height in inches − 60])

3. Select respiratory rate (RR) to achieve preventilator minute ventilation, but do not exceed RR = 35/min

4. Add PEEP at 5 to 7 cm H_2O

5. Reduce Vt by 1 mL/kg every 2 hours until Vt = 6 mL/kg

6. Adjust FIO_2 and PEEP to keep PaO_2 greater than 55 mm Hg or arterial oxygen saturation greater than 88%

7. When Vt is decreased to 6 mL/kg, measure

    a. Plateau pressure

    b. Arterial PCO_2 and pH

Remember that this is a general guideline. Each patient has a unique pathologic profile and will need ventilator adjustments specific for their pathologic condition (ie, asthmatic intubations will need to have a lower respiratory rate to allow exhalation of an obstructive lung disease process).

Data from Marino PL. The ICU book. 3rd edition. Philadelphia: Lippincott Williams and Wilkins; 2007.

Table 5
Sedation choices for mechanical ventilation

Drug	Characteristics	Indications	Precautions
Midazolam	Dosage: 1–5 mg Onset: 1–4 min Duration: 30–60 min Maintenance dosage: 1–8 mg/h Drip titration: 1 mg/h	Typically used with fentanyl for sedation; medical patients who are hypotensive (may need to start pressors); patients with delirium tremens if propofol is not available	May cause hypotension with drug bolus; prolonged duration in renal and hepatic failure
Propofol	Dosage: Bolus not recommended Onset: 1–2 min Duration: 30 min Maintenance dosage: 25–50 mcg/kg/min Drip titration: 10 mcg/kg/min	Typically used with fentanyl for sedation; good for critically ill patients with neurological problems	Possible hypotension with bolus, bradycardia, hypertriglyceridemia, pancreatitis, and propofol-related infusion syndrome
Ketamine	Dosage: 25–50 mg Onset: 30 sec Duration: 5–10 min Maintenance dosage: 1–3 mg/kg/min Drip titration: 0.25–0.5 mg/kg/min	Typically used with fentanyl for sedation; good for trauma patients who are hypotensive	Possible emergence reaction; purposeless and tonic-clonic movements may occur

Abbreviation: IV, intravenous.

Data from Casabar E, Portell J. Barnes Jewish Hospital the tool book for drug dosage and usage guidelines. St Louis (MO): The Department of Pharmacy Barnes Jewish Hospital; 2011.

SUMMARY

Airway management is a critical skill for emergency physicians. Careful airway assessment and preplanning are essential in determining which patients require invasive airway management and what equipment will be required to successfully manage that patient's airway. Airway management is a team-based procedure, and the emergency physician must be receptive and responsive to team input to maximize the safety of the procedure.

REFERENCES

1. Walls RM. The emergency airway algorithms. In: Walls RM, Murphy MF, editors. Manual of emergency airway management. 4th edition. Philadelphia: Lippincott Williams and Wilkins; 2012. p. 22–34.
2. Murphy MF, Doyle DJ. Airway evaluation. In: Hung OR, Murphy MF, editors. Management of the difficult and failed airway. New York: McGraw-Hill; 2008. p. 1–14.
3. Langeron O, Masso E, Huraux C, et al. Prediction of difficult mask ventilation. Anesthesiology 2000;92(5):1229–36.
4. Yildiz TS, Solak M, Toker K. The incidence and risk factors of difficult mask ventilation. J Anesth 2005;19(1):7–11.
5. Murphy MF, Walls RM. Identification of the difficult and failed airway. In: Walls RM, Murphy MF, editors. Manual of emergency airway management. 4th edition. Philadelphia: Lippincott Williams and Wilkins; 2012. p. 81–93.
6. Reed MJ, Rennie LM, Dunn MJ, et al. Is the 'LEMON' method an easily applied emergency airway assessment tool? Eur J Emerg Med 2004;11(3):154–7.
7. Callahan J. Pulse oximetry in emergency medicine. Emerg Med Clin North Am 2008;26(4):869–79.
8. Howell M. Pulse oximetry: an audit of nursing and medical staff understanding. Br J Nurs 2002;11(3):191–7.
9. Elliot M, Tate R, Page K. Do clinicians know how to use pulse oximetry? A literature review and clinical implications. Aust Crit Care 2006;19(4):139–44.
10. Nagler J, Baruch K. Capnography: a valuable tool for airway management. Emerg Med Clin North Am 2008;26(4):881–97.
11. Taryle DA, Chandler JE, Good JT, et al. Emergency room intubations - complications and survival. Chest 1979;75(5):541–3.
12. Sakles JC, Laurin EG, Rantapaa AA, et al. Airway management in the emergency department: a one-year study of 610 tracheal intubations. Ann Emerg Med 1998;31(3):325–32.
13. Wongyingsinn M, Songarj P, Assawinvinijkul T. A prospective observational study of tracheal intubation in an emergency department in a 2300-bed hospital of a developing country in a one-year period. Emerg Med J 2009;26(8):604–8.
14. Antonescu-Turcu A, Parthasarathy S. CPAP and Bi-level PAP therapy: new and established roles. Respir Care 2010;55(9):1216–28.
15. Drinker PA, McKhann CF. The iron lung: first practical means of respiratory support. JAMA 1986;255(11):1476–80.
16. Kosowsky JM, Storrow AB, Carleton SC. Continuous and bi-level positive airway pressure in the treatment of acute cardiogenic pulmonary edema. Am J Emerg Med 2000;18(1):91–5.
17. Marik PE. Handbook of evidence-based critical care. 2nd edition. Springer Science and Business Media, New York: LLC; 2010.

18. Keenan SP, Sinuff T, Cook DJ, et al. Which patients with acute exacerbation of chronic obstructive pulmonary disease benefit from noninvasive positive-pressure ventilation? A systematic review of the literature. Ann Intern Med 2003;138(11):861–70.

19. Ram FS, Picot J, Lightowler J, et al. Non-invasive positive pressure ventilation for treatment of respiratory failure due to exacerbations of chronic obstructive pulmonary disease. Cochrane Database Syst Rev 2004;(3):CD004104.

20. Brochard L, Mancebo J, Wysocki M, et al. Noninvasive ventilation for acute exacerbations of chronic obstructive pulmonary disease. N Engl J Med 1995; 333(13):817–22.

21. Kramer N, Meyer TJ, Meharg J, et al. Randomized, prospective trial of noninvasive positive pressure ventilation in acute respiratory failure. Am J Respir Crit Care Med 1995;151(6):1799–806.

22. Wysocki M, Tric L, Wolff MA, et al. Noninvasive pressure support ventilation in patients with acute respiratory failure: a randomized comparison with conventional therapy. Chest 1995;107(3):761–8.

23. Mehta S, Jay GD, Woolard RH, et al. Randomized, prospective trial of bilevel versus continuous positive airway pressure in acute pulmonary edema. Crit Care Med 1997;25(4):620–8.

24. Lin M, Yang YF, Chiang HT, et al. Reappraisal of continuous positive airway pressure therapy in acute cardiogenic pulmonary edema: short-term results and long-term follow-up. Chest 1995;107(5):1379–86.

25. Winck JC, Azevedo LF, Costa-Pereira A, et al. Efficacy and safety of non-invasive ventilation in the treatment of acute cardiogenic pulmonary edema – a systematic review and meta-analysis. Crit Care 2006;10(2):R69.

26. Ho KM, Wong K. A comparison of continuous and bi-level positive airway pressure non-invasive ventilation in patients with acute cardiogenic pulmonary oedema: a meta-analysis. Crit Care 2006;10(2):R49.

27. Weng CL, Zhao YT, Liu QH, et al. Meta-analysis: noninvasive ventilation in acute cardiogenic pulmonary edema. Ann Intern Med 2010;152(9):590–600.

28. Hilbert G, Gruson D, Vargas F, et al. Noninvasive ventilation in immunosuppressed patients with pulmonary infiltrates, fever, and acute respiratory failure. N Engl J Med 2001;344(7):481–7.

29. Marik PE. Non-invasive positive-pressure ventilation in patients with malignancy. Am J Hosp Palliat Care 2007;24(5):417–21.

30. Nava S, Ambrosino N, Clini E, et al. Noninvasive mechanical ventilation in the weaning of patients with respiratory failure due to chronic obstructive pulmonary disease: a randomised, controlled trial. Ann Intern Med 1998;128(9):721–8.

31. Girault C, Daudenthun I, Chevron V, et al. Non-invasive ventilation as a systematic extubation and weaning technique in acute-on-chronic respiratory failure: a prospective, randomized controlled study. Am J Respir Crit Care Med 1999; 160(1):86–92.

32. Ferreyra GP, Baussano I, Squadrone V, et al. Continuous positive airway pressure for treatment of respiratory complications after abdominal surgery: a systematic review and meta-analysis. Ann Surg 2008;247(4):617–26.

33. Squadrone V, Coha M, Cerutti E, et al. Continuous positive airway pressure for treatment of postoperative hypoxemia: a randomized controlled trial. JAMA 2005;293(5):589–95.

34. Gupta D, Nath A, Agarwal R, et al. A prospective randomized controlled trial on the efficacy of noninvasive ventilation in severe acute asthma. Respir Care 2010; 55(5):536–43.

35. Ram FS, Wellington S, Rowe B, et al. Non-invasive positive pressure ventilation for treatment of respiratory failure due to severe acute exacerbations of asthma. Cochrane Database Syst Rev 2005;(3):CD004360.

36. Mehta S, Hill NS. Noninvasive ventilation: state of the art. Am J Respir Crit Care Med 2001;163(2):540–77.

37. Confalonieri M, Garuti G, Cattaruzza M, et al. A chart of failure risk for noninvasive ventilation in patients with COPD exacerbation. Eur Respir J 2005;25(2): 348–55.

38. Davies AE, Stone SP, Kidd D, et al. Pharyngeal sensation and gag reflex in healthy subjects. Lancet 1995;345(8948):487–8.

39. Sexton JB, Berenholtz SM, Goeschel CA, et al. Assessing and improving safety climate in a large cohort of intensive care units. Crit Care Med 2011;39(5):934–9.

40. Jaber S, Jung B, Corne P, et al. An intervention to decrease complications related to endotracheal intubation in the intensive care unit: a prospective, multiple-center study. Intensive Care Med 2010;36(2):248–55.

41. Cook TM, Woodall N, Harper J, et al. Major complications of airway management in the UK: results of the Fourth National Audit Project of the Royal College of Anaesthetists and the Difficult Airway Society. Part 2: intensive care and emergency departments. Br J Anaesth 2011;106(5):632–42.

42. Rall M. Safety culture and crisis resource management in airway management: general principles to enhance patient safety in critical airway situations. Best Pract Res Clin Anaesthesiol 2005;19(4):539–57.

43. Carleton SC, Reardon RF, Brown CA. Bag-mask ventilation. In: Walls RM, Murphy MF, editors. Manual of emergency airway management. 4th edition. Philadelphia: Lippincott Williams and Wilkins; 2012. p. 79–91.

44. Chandler M, Crawley BE. Rationalization of the selection of tracheal tubes. Br J Anaesth 1986;58(1):111–6.

45. Luten RC, Wears RL, Broselow J, et al. Length-based endotracheal tube and emergency equipment in pediatrics. Ann Emerg Med 1992;21(8):900–4.

46. Griesdale DE, Liu D, McKinney J, et al. Glidescope(®) video-laryngoscopy versus direct laryngoscopy for endotracheal intubation: a systematic review and meta-analysis. Can J Anaesth 2012;59(1):41–52.

47. Sternbach G. Ivan Magill: forceps for intratracheal anesthesia. J Emerg Med 1984;1(6):543–5.

48. Arthur W, Bennett W, Stanush P, et al. Factors that influence skill decay and retention: a quantitative review and analysis. Hum Perform 1998;11(1):57–101.

49. Bond WF, Lammers RL, Spillane LL, et al. The use of simulation in emergency medicine: a research agenda. Acad Emerg Med 2007;14(4):353–63.

50. McLaughlin SA, Doezema D, Sklar DP. Human simulation in emergency medicine training: a model curriculum. Acad Emerg Med 2002;9(11):1310–8.

51. Batra YK, Mathew P. Airway management with endotracheal intubation (including awake intubation and blind intubation). Indian J Anaesth 2005; 49(4):263–8.

52. Reardon RF, Carelton SC, Brown CA. Direct laryngoscopy. In: Walls RM, Murphy MF, editors. Manual of emergency airway management. 4th edition. Philadelphia: Lippincott Williams and Wilkins; 2012. p. 121–38.

53. Adnet F, Baillard C, Borron SW, et al. Randomized study comparing the "sniffing position" with simple head extension for laryngoscopic view in elective surgery patients. Anesthesiology 2001;95(4):836–41.

54. Butler J, Sen A. Best evidence topic report. Cricoid pressure in emergency rapid sequence induction. Emerg Med J 2005;22(11):815–6.

55. American Heart Association. ACLS provider manual supplementary material. In: Sinz E, Navarro K, editors. Advanced cardiovascular life support provider manual. Dallas(TX): American Heart Association; 2011. p. 1–86.

56. Hirabayashi Y, Otsuka Y. The BURP manoeuvre for better glottic view using the paediatric GlideScope. Anaesthesia 2010;65(8):862–3.

57. Takahata O, Kubota M, Mamiya K, et al. The efficacy of the "BURP" maneuver during a difficult laryngoscopy. Anesth Analg 1997;84(2):419–21.

58. Levitan RM, Kinkle WC, Levin WJ, et al. Laryngeal view during laryngoscopy: a randomized trial comparing cricoid pressure, backward-upward-rightward pressure, and bimanual laryngoscopy. Ann Emerg Med 2006; 47(6):548–55.

59. Li J, Murphy-Lavoie H, Bugas C, et al. Complications of emergency intubation with and without paralysis. Am J Emerg Med 1999;17(2):141–3.

60. Finucane BT, Tsui BCH, Santora AH. Complications of airway management. In: Finucane BT, Tsui BC, Santora AH, editors. Principles of airway management. New York: Springer; 2011. p. 683–730.

61. Li J. Capnography alone is imperfect for endotracheal tube placement confirmation during emergency intubation. J Emerg Med 2001;20(3):223–9.

62. Stone DJ, Gal TJ. Airway management. In: Miller RD, editor. Anesthesia. New York: Churchill Livingstone; 2000. p. 1414–51.

63. Grmec S. Comparison of three different methods to confirm tracheal tube placement in emergency intubation. Intensive Care Med 2002;28(6):701–4.

64. Deiorio NM. Continuous end-tidal carbon dioxide monitoring for confirmation of endotracheal tube placement is neither widely available nor consistently applied by emergency physicians. Emerg Med J 2005;22(7):490–3.

65. Sim SS, Lien WC, Chou HC, et al. Ultrasonographic lung sliding sign in confirming proper endotracheal intubation during emergency intubation. Resuscitation 2012;83(3):307–12.

66. Brun PM, Bessereau J, Cazes N, et al. Lung ultrasound associated to capnography to verify correct endotracheal tube positioning in prehospital. Am J Emerg Med 2011. [Epub ahead of print].

67. Pfeiffer P, Rudolph SS, Børglum J, et al. Temporal comparison of ultrasound vs. auscultation and capnography in verification of endotracheal tube placement. Acta Anaesthesiol Scand 2011;55(10):1190–5.

68. Weaver B, Lyon M, Blaivas M. Confirmation of endotracheal tube placement after intubation using the ultrasound sliding lung sign. Acad Emerg Med 2006;13(3):239–44.

69. Shah KH, Kwong BM, Hazan A, et al. Success of the gum elastic bougie as a rescue airway in the emergency department. J Emerg Med 2011;40(1):1–6.

70. Arora MK, Karamchandani K, Trikha A. Use of a gum elastic bougie to facilitate blind nasotracheal intubation in children: a series of three cases. Anaesthesia 2006;61(3):291–4.

71. Arisaka H, Sakuraba S, Furuya M, et al. Application of gum elastic bougie to nasal intubation. Anesth Prog 2010;57(3):112–3.

72. Marciniak D, Smith CE. Emergent retrograde tracheal intubation with a gum-elastic bougie in a trauma patient. Anesth Analg 2007;105(6):1720–1.

73. Smith MD, Katrinchak J. Use of a gum elastic bougie during surgical crichothyrotomy. Am J Emerg Med 2008;26(6):738.

74. Nolan JP, Wilson ME. Orotracheal intubation in patients with potential cervical spine injuries. An indication for the gum-elastic bougie. Anaesthesia 1993; 48(7):630–3.

75. Sime J, Bailitz J, Moskoff J. The bougie: an inexpensive lifesaving airway device. J Emerg Med 2011. [Epub ahead of print].
76. Kidd JF, Dyson A, Latto IP. Successful difficult intubation. Use of the gum elastic bougie. Anaesthesia 1988;43(6):437–8.
77. Phelan MP. Use of the endotracheal bougie introducer for difficult intubations. Am J Emerg Med 2004;22(6):479–82.
78. Hernandez MR, Klock PA Jr, Ovassapian A. Evolution of the extraglottic airway: a review of its history, applications, and practical tips for success. Anesth Analg 2012;114(2):349–68.
79. Parmet JL, Colonna-Romano P, Horrow JC, et al. The laryngeal mask airway reliably provides rescue ventilation in cases of unanticipated difficult tracheal intubation along with difficult mask ventilation. Anesth Analg 1998;87(3):661–5.
80. Jones JR. Laryngeal mask airway: an alternative for the difficult airway. AANA J 1995;63(5):444–9.
81. Schälte G, Stoppe C, Aktas M, et al. Laypersons can successfully place supraglottic airways with 3 minutes of training. A comparison of four different devices in the manikin. Scand J Trauma Resusc Emerg Med 2011;19:60.
82. Gerstein NS, Braude DA, Hung O, et al. The Fastrach Intubating Laryngeal Mask Airway: an overview and update. Can J Anaesth 2010;57(6):588–601.
83. Fukutome T, Amaha K, Nakazawa K, et al. Tracheal intubation through the intubating laryngeal mask airway (LMA-Fastrach) in patients with difficult airways. Anaesth Intensive Care 1998;26(4):387–91.
84. Rosenblatt WH, Murphy M. The intubating laryngeal mask: use of a new ventilating-intubating device in the emergency department. Ann Emerg Med 1999;33(2):234–8.
85. Levitan RM, Ochroch EA, Stuart S, et al. Use of the intubating laryngeal mask airway by medical and nonmedical personnel. Am J Emerg Med 2000;18(1):12–6.
86. Young B. The intubating laryngeal-mask airway may be an ideal device for airway control in the rural trauma patient. Am J Emerg Med 2003;21(1):80–5.
87. Ferson DZ, Rosenblatt WH, Johansen MJ, et al. Use of the intubating LMA-Fastrach in 254 patients with difficult-to-manage airways. Anesthesiology 2001;95(5):1175–81.
88. Wakeling HG, Bagwell A. The intubating laryngeal mask (ILMA) in an emergency failed intubation. Anaesthesia 1999;54(3):305–6.
89. Murdoch JA. Emergency tracheal intubation using a gum elastic bougie through a laryngeal mask airway. Anaesthesia 2005;60(6):626–7.
90. Hubble MW, Wilfong DA, Brown LH, et al. A meta-analysis of prehospital airway control techniques part II: alternative airway devices and cricothyrotomy success rates. Prehosp Emerg Care 2010;14(4):515–30.
91. Deakin CD, Nolan JP, Soar J, et al. European resuscitation council guidelines for resuscitation 2010 section 4. Adult advanced life support. Resuscitation 2010;81(10):1305–52.
92. Russi CS, Miller L, Hartley MJ. A comparison of the King-LT to endotracheal intubation and Combitube in a simulated difficult airway. Prehosp Emerg Care 2008;12(1):35–41.
93. Guyette FX, Wang H, Cole JS. King airway use by air medical providers. Prehosp Emerg Care 2007;11(4):473–6.
94. Hagberg C, Bogomony Y, Gilmore C, et al. An evaluation of the insertion and function of a new supraglottic airway device, the King LT, during spontaneous ventilation. Anesth Analg 2006;102(2):621–5.

95. Genzwuerker HV, Vollmer T, Ellinger K. Fibreoptic tracheal intubation after placement of the laryngeal tube. Br J Anaesth 2002;89(5):733–8.
96. Lutes M, Worman DJ. An unanticipated complication of a novel approach to airway management. J Emerg Med 2010;38(2):222–4.
97. Bentsianov BL, Parhiscar A, Azer M, et al. The role of fiberoptic nasopharyngoscopy in the management of the acute airway in angioneurotic edema. Laryngoscope 2000;110(12):2016–9.
98. Agrawal P, Gupta B, D'souza N, et al. Fiberoptic bronchoscope assisted difficult airway management in maxillofacial trauma. Ann Maxillofac Surg 2011;1(1): 95–6.
99. Wang HE, Kupas DF, Greenwood MJ, et al. An algorithmic approach to prehospital airway management. Prehosp Emerg Care 2005;9(2):145–55.
100. Godwin SA. Blind intubation techniques. In: Walls RM, Murphy MF, editors. Manual of emergency airway management. 4th edition. Philadelphia: Lippincott Williams and Wilkins; 2012. p. 185–92.
101. Rosen CL, Wolfe RE, Chew SE, et al. Blind nasotracheal intubation in the presence of facial trauma. J Emerg Med 1997;15(2):141–5.
102. Murphy MF, DeBlieux PMC. Flexible endoscopic intubation. In: Walls RM, Murphy MF, editors. Manual of emergency airway management. 4th edition. Philadelphia: Lippincott Williams and Wilkins; 2012. p. 166–73.
103. Gwinnutt CL. The interface between anaesthesia and emergency medicine. Emerg Med J 2001;18(5):325–6.
104. Walls RM. Rapid sequence intubation. In: Walls RM, Murphy MF, editors. Manual of emergency airway management. 4th edition. Philadelphia: Lippincott Williams and Wilkins; 2012. p. 220–32.
105. Baraka AS, Taha SK, Aouad MT, et al. Preoxygenation: comparison of maximal breathing and tidal volume breathing techniques. Anesthesiology 1999;91(3): 612–6.
106. Farmery AD, Roe PG. A model to describe the rate of oxyhaemoglobin desaturation during apnoea. Br J Anaesth 1996;76(2):284–91.
107. Mort TC. Preoxygenation in critically ill patients requiring emergency tracheal intubation. Crit Care Med 2005;33(11):2672–5.
108. Weingart SD, Levitan RM. Preoxygenation and prevention of desaturation during emergency airway management. Ann Emerg Med 2012;59(3):165–75.
109. Baker PA, Weller JM, Greenland KB, et al. Education in airway management. Anaesthesia 2011;66(Suppl 2):101–11.
110. Singh H, Vichitvejpaisal P, Gaines GY, et al. Comparative effects of lidocaine, esmolol, and nitroglycerin in modifying the hemodynamic response to laryngoscopy and intubation. J Clin Anesth 1995;7(1):5–8.
111. Donegan MF, Bedford RF. Intravenously administered lidocaine prevents intracranial hypertension during endotracheal suctioning. Anesthesiology 1980; 52(6):516–8.
112. Chraemmer-Jørgensen B, Høilund-Carlsen PF, Marving J, et al. Lack of effect of intravenous lidocaine on hemodynamic responses to rapid sequence induction of general anesthesia: a double-blind controlled clinical trial. Anesth Analg 1986;65(10):1037–41.
113. Walls RM. Management of the difficult airway in the trauma patient. Emerg Med Clin North Am 1998;16(1):45–61.
114. de Nadal M, Munar F, Poca MA, et al. Cerebral hemodynamic effects of morphine and fentanyl in patients with severe head injury: absence of correlation to cerebral autoregulation. Anesthesiology 2000;92(1):11–9.

115. McAuliffe G, Bissonnette B, Boutin C. Should the routine use of atropine before succinylcholine in children be reconsidered? Can J Anaesth 1995;42(8):724–9.

116. Fastle RK, Roback MG. Pediatric rapid sequence intubation: incidence of reflex bradycardia and effects of pretreatment with atropine. Pediatr Emerg Care 2004;20(10):651–5.

117. Reynolds SF, Heffner J. Airway management of the critically ill patient: rapid-sequence intubation. Chest 2005;127(4):1397–412.

118. Sivilotti ML, Filbin MF, Murray HE, et al. Does the sedative agent facilitate emergency rapid sequence intubation? Acad Emerg Med 2003;10(6):612–20.

119. Bergen JM, Smith DC. A review of etomidate for rapid sequence intubation in the emergency department. J Emerg Med 1997;15(2):221–30.

120. Yeung JK, Zed PJ. A review of etomidate for rapid sequence intubation in the emergency department. CJEM 2002;4(3):194–8.

121. Sih K, Campbell SG, Tallon JM, et al. Ketamine in adult emergency medicine: controversies and recent advances. Ann Pharmacother 2011;45(12):1525–34.

122. Sehdev RS, Symmons DA, Kindl K. Ketamine for rapid sequence induction in patients with head injury in the emergency department. Emerg Med Australas 2006;18(1):37–44.

123. Hudetz JA, Pagel PS. Neuroprotection by ketamine: a review of the experimental and clinical evidence. J Cardiothorac Vasc Anesth 2010;24(1):131–42.

124. Bourgoin A, Albanèse J, Léone M, et al. Effects of sufentanil or ketamine administered in target-controlled infusion on the cerebral hemodynamics of severely brain-injured patients. Crit Care Med 2005;33(5):1109–13.

125. Bar-Joseph G, Guilburd Y, Tamir A, et al. Effectiveness of ketamine in decreasing intracranial pressure in children with intracranial hypertension. J Neurosurg Pediatr 2009;4(1):40–6.

126. Martyn JA, Richtsfeld M. Succinylcholine-induced hyperkalemia in acquired pathologic states: etiologic factors and molecular mechanisms. Anesthesiology 2006;104(1):158–69.

127. Burkle CM, Walsh MT, Harrison BA, et al. Airway management after failure to intubate by direct laryngoscopy: outcomes in a large teaching hospital. Can J Anaesth 2005;52(6):634–40.

128. Agro F, Hung OR, Cataldo R, et al. Lightwand intubation using the Trachlight: a brief review of current knowledge. Can J Anaesth 2001;48(6):592–9.

129. Hung OR, Pytka A, Morris I, et al. Clinical trial of a new lightwand device (Trachlight) to intubate the trachea. Anesthesiology 1995;83(3):509–14.

130. Kovacs G, Law JA, McCrossin C, et al. A comparison of a fiberoptic stylet and a bougie as adjuncts to direct laryngoscopy in a manikin-simulated difficult airway. Ann Emerg Med 2007;50(6):676–85.

131. Dhara SS. Retrograde tracheal intubation. Anaesthesia 2009;64(10):1094–104.

132. Elliott DS, Baker PA, Scott MR, et al. Accuracy of surface landmark identification for cannula cricothyroidotomy. Anaesthesia 2010;65(9):889–94.

133. Bennett JD, Guha SC, Sankar AB. Cricothyrotomy: the anatomical basis. J R Coll Surg Edinb 1996;41(1):57–60.

134. Murphy MF. Applied functional anatomy of the airway. In: Walls RM, Murphy MF, editors. Manual of emergency airway management. 4th edition. Philadelphia: Lippincott Williams and Wilkins; 2012. p. 36–44.

135. Won HS, Han SH, Oh CS, et al. Superior and middle thyroid arteries arising from the common carotid artery. Surg Radiol Anat 2011;33(7):645–7.

136. Farcy DA, Chiu MC, Flaxman A, et al. Critical care emergency medicine. New York: McGraw Hill Professional; 2011.

137. Isaacs JH Jr, Pedersen AD. Emergency cricothyroidotomy. Am Surg 1997;63(4): 346–9.
138. Schaumann N, Lorenz V, Schellongowski P, et al. Evaluation of Seldinger technique emergency cricothyroidotomy versus standard surgical cricothyroidotomy in 200 cadavers. Anesthesiology 2005;102(1):7–11.
139. Richard JD, Dreyfuss D, Saumon G. Ventilation-induced lung injury. Eur Respir J 2003;22(Suppl 42):2s–9s.
140. The Acute Respiratory Distress Syndrome Network. Ventilation with lower tidal volumes as compared with traditional tidal volumes for acute lung injury and the acute respiratory distress syndrome. N Engl J Med 2000;342(18):1301–8.
141. Brower RG, Lanken PN, MacIntyre N, et al. Higher vs. lower positive end-expiration pressures in patients with the acute respiratory distress syndrome. N Engl J Med 2004;351(4):327–36.
142. NHLBI ARDS Network. Ventilator protocol card. Available at: http://www.ardsnet. org/node/77791. Accessed January 24, 2012.
143. Marino PL. The ICU book. 3rd edition. Philadelphia: Lippincott Williams and Wilkins; 2007.
144. Strom T, Martinussen T, Toft P. A protocol of no sedation for critically ill patients receiving mechanical ventilation: a randomised trial. Lancet 2010;375(9713): 475–80.

Critical ENT Skills and Procedures in the Emergency Department

Jorge L. Falcon-Chevere, MD[a],*, Laureano Giraldez, MD[b],
Jose O. Rivera-Rivera, MD[a], Tito Suero-Salvador, MD[a]

KEYWORDS

- Ear laceration • Foreign body • Epistaxis • Peritonsilar abscess
- Nasal septal hematoma

KEY POINTS

- Emergency physicians (EPs) must be familiar with otolaryngologic emergencies.
- They must be dexterous while performing otolaryngologic (ear, nose, and throat [ENT]) procedures to maintain function while avoiding complications.
- Among critical skills needed and procedures performed by the emergency practitioner are complex auricular lacerations repair, auricular hematoma incision and drainage, epistaxis management, and peritonsillar abscess incision and drainage.

AURICLE AND EAR CANAL ANATOMY

Knowledge of the anatomy of the external ear is essential to the emergency provider; from laceration repair to foreign bodies removal, it is fundamental for the success of the procedures to be performed. The auricle (pinna) consists of the visible and convoluted external part of the ear, it is a thin cartilage surrounded by thin skin. **Fig. 1** shows in detail the external anatomy of the ear. The auditory canal measures about 2.5 cm, it extends from the external side at the concha to the internal portion at the level of the tympanic membrane. The canal is lined by squamous and hairy epithelium that produces cerumen. Its arterial supply is derived from the external carotid artery via superficial branches such as the maxillary, superficial temporal, and posterior. The greater auricular, auriculotemporal, and auricular branch of the vagus nerve provide innervation to the ear.[1] The external ear canal has two anatomical narrowing areas. The first one is found at the junction of cartilage and bone, while the second one is lateral to the tympanic membrane. The emergency physician must consider these narrowing areas when attempting to remove foreign bodies.[2]

None of the authors have any disclosure.

[a] Department of Emergency Medicine, University of Puerto Rico School of Medicine, 65th Inf. Station, San Juan, PR 00929, USA; [b] Department of Otolaringology, University of Puerto Rico School of Medicine, 65th Inf. Station, San Juan, PR 00929, USA

* Corresponding author. Department of Emergency Medicine, University of Puerto Rico School of Medicine, PO Box 29207, 65th Inf. Station, San Juan, PR 00929.

E-mail address: jfalconc@gmail.com

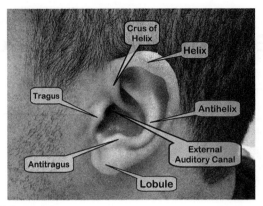

Fig. 1. Anatomy of the auricle.

ANESTHESIA OF THE EAR
Field Blocks of the Auricle

The term field block is used to describe the technique in which anesthesia is infiltrated to the subcutaneous tissue surrounding the operative field.[3] It is indicated when large lacerations, hematomas, and incision and drainage (I & D) of the auricle are to be performed, because extensive local infiltration is not desired.[4] Among the advantages of field blocks are longer duration of anesthesia and less swelling and anatomic disruption when compared with local infiltration.[5] The use of small needles and stretching the skin is found to be effective in decreasing injection site pain.[3] Local care must be provided with cleansing solution to the injection site. There are various approaches to provide anesthesia to the auricle. The procedure consists of 2 simple anesthetic injections. The first injection site is located about 1 cm over the superior pole of the ear. The needle (25–27 gauge) with lidocaine or bupivacaine[2] is directed toward the anterior portion of the tragus up to the middle of the ear infiltrating anesthesia (2–3 mL) as the needle is withdrawn to the insertion point; then the ear is infiltrated posteriorly. The second infiltration site is located at the inferior pole of the ear to the remaining portion of the anterior and posterior ear. A diamond-shaped area is anesthetized around the ear (**Fig. 2**), but changing the number and direction of the anesthetic walls could modify the shape.[3] Another alternative method uses approximately 3 to 4 mL of anesthetic, both at a point anterior to the tragus and in the posterior ear sulcus. If only the central concha and/or ear canal anesthesia is desired, a series of 0.5- to 1.0-mL injections of 1% lidocaine to the external ear meatus are performed. Complications could arise if epinephrine is used in conjunction with local anesthesia, because often the patient's auricular vascular area is already compromised and there is an existent risk of necrosis to inject epinephrine to the terminal arterial branches in the ear lobes.[5]

EAR LACERATION

When dealing with ear lacerations, the primary goals are repair of the structure, early management of the cartilage exposure, and prevention of complications. The EP should assess the need for immediate evaluation, approximate wound the margins to evaluate large gapping areas or anticipate gross deformities. Preserving the skin is a major concern because of the need for stretching it to cover the cartilage. No cartilage should be left exposed; if needed, up to 5 mm of cartilage can be excised before

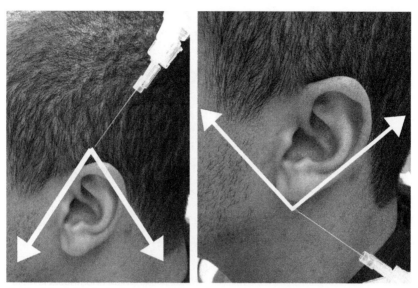

Fig. 2. Auricle field block. A diamond-shaped area is anesthetized around the ear.

the ear starts to show a deformed appearance.[1] Local care to the affected area is vital; it is prepared in the usual fashion. When suturing the cartilage, the anatomic areas and landmarks of the ear are approximated first at the areas of the ridge and the pinna to preserve the anatomy of the ear. Suturing the cartilage is done in a gentle manner and with the amount of force necessary to touch the borders of the cartilages to avoid ripping. The suture must include the anterior and posterior perichondrium using 4-0 and 5-0 absorbable sutures. After managing the cartilage, the skin is sutured using 5-0 to 6-0 nonabsorbable synthetic sutures, taking into consideration the landmarks of the ear and using it as anchors to maintain the anatomy of the ear (**Fig. 3**).

The use of oral antibiotics is highly advised on scenarios that involve cartilage debridement, dirty wound, and injuries that raise concern for infection. Finally, after suturing the laceration, the use of compression dressing over the ear (**Fig. 4**) ora bolster for 7 days is highly advised to prevent the formation of ear hematoma. Both methods are discussed in detail in the section dealing with auricular hematoma management.

Complications (**Box 1**) that might compromise the normal anatomy of the ear could arise, resulting in a hematoma formation, which separates the skin from the cartilage, resulting in the interruption of the vascular supply to the cartilage.[1,2]

AURICULAR HEMATOMA

Auricular hematomas (**Fig. 5**) are commonly encountered in wrestlers and boxers and people involved in other unprotected contact sports.[6] Usually, hematomas occur as a result of blunt trauma to the ear, whereby shearing forces separate the skin, subcutaneous tissue, and perichondrium of the ear from the underlying cartilage, forming pockets where blood can accumulate. Disruption of the perichondrium–cartilage interface disrupts the vascular anatomy of the ear, leading to deficient nutrient transport causing devitalized cartilage. This cartilage has a propensity for fibrosis formation and results in "cauliflower ear" (**Fig. 6**).[7] Cauliflower ear is also known as "wrestler's

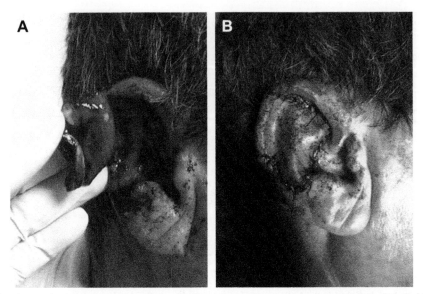

Fig. 3. Ear laceration suture repair. Cartilage is repaired using 4-0 and 5-0 absorbable sutures. Skin is sutured using 5-0 to 6-0 nonabsorbable synthetic sutures. (*A*) Complex ear laceration. (*B*) Ear laceration repaired using 5–0 to 6–0 nonabsorbable synthetic sutures, taking into consideration the landmarks of the ear and using it as anchors to maintain the anatomy of the ear.

ear." Hence, auricular hematoma requires prompt treatment because it may lead to cartilage necrosis, contracture, new cartilage formation, and ultimately ear deformity.[8]

Auricular hematomas are treated with evacuation of fluid collection and subsequent bolster of the ear. Indications and contraindications of the procedure are mentioned in **Box 2**. There are many approaches to addressing hematomas and subsequently

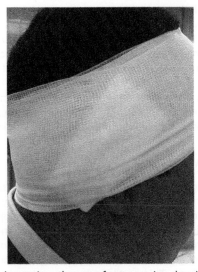

Fig. 4. After suturing the laceration, the use of compression dressing over the ear for 7 days is advised to prevent the formation of ear hematoma.

Box 1
Auricular laceration repair complications
Complications
Chondritis
Auricular hematomas including cauliflower hematoma (chronic)
Keloid

restoring the anatomy of the ear. For small hematomas of the ear, needle aspiration and subsequent bolster dressing or splint is recommended. Larger hematomas require aggressive incision and drainage and also bolster dressing placement. If there are accompanying lacerations, then they must be primarily repaired.

Needle aspiration is usually done with hematomas that are less than 1.5 cm in diameter. Equipment recommended to perform this procedure is mentioned in **Box 3**. An 18-gauge needle is used with a 5-mL syringe to evacuate the contents of the hematoma. If small hematomas do not resolve because the blood clot is not completely evacuated with the needle, incision and drainage must be done. Nonetheless, even if the hematoma is small, it is recommended to leave a bolster dressing on for 5 to 7 days. The technique of bolster dressing placement is explained later.

Larger hematomas usually require incision and drainage (see **Box 3**). Lidocaine/epinephrine solution is used to infiltrate the skin over the hematoma. Parallel vertical incisions are made with a number. 15 blade on the anterior and, if necessary, posterior skin of the auricle. The hematoma is evacuated. Penrose drainage is inserted at this point for large hematomas and secured with prolene sutures. Penrose drainages are removed when serous fluid and bloody drainage stop within 2 to 3 days of placement; if left in place, they need close follow-up in the outpatient setting. Otolaryngology consult is recommended for evaluation of these patients.

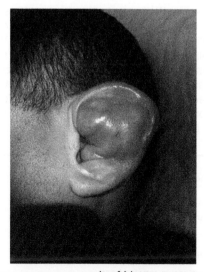

Fig. 5. Auricular hematomas occur as a result of blunt trauma to the ear. Shearing forces separate the skin, subcutaneous tissue, and perichondrium of the ear from the underlying cartilage, forming pockets where blood can accumulate.

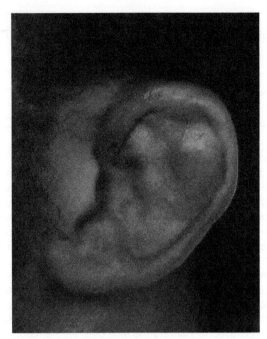

Fig. 6. Cauliflower ear or wrestler's ear is a chronic deformity that results from fibrosis due to unsolved or recurrent auricular hematoma.

Complications of auricular hematoma include hematoma reaccumulation, infection, and cosmetic deformity, among others (**Box 4**).

COMPRESSION DRESSING AND EAR BOLSTER

After hematoma aspiration or drainage, a compression dressing is applied to avoid hematoma reaccumulation. Dry cotton is placed into the external canal. All external auricular crevices are filled with moist gauzes. Alternatively, Vaseline gauze may be used. A gauze pack is placed posterior to the auricle. The ear is covered with multiple layers of gauzes. An elastic bandage is used to keep the gauzes in place. An alternative to compression dressing is the ear bolster (**Fig. 7**). A 14F or 16F suction catheter is cut into 1.5- to 2-cm pieces. These pieces are used as anterior and posterior bolster dressings. Prolene 2-0 or 3-0 sutures are usually used for this procedure. A horizontal mattress suture is used to hold the French catheters against the skin of the auricle in

---

Box 2
Auricular hematomas—indications and contraindications

Indications

Subperichondrial auricular hematoma less than 7 days old

Contraindications

Subperichondrial auricular hematoma older than 7 days

Severe trauma requiring extensive repair of ear

Physician unrelated to procedure

Box 3
Equipment recommended to perform an auricular hematoma evacuation
Equipment
Sterile gloves
Local anesthetics
Antiseptic topical solution
Needle (27 gauge) for local anesthesia infiltration
Needle (18 gauge) for drainage
Syringes (2)
Suction catheter
Scalpel with number 15 blade
Sterile rubber drain for bolsters
Sterile gauze pads
Normal saline solution
Compression dressings

the area of the drained hematoma. This procedure results in eliminating the pocket of blood accumulation and obliterating the subperichondral space. Bolster splints are usually removed 7 days after being sutured. Bolsters have been made of cotton dressings, silicone rubber splints, and removable auricular stents, among other things.[7] A recent Cochrane review of the literature revealed that there is no consensus on how to treat auricular hematomas and no advantage of one technique over another.[9]

Patients who undergo auricular soft-tissue trauma with associated immunocompromise are prophylactically administered antipseudomonal and antistaphylococcal antibiotic to avoid posttraumatic chondritis. Patients without marked leukocytosis, altered vital signs, or associated head trauma are discharged home and followed up as outpatients. The bolster dressing is removed in 7 days. If persistent fluid, auricular edema, erythema, or pain is still present when the bolster dressing is removed, then evaluation by an otolaryngologist is needed.

CERUMEN IMPACTION

Cerumen is a natural product of the ear canal, composed of epithelial cells, hair,[10] and sebaceous glands. The glands produce sebum and sweat to protect, lubricate, and clean the ear canal.[11] Cerumen can occlude the ear canal easily as a result of

Box 4
Auricular hematoma drainage complications
Complications
Hematoma reaccumulation
Cellulitis
Abscess formation
Cosmetic deformity
Cartilage necrosis

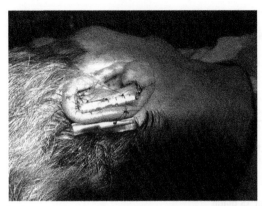

Fig. 7. Ear bolster eliminates blood reaccumulation, obliterating the subperichondral space.

excessive accumulation, causing tinnitus, pain, external ear infection, hearing loss, fullness, itching, and even cough.[12,13] About 8 million ear irrigations are performed annually for this condition.[12,14] The 2 most common populations affected are the elderly (up to 57%) and patients with mental retardation (up to 36%).[11,12] Available techniques for cerumen removal are manual removal, irrigation, and ceruminolytics. Cerumen removal is indicated in symptomatic patients and those who require an evaluation of the tympanic membrane.

Manual removal of cerumen has the benefit of being faster to perform as it allows the physician to have direct visualization of the anatomic area. However, the required equipment for the procedure is not readily available in most emergency departments.[10,12] The need for a cooperative patient and a skilled physician are also important considerations for successful removal and therefore can become contraindications. The common complications are tympanic membrane perforation and trauma to the external ear canal[10] that could lead to secondary infection. If cerumen cannot be removed manually, then the irrigation technique is performed or the patient referred to an outpatient evaluation by the otorhinolaryngologist.

Irrigation for cerumen removal is often used alone or with a ceruminolytic pretreatment.[10] Even though there are no randomized controlled clinical trials of ear irrigation versus no treatment, there is a consensus that aural irrigation is effective in removing cerumen.[12] Because ear syringes and oral jet irrigators are widely available and inexpensive, they are great alternatives for performing this procedure,[10,14] although there still exists the risk of tympanic membrane perforation especially with the use of oral jet irrigators.[15] There are commercially available kits, but a 20- to 30-mL syringe with an 18-gauge plastic intravenous (IV) catheter or the plastic portion of a butterfly needle is an acceptable instrument for irrigating the ear (**Fig. 8**).[2,10]

The procedure is simple and involves applying soft traction up and back to make a straighter canal and equal soft irrigation to the ear, checking sporadically for the cerumen. Contraindications include recent ear surgery, any concern for tympanic membrane perforation, myringotomy tube presence, a history of middle-ear disease, radiation therapy to the area, severe otitis externa, sharp foreign objects in the external auditory canal, or vertigo.[2,10]

Topical therapy for ceruminolytic agents is regularly used to manage cerumen impactions either alone or in combination with other techniques, including irrigation of the ear canal and manual removal of cerumen. Water-based agents act by inducing hydration and fragmentation, whereas oil-based products lubricate and soften

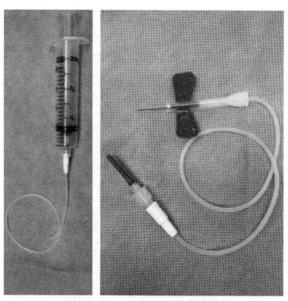

Fig. 8. Use a 20- to 30-mL syringe with a plastic angiocatheter (18 gauge) or a butterfly cannula without the needle to irrigate the ear for foreign body removal.

cerumen without decomposing it. The exact mechanism of the non–oil-based or non–water-based agents has not been completely defined yet (**Table 1**).[10,12] Evidence shows that any type of agent seems to be superior to no treatment, but it is not shown that any particular agent is superior to any other. Evidence exists that supports a true ceruminolytic rather than an oil-based lubricant for dissolution of cerumen for a longer period of treatment. The use of these agents improves success of irrigation, but no agent has been shown to be better than the other. Using an agent immediately before irrigation has not been shown to be superior or inferior to using one several days before irrigation either. As with other procedures, there are complications related to the use of ceruminolytic agents, such as dermatitis, allergic reactions, and otitis externa.[12]

Ear Foreign Bodies Removal

There is a wide range of foreign bodies that could be trapped in the external auditory canal because of its anatomic narrowings: from small objects in children, such as organic material like popcorn kernels,[16] toys and beads, food and inorganic objects, to small living insects in adults.[2] Even though many foreign bodies are successfully removed, the procedure has a wide range of complications.[16]

To manage foreign bodies in the ear, physicians should be aware of their skills and expertise of the anatomic area, the number of attempts to be performed with a realistic goal, and the need for consultation with the otolaryngology service.[2] There is little evidence of which intervention is the best method for foreign body removal.[17] There are many factors that contribute to higher failure rates such as patient's young age and the period the foreign body was in the external ear canal.[18,19]

There are many options for ear foreign body removal (**Box 5**), which include water irrigation, forceps removal, and use of cerumen loops, cyanoacrylate, and even suction catheters. The EP should be cautious if there is concern of tympanic membrane rupture. The first attempt of removal of a foreign body is the most critical because it is related to higher success and further attempts are related to failure.[19–21]

Table 1
Cerumen removal agents

Agent	Use	Dosing
Water based		
Water	Soften cerumen	Instill water to area to achieve softening of the cerumen
10% Sodium bicarbonate	Soften cerumen	Fill ear with 2–3 mL 15–30 min before irrigation or, alternatively, for 3–14 d at home with or without irrigation
Docusate sodium	Soften cerumen	Fill ear canal with 1 mL 15–30 min before irrigation
10% Triethanolamine polypeptide oleate condensate	Soften cerumen	Fill ear canal 15–30 min before irrigation
3% Hydrogen peroxide	Soften cerumen	Fill ear canal 15–30 min before irrigation
2.5% Acetic acid	Outpatient treatment	Fill ear with 2–3 mL twice daily for up to 14 d
Non–water based/non–oil based		
Carbamide peroxide	Soften cerumen before irrigation or as an alternative to irrigation	Put 5–10 drops into the affected ear twice daily
50% Choline salicylate and glycerol; ethylene oxide polyoxypropylene glycol; propylene glycol; 0.5% chlorbutol	Soften cerumen	Put 3 drops into the affected ear twice daily
Oil based		
57.3% Arachis oil, 5% chlorbutol, 2% paradicholorbenzene, 10% oil of turpentine	Soften cerumen	Fill ear with 5 mL twice daily for 2–3 d
Mineral oil	Soften cerumen	Put 3 drops into the affected ear at bedtime for 3 or 4 d

Adapted from McCarter DF, Courtney AU, Pollart SM. Cerumen impaction. Am Fam Physician 2007;75(10):1523–8.

Box 5
Equipment recommended for ear foreign body removal

Equipment

Curette

Probe

Hook

Forceps

Suction under direct visualization with headlight

Otoscopy or microscopy

Consultations to an ENT specialist include tympanic membrane perforation or trauma to the canal, a nongraspable object, and objects with sharp edges, or unsuccessful attempts to remove it.[16,22,23] Visualization of the foreign body has been associated with a low complication rate, and the rate of lacerations of the canal was as low as 4% when a microscope was used versus a 48% when a microscope was not used (**Fig. 9**).[17,24]

Irrigation technique is the preferred method to retrieve small objects. The procedure is simple; a 30- to 60-mL syringe with a plastic angiocatheter (18 gauge) or a butterfly cannula without the needle is used as previously described. It is introduced in the ear with water at room temperature to achieve the extraction of the object. The stream is directed toward the superior aspect of the ear canal.[25] This is a simple procedure that has a low complication rate but is contraindicated in patients with foreign bodies that could swell or are made of vegetable material.[24]

Another available technique is suction of the foreign body, which is easily available at the emergency department. It is effective for round objects. Negative pressures about 100 to 140 mm Hg are used.[17,26,27] Often it could be performed with soft catheters such as the ones used for endotracheal tube suctioning.[25] A pitfall of this procedure is the noise that is generated; it could easily increase the fear and anxiety in patients, especially among pediatric population.

The glue technique was first described in India in 1977 using gum-based glue.[17,28] Now it has been replaced with a faster-acting material called cyanoacrylate or the so-called superglue.[17,29,30] Its use is indicated to remove smooth, round, dry, and easily visualized foreign bodies that are hard to grasp. It is recommended to use a small amount of glue preferentially on a tip of a paper clip or a wooden stick with a cotton tip to limit the amount of glue inside the ear and decrease the risk for new material trapped in the ear canal. Even though it is a simple technique, it requires patient compliance and is generally an acceptable method for children.[17]

The manual technique is the most related to complications and highly associated with abrasions, lacerations of ear canal, bleeding, and tympanic membrane perforation. This technique requires the direct visualization of the foreign body. The choice of the instrument to use varies depending on the foreign body. Recommended instruments are alligator forceps, hooks, curettes, and loops. This technique is not the best option with foreign bodies that could easily tear apart while removing or with uncooperative patients.[17]

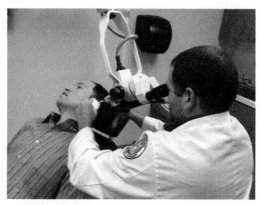

Fig. 9. Foreign body removal through a microscope has been associated with low complications rate.

An alternative method uses a Foley or Fogarty balloon catheter. The literature shows that its use has been successful for both nasal and ear foreign bodies retrieval.[31,32] The noninflated balloon tip is passed beyond the object. The balloon is filled with 3 mL of air, then the catheter is pulled back to recover the object.[17]

Insects inside the ear canal raise a concern, because a living insect is disturbing to the patient. The first step in removing the insect is killing it. The best way to accomplish this is filling the ear canal with mineral oil or lidocaine 2% solution.[25] The mineral oil is the fastest way to kill the insect as compared with lidocaine.[33] Mineral oil becomes more viscous in the ear than lidocaine. After the insect is dead, extraction can proceed with one of the above-described methods. If the physician is unable to remove the dead insect, the patient is referred for outpatient removal.

Complications could arise from ear foreign body removal, including simple abrasions, lacerations, infection, bleeding, and tympanic membrane perforation.[17,25] Most of the ear foreign bodies could be referred to outpatient management. The only case that requires immediate management would be a button battery because of complications such as ulceration and necrosis of the ear canal.[17,34] There is no routine follow-up needed in uncomplicated cases except for the above-mentioned condition.[17]

Nose

The nose is the external portion of the respiratory system and is found at the entrance of the airway, where it acts as a filter, a humidifier, and a chemosensor. It should not be considered as 1 single airway but rather 2 separate nasal passages, each with its own blood supply and nervous pathways. Considering the position of the nose in relation to the rest of the structures in the face, one could be at great risk to injure the nose when trauma occurs.

Anatomy of the Nose

Understanding the basic anatomy of the nose is of great importance when it comes to treating the most common encounters in the emergency department. The structural composition of the nose is essentially of cartilage and bone covered by skin, with mucosa lining the inner surface. The nose consists of the vestibule, nasal septum, lateral wall, and nasopharynx.[2] The most ventral portion of the nares is composed of the vestibule. The midline structure is formed by the septum, and the lateral wall is formed by the turbinates.

Three major arteries provide blood supply to the nose (**Fig. 10**). The ophthalmic artery divides into the ethmoidal artery to supply the superior nasal mucosa. The sphenopalatine artery supplies the posterior septum and the lateral turbinates. To complete the triad, the superior labial artery supplies the nasal septum and vestibule. The terminal branches of these major arteries supply an arterial anastomotic triangle known as Kiesselbach plexus; 90% to 95% of episodes of epistaxis arise from the anterior nasal septum.[35] The most common arterial source of posterior nosebleeds is the sphenopalatine artery.

The sensation of the nose is divided into the internal and external innervation.[36] The ophthalmic and maxillary branches of the trigeminal nerve innervate the external aspect of the nose. The infratrochlear and supratrochlear nerves and a branch of the anterior ethmoid nerve, the external nasal nerve, supply the superior aspect of the nose, including the tip. The infraorbital nerve innervates the inferior and lateral aspects of the nose.

To better understand the innervations of the internal nasal cavity, it is subdivided into the nasal septum, the lateral walls, and the cribriform plate. The ethmoid nerves supply the inner aspect of the lateral nasal wall. The sphenopalatine ganglion

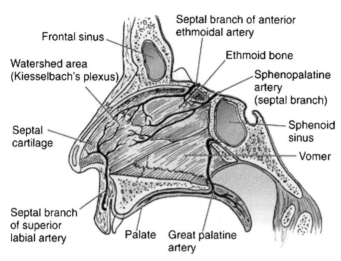

Fig. 10. Nasal vascular supply. The most common site of anterior epistaxis is within the area labeled Kiesselbach plexus. (*From* Maceri DR. Epistaxis and nasal trauma. In: Cummings CW, editor. Otolaryngology—head and neck surgery. 2nd edition. St Louis (MO): Mosby–Year Book; 1993. p. 728.)

innervates the posterior nasal cavity. Fibers of the previously mentioned ethmoid nerves and the sphenopalatine ganglion provide sensation to most of the septum.

Physical Examination

When examining the nose, some important points are to be taken into consideration. Both the internal and external anatomy should be assessed. Both the ability to smell and the sensation in the nasal region should be assessed, but it is considered as part of the neurologic examination instead of as part of the nose examination itself. When preparing the instruments for the procedure, a light source, suction, and a nasal speculum can all be of aid in the examination of the anterior nasal cavity. Topical sprays of anesthetics may also assist in the examination.

Epistaxis

Epistaxis is the most common otolaryngologic emergency. It is idiopathic in most patients, but it is also caused by neoplasm or trauma. Hypertension and coagulopathy are frequent comorbidities (ie, liver disease and renal dysfunction) seen in these patients. Many patients with epistaxis use either prescription anticoagulation medication (ie, coumadin, enoxaparin, acetylsalicylic acid, and clopidrogel) or natural herbal supplements with anticoagulation properties (ie, garlic, ginkgo, ginseng, and vitamin E).

The nasal cavity is highly vascular; branches of the internal and external carotid arteries that frequently anastomose with each other supply it. The internal carotid system supplies the ethmoidal arteries, whereas the external carotid system supplies the sphenopalatine artery, a branch of the internal maxillary artery. The area of more frequent bleeding is in the anterior nasal septum, called Kiesselbach or Little area.[37] It is a confluence of the internal and external carotid system.

Blood loss in epistaxis can range from mild bleeding to massive life-threatening hemorrhage. The amount of blood loss is quantified, and a complete blood count, type and group, and coagulation parameters are obtained. The patient is asked if bleeding was enough to fill a spoon, a teacup, or a larger container. The EP should ask if the bleeding was enough to soak a napkin or a towel. Melena is also a sign of excessive bleeding and should be warranted during taking of patient history. A clinical assessment of the patient's overall blood volume is established. Signs of tachycardia and hypotension cause worry especially in young individuals, as these are signs of significant blood loss.

Physical examination aims at identifying the type of bleeding. If the patient has intermittent episodes of bleeding and is not actively bleeding at the time, then anterior rhinoscopy is performed to identify areas of vessel exposure in the anterior septum. In the emergency room (ER), the aim is to control the bleeding with pressure in the anterior portion of the nose. If this technique does not control bleeding, 4% lidocaine with a vasoconstrictive agent (**Fig. 11**) such as cocaine or oxymetazoline is used. This method aids in 2 ways: it decongests the nasal cavity, leading to better visualization, and anesthetizes the nasal cavity to reduce patient discomfort and to better manage heavy bleeding.[38] If bleeding continues despite the previously described interventions, then nasal packing is immediately warranted.

Management aims at stopping the bleeding and addressing any underlying comorbidities that may precipitate epistaxis. Anticoagulation medication and natural supplements are discontinued. Hypertension is controlled. Renal and hepatic dysfunctions are identified. History of nasal obstruction, pain, or unilateral hearing loss associated with epistaxis may represent a nasal tumor.

Direct Pressure

Direct pressure is indicated for initial mild to moderate bleeding. Patients are instructed to sit upright to decrease venous return. They should pinch the nose with the thumb and index finger for at least 20 minutes; this exerts pressure on the septal

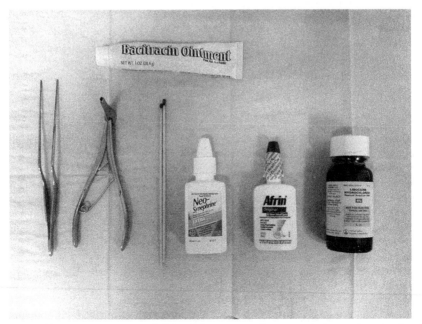

Fig. 11. Mild epistaxis tray. From left to right: Bayonet forceps, nasal speculum, bacitracin ointment, silver nitrate sticks, oxymetazoline 0.05% solution, lidocaine topical solution.

vasculature and stops the bleeding. If bleeding is associated with trauma, coagulation disorders, anticoagulation medication, or renal or hepatic disorder, then the patient is referred to a specialist.[39]

Silver Nitrate Cauterization

Silver nitrate cauterization is indicated in patients who have recurrent episodes of mild epistaxis without other comorbidities or a history of use of anticoagulation medications. Patients with recurrent epistaxis usually rebleed from vessels in the anterior portion of the septum. This bleeding is frequent during cold months when there is less humidity of the nasal cavity, leading to mucosal irritation and vessel exposure. A light source, nasal speculum, and silver nitrate stick are needed for this procedure. Using a nasal speculum with the nondominant hand helps to identify the area of bleeding. Then, gentle pressure is applied on the nasal septum with a silver nitrate cautery stick over the hyperemic blood vessel. This procedure is done in patients who have subtle active bleeding from the anterior septum. Suction instruments may be required if bleeding or a clot obliterates the vestibule. After cauterization, the patient is advised against nose blowing, lifting heavy objects, or any activity that involves a Valsalva maneuver. If moderate to heavy bleeding is present, then the patient may need anterior or posterior nasal packing.

Anterior Nasal Packing

Anterior nasal packing is usually used when epistaxis is unrefractory to the treatments described earlier. The purpose of anterior nasal packing is to collapse the bleeding vessel or vessels to cause clot and thrombus formation and eventually vessel obliteration. Nasal packing of all types requires broad-spectrum antibiotic coverage for prophylaxis against toxic shock syndrome. The traditional approach to packing involves ribbon gauze packing, but with the widespread availability of prefabricated nasal packings (**Fig. 12**), this has fallen into less usage. Both methods of packing are discussed later.

First, the nose is decongested and anesthetized. One must be careful about the amount of decongestant used, especially in patients with a history of arrhythmias or cardiac conditions. Prefabricated anterior packings are dressed in ointment and aligned with the floor of the nasal cavity on insertion. Sometimes the addition of another pack is needed to exert more pressure on the nasal cavity, and, although discomforting, it is well tolerated by the patient. Anterior ribbon gauze packing requires

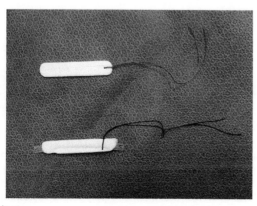

Fig. 12. Nasal packings.

the availability of 3% bismuth tribromophenate (Xeroform) gauze or Adaptic strip impregnated with petroleum jelly or antibiotic ointment. The procedure is performed using bayonet forceps, and packing should proceed from posterior to anterior and inferior to superior. Packing continues with additional ribbon gauze until the nasal cavity is completely packed (**Fig. 13**). A gauze drip pad is taped against the nose and changed periodically when necessary. Patients with any nasal packing are admitted for laboratory workup, observation for 24 hours, and otolaryngology consult. If no rebleeding occurs for 24 hours, the patient is discharged home with broad-spectrum antibiotics and followed up in 5 days for nasal packing removal.

Posterior Packing

Posterior packing requires evaluation by an otolaryngologist. Posterior bleeding is rare and is reported in less than 15% of patients with epistaxis. The usual source of bleeding is the posterior septal branch of the sphenopalatine artery. In recent years, the paradigm has shifted to perform transnasal sphenopalatine artery ligation to avoid the morbidity of posterior nasal packing. Various prefabricated posterior packing is also available in the form of balloons. The purpose is to completely fill the posterior nasal cavity. Alternatively, Foley catheters are used for posterior nasal cavity packing until the patient is stabilized and transferred to an institution with an on-call otolaryngologist. Traditional posterior nasal cavity packing required the availability of gauze, Foley or any other plastic catheter, umbilical tapes, sponge metal instrument or any type of forceps, and an excellent light source. This procedure is morbid and used in patients with severe epistaxis that has not been controlled with any of the methods described earlier.

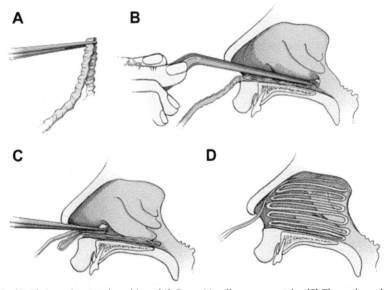

Fig. 13. (*A–D*) Anterior nasal packing. (*A*) Grasp Vaseline gauze strip. (*B*) Then place the first layer on the floor of the nose through the nasal speculum. Withdraw the bayonet forceps and nasal speculum. (*C*) Reintroduce the nasal speculum on top of the first layer of packing, and place a second layer in an identical manner. Apply several layers. (*D*) A complete anterior nasal pack can tamponade a bleeding point.

The patient is made to sit upright. The nose is thoroughly anesthetized and decongested. Gauze packing should be prepared beforehand. Three umbilical tapes are tied to the rolled gauze. The 2 lateral umbilical tapes should be facing toward one side; these are the tapes that come out of the nose. The other umbilical tape is tied at the middle and facing toward one side. This umbilical tape ultimately comes out through the mouth and is used for packing removal. Two 14F catheters are inserted, one through each nostril, and the tip of the catheters should be pulled through the oropharynx toward the oral cavity. The ends of the 2 lateral umbilical tapes are tied to the end of the catheters firmly. Then, the catheters are pulled through the nose so that the gauze traverses the oral cavity and the oropharynx and is pulled tightly into the nasopharynx. The umbilical tapes are tied with care not to exert pressure on the columella and cause columellar necrosis. The middle umbilical tape is brought through the mouth and secured to the cheek skin with tape. Otolaryngologist consult is warranted. If no otolaryngologist is available, then the patient is admitted and observed with constant cardiac monitoring and constant O_2 saturometry. Packing is removed in 7 days and the patient discharged home.

NASAL ANESTHESIA

Nasal anesthesia is required for the management of common emergency procedures such as nasal inspection after trauma, laceration repair, closed nasal bone reduction, and nasal or facial abscesses drainage. The choice of anesthesia depends on the complexity of the lesion and procedure, as well as the area to be anesthetized. To achieve an adequate internal and external nasal anesthesia, a combination of 3 different methods is used; these include application of topical solutions (applied to the internal mucosa of nares), nerve block, and/or local infiltration. The clinical presentation of the patient determines which type is most appropriate for the resolution of pain. Conscious sedation must be considered as an adjunct in pediatric and noncooperative adults. The emergency medicine provider must know the different methods to provide nasal anesthesia, its indications, contraindications (**Table 2** and **3**), and complications.

Contraindications

True allergy to local anesthetics is the only absolute medical contraindication to both topical and peripheral nerve blocks of the nose.[40] Regional blocks should be avoided when cutaneous or subcutaneous lesions are present at the contemplated site of puncture. If coagulation disorders are either known or suspected, it is prudent to avoid

Table 2	
Indications and contraindications for internal nasal anesthesia	
Indications	**Contraindications**
Nasal endoscopy	Allergy to anesthetic topical solutions
Nasal evaluation with speculum	Uncontrolled hypertension, coronary artery disease
Nasal abscess incision and drainage	Uncooperative patient
Septal hematoma evacuation	
Nasotracheal intubation	
Nasogastric tube	
Foreign body removal	
Nasal packing placement	

Table 3
Indications and contraindications for external nasal anesthesia

Indications	Contraindications
Laceration repair	Allergy to anesthetic agents
Nasal wound evaluation	Signs of infection
Abscess incision and drainage	Uncooperative patient
Septal hematoma evacuation	
Nasal bone fracture	
Nasal debridement	

techniques in which compression is difficult (an infraorbital nerve block by intraoral approach). The use of vasoconstrictors is a relative contraindication in patients with coronary artery disease or uncontrolled hypertension.

Topical Nasal Anesthesia

Oxymetazoline 0.05% solution or a topical decongestant is sprayed into the nasal cavity to decrease bleeding during the procedure; it also decreases the systemic absorption of topical anesthesia.

Topical agents (**Table 4**) are sprayed into the nasal cavity, followed by the placement of cotton pledgets soaked in topical agents for 5 to 10 minutes. Branches of the anterior and posterior ethmoid, sphenopalatine, and nasopalatine nerves are anesthetized by these pledgets. If copious nasal secretions are suspected to hinder the topical anesthesia procedure, then the use of intramuscular glycopyrrolate is highly advised. The pledgets are removed, and swabs containing topical anesthesia are inserted for blockage of the ethmoidal nerves branches, which are located in an anterior–superior aspect of the internal nose; the swabs are then moved posteriorly along the medial meatus for blockage of the sphenopalatine nerve. This process is repeated after 5 minutes if no adequate anesthesia is achieved.

Table 4
Dosage and mechanism of action of topical anesthetic agents

Medication	Dosage	Mechanism of Action
Topical anesthesia		
Oxymetazoline 0.05% nasal solution	2–3 sprays in nostril	Produce nasal mucosa vasoconstriction
Glycopyrrolate	0.004 mg/kg Intramuscular, 30–60 min before intervention	Preoperative, reduces secretions, and blocks cardiac vagal reflexes
Lidocaine 4% topical	Apply with cotton swab to affected area	Local anesthetic. Inhibits nerve impulse initiation and conduction
Tetracaine 2%	Apply with cotton swab to affected area	Local anesthetic. Inhibits nerve impulse initiation and conduction
Cocaine 4%	Apply with a cotton swab directly to affected area	Local anesthetic. Inhibits nerve impulse initiation and conduction

Field Blocks of the Nose

The physician should be familiar with the medications to be used when a regional block is being considered. The safety, dosages, and adverse effects of any local anesthetic agent used should be known (**Table 5**).[41–43]

Field Block Technique

After explaining the technique to the patient and discussing the risks and benefits of the procedure, the patient is positioned depending on the area to be infiltrated. Before preparing the puncture site, the area of interest is examined for any overlying breaks in the skin, signs of infection, or superficial lesions. Once a technique is decided, the area is cleaned and prepared using a cleaning solution.

The infraorbital nerve block has shown to be an effective way to produce anesthesia of the ipsilateral side of the nose, and it is often used for surgical procedures and postoperative pain.[44–46] However, the nasal mucosa is not anesthetized by this technique.

Two different approaches are used for an infraorbital nerve block, the intraoral and the extraoral (**Fig. 14**). Their use is basically based on personal preferences; however, the intraoral approach has been associated with a longer duration of anesthesia.[47] When performing either technique, the infraorbital foramen is located by palpating the infraorbital rim. It is found directly below the pupil as the patient stares straight ahead when no strabismus is present. For the intraoral approach, the needle is inserted just anterior to the apex of the first premolar into the mucolabial fold and directed parallel to the axis of the tooth until it is palpated near the foramen, to a depth of approximately 2 cm. When proper needle location has been determined and aspiration performed, about 2 mL of solution is injected adjacent to, but not within, the foramen.[48]

As mentioned previously, the infraorbital foramen is also located when performing the extraoral approach. The skin is prepared, and the injection site is at the same point where the foramen was previously located. The needle is directed toward the foramen, and the solution is injected adjacent to it but not within it.

Complications

Complications associated with the regional block in the area of the nose are due to the solution used as well as the structural injury to the tissue adjacent to the puncture wound and infiltration. When epinephrine and cocaine are used, tachycardia, seizures, hypertension, and hyperpyrexia are seen.[43] Structural complications include orbit injury, bleeding, infection, neuropraxia, needle breakage, and pain at the injection site.

Table 5	
Local anesthetic agents and equipment used during nasal field blocks	
Anesthetic Agents	**Dosage**
Lidocaine	20–100 mg of 2% solution
Bupivacaine	12.5–25 mg of 0.25%–0.5% solution, to a maximum of 400 mg
Mepivacaine	50–400 mg of 1% solution or 100–400 mg of 2% solution
Other equipment	
Sterile gauze	
27-Gauge needle	
5-mL Sterile syringe	

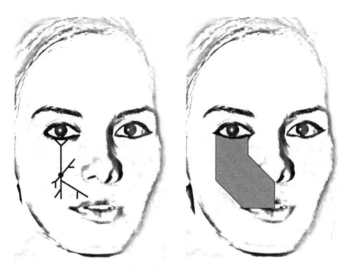

Fig. 14. Infraorbital nerve block. Two different approaches are used for an infraorbital nerve block, the intraoral and the extraoral. The intraoral approach has been associated with a longer duration of the anesthesia.

NASAL SEPTAL HEMATOMA

A nasal septal hematoma (**Fig. 15**) is the accumulation of blood between the mucoperichondrium and the septal cartilage. The most common cause is direct trauma to the nose.[49] Blood in the confined space is a perfect medium for bacterial overgrowth and cartilaginous destruction, with resultant saddle-nose deformity if left untreated.

Treatment of a septal hematoma consists of incision and drainage of the stagnant blood and clot with immediate septal pressure to approximate the perichondrium to the cartilage (**Fig. 16**).[35] The indication to proceed with this procedure is

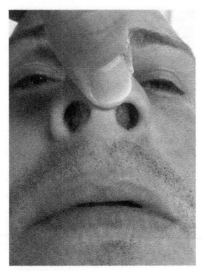

Fig. 15. Left nasal septal hematoma. Notice the accumulation of blood between the mucoperichondrium and the septal cartilage.

straightforward; any nasal septal hematomas should be drained in an urgent manner.[50] No absolute contraindications exist with nasal septal hematoma. Appropriate anesthesia can effectively be achieved in a topical manner with lidocaine. If injectable lidocaine is used, epinephrine is not recommended.

Incision and Drainage

The equipment needed to drain a nasal septal hematoma is described in **Box 6**. Anesthesia is achieved with local infiltration of 2% lidocaine or topical application of 4% cocaine solution and packing the affected nostril with soaked gauze for 3 to 5 minutes.[51] To drain the hematoma, blade number 11 is used to incise the mucosa over the hematoma in a horizontal direction. The procedure is done by starting with a small incision and increasing the diameter as needed to achieve complete extraction of the blood. The content is then suctioned out, followed by copious irrigation with normal saline. A small amount of mucosa is excised to prevent premature closure of the incision. After irrigation, a drain is left in place that also helps in preventing

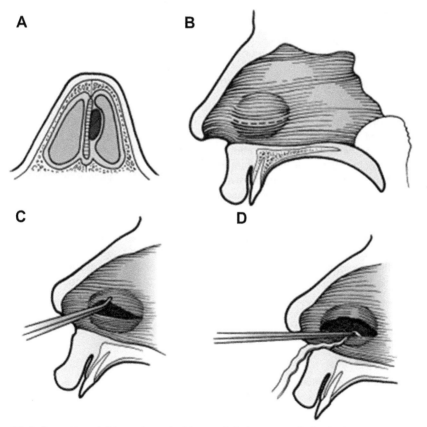

Fig. 16. Left nasal septal hematoma incision and drainage. To drain the hematoma, blade number 11 is used to incise the mucosa over the hematoma in a horizontal direction. (*A*) Left nasal septal hematoma. (*B*) Apply anesthesia (topical/infiltrate). (*C*) To drain the hematoma, use a blade number 11 to incise the mucosa over the hematoma horizontally. (*D*) Place a drain and packing.

Box 6
Nasal septal hematoma I & D equipment

Equipment

Topical/infiltration anesthesia

Scalpel/blade #11

Forceps

Suction

Packing materials

---

premature closure. It may take up to 3 days for drainage to stop.[52–54] When there is no further hematoma formation for a 24-hour period, the drain is removed.

A critical step of the procedure is to approximate the perichondrium to the cartilage by packing the nostril, as in anterior epistaxis. The nose pack is left in place for 24 hours.

Disposition consists of home discharge with prescription of oral antibiotics to cover *Streptococcus pneumoniae* and beta-lactamase producing organisms and early follow-up with an otolaryngologist.

As with any surgical procedure, complications may occur with this procedure also; among them are hematoma reaccumulation, bleeding, and infection (**Box 7**).

NECK ANATOMY/PHYSICAL EXAMINATION

The anatomy of the neck is often simplified into triangles for the purpose of organizing the components of this complex area of the body. These triangles are multilayered, consisting of a superficial cervical fascia and 3 layers of deep fascia.[55] For clinical purposes, the neck is partitioned into 3 zones.[56] An understanding of the layers of the deep fascia of the neck is important because these layers form planes that provide routes of surgical procedures, or pathways for hemorrhage and infection. The deepest layer, known as the prevertebral fascia, encloses the C1–C7 vertebrae and the muscles that flex them. It also contains the carotid and jugular vessels. The external and internal jugular veins return blood from the head and face. The triangles mentioned previously are 3-dimensional spaces composed of blood vessels, nerves, lymphatic vessels, and lymph nodes and bounded by bone and muscles.

The sternocleidomastoid muscle, the anterior border of the trapezius muscle, and the middle portion of the clavicle form the first of the triangles, the posterior cervical

---

Box 7
Nasal septal hematoma I & D complications

Complications

Septum injury

Hematoma reaccumulation

Bleeding

Abscess

Cartilage necrosis

Nasal deformity

Infection

---

triangle. It contains numerous lymph nodes, branches of the cervical plexus, the accessory or cranial nerve XI, and 2 arterial branches of the thyrocervical trunk.

The second triangle, the anterior cervical triangle, runs alongside the posterior triangle, sharing the sternocleidomastoid muscle. The remaining 2 sides of the anterior triangle are formed by the body of the mandible superiorly and midline of the neck anteriorly. Most of the important vascular and visceral organs lie within the anterior triangle, including the major vascular structures of the neck and glandular structures including the thyroid, parathyroid, submandibular, and parotid glands.

Peritonsilar Abscess

If bacterial pharyngitis is left untreated or partially treated, cellulitis of the pharyngeal space with phlegmon and ultimately abscess formation between the tonsillar capsule, the superior constrictor muscle, and the palatopharyngeus muscle could develop. A capsule surrounds the tonsils, and it is within this potential space between the tonsils and the capsule that peritonsilar abscesses form.[57] It remains the most common head and neck abscess in children and adults.[2]

The clinical presentation consists of an ill-appearing patient presenting with a sore throat, odynophagia, dysphagia, neck pain, low-grade fever, trismus, and ipsilateral otalgia. On physical examination, bulging of the superior tonsillar pole and soft palate and deviation of the uvula away from the abscess are often seen.[58]

Together with the clinical diagnosis, the use of the ultrasound for the diagnosis of peritonsilar abscess in the emergency department is of considerable benefit in emergency medicine practice. In a cooperative patient, this method is cost-effective, safe, and fast. Although most studies involve small numbers of subjects, intraoral ultrasonography has been reported to have a sensitivity of 89% to 92% and a specificity of 80% to 100%.[59,60] A 5.0- to 10.0-MHz curved array endovaginal probe is used for intraoral ultrasonography. Preapplication of a topical anesthetic spray is recommended to reduce gagging and overcome trismus. During the ultrasound evaluation of a peritonsilar abscess, the carotid artery and its relationship to the abscess cavity

---

Physical examination findings

Ill appearing

Fever, tachycardia

Dehydration

    Poor oral intake

Lymphadenopathy

    Anterior chain cervical/submandibular

Sore throat

    Worsens, becomes unilateral

Trismus

Internal pterygoid muscle spasm

    Present in peritonsilar abscess

    Absent in severe pharyngitis

Muffled voice ("hot potato")

Drooling

Halitosis

should be identified. It is generally located posterolateral to the tonsil and within 5 to 25 mm from the abscess. Sonographically, its anechoic and tubular shape identifies the internal carotid artery. Its location should be evident with systematic scanning of the peritonsillar area in both the sagittal and transverse planes. A peritonsillar abscess most commonly appears as a hypoechoic or complex cystic mass.

Peritonsilar Abscess Drainage

When a peritonsilar abscess is suspected, either based on history plus physical examination or on ultrasonographic findings, drainage is indicated. For the successful and safe drainage of a peritonsilar abscess, it is required that the patient does not have severe trismus because drainage is achieved with the intraoral approach and adequate opening of the mouth is necessary. Cooperation is also required to decrease the risks associated with the procedure. Sedation is recommended before attempting aspiration. Local infiltration of 1 to 2 mL of 1% lidocaine with epinephrine via a 27-gauge needle in the area of major fluctuance provides anesthesia and decreases discomfort.[2]

Start by preparing the equipment. Take a 16- to 18-gauge needle attached to a 5-mL syringe. Cut the plastic needle cover into 2, and slide the proximal half back over the needle. Tape the cover to the syringe, and it functions as a "depth gauge," preventing deep tissue penetration to avoid puncturing the carotid arteries, which are located 2.5 cm behind and lateral to the tonsil.

After appropriate anesthesia and preparation, the abscess is better reached by having the patient sit upright with a support behind the head and with the help of an assistant to pull the ipsilateral cheek laterally to increase the visual field.[61] Next, find the point of maximal bulging, which is usually near the top of the tonsil, lateral to uvula consistent with the 10 to 11 o'clock position when facing the patient (**Fig. 17**). When inserting the needle, advance it in the sagittal and medial planes only, avoiding lateral angulation toward the carotid artery. Aspirate as much pus as possible (on average only 3–5 mL of pus). If no pus is collected, try again 1 cm lower. The inability to get pus may indicate peritonsillar cellulitis only, but it does not fully rule out abscess. If bedside ultrasound machine is available and the physician is experienced with its use, it is preferable to do the procedure with the help of sonographic imaging.

For ultrasound-guided drainage, as explained earlier, once the abscess is identified on the screen as a hypoechoic or complex cystic mass, insert the needle adjacent to

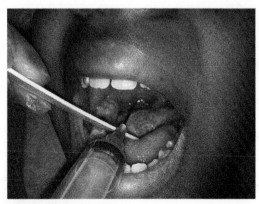

Fig. 17. Peritonsillar abscess drainage. Find the point of maximal bulging, which is usually near the top of the tonsil, lateral to uvula consistent with the 10 to 11 o'clock position when facing the patient.

the probe head and direct into the abscess cavity. The ability to simultaneously image and introduce the needle allows the EP to track the course of needle and prevent complications such as puncturing the carotid artery.[62–64]

Larger abscesses may require incision and drainage, and if the emergency provider is not comfortable with this procedure or the patient presents with severe trismus, an otolaryngologist must be consulted.

If incision and drainage are required, a small incision is made using preferably a guarded scalpel above the tonsil, in the soft palate. The best approach to avoid injury to the internal carotid artery is to make medial and superior incisions. The incision is then blunt dissected using a curved Kelly clamp, which is gently directed inferiorly, posteriorly, and slightly laterally. Gentle dissection in the area of fluctuance is usually sufficient to penetrate the abscess cavity, and once in there, dissection is continued with the clamp to break up any septation inside the abscess.

Caution has to be taken in the uncooperative patient, and it is for this reason that sedation and good pain management are important when attempting the procedure in a patient with significant apprehension or in the pediatric population, which make these 2 scenarios contraindications.

Contraindications

There are cases when incision and drainage are absolutely contraindicated in the emergency department. One of these special situations is when the patient has a known vascular malformation that could have altered the anatomy around the abscess, increasing the risk for vascular damage. Another absolute contraindication is for patients with malignancy in the periphery of the peritonsilar abscess.

Complications

After successful drainage, the patient might complain of bad taste, as the abscess continues to empty the pus. This condition puts the patient at risk for aspiration of the content into the lungs, which can complicate the procedure. Another complication of peritonsilar abscess drainage is severe bleeding, which may or may not be related to the puncture of the carotid artery.

Disposition

Both needle aspiration and incision and drainage can be done in combination with hospital admission and administration of intravenous antibiotics or as an outpatient treatment with oral antibiotics.[2] Studies have shown that adjuvant steroids therapy has demonstrated benefit for severe, acute pharyngitis.[65]

For patients who appear toxic and dehydrated with severe trismus or who have any signs of airway compromise, admission is indicated for the administration of intravenous antibiotics and surgical evaluation in case drainage in the operating room is necessary. If patients are nontoxic and are able to take medications by mouth, with adequate oral intake and managing secretions well, they could be discharged home with antibiotic coverage. Clear instructions are given to follow up with the primary care physician or ENT on an urgent basis. Patients are also instructed to return to the emergency department if increasing dyspnea occurs, sore throat worsens, or there is enlarging of the mass and even persistent high fever.

POSTTONSILLECTOMY HEMORRHAGE

Posttonsillectomy bleeding is one of the most feared surgical complications by otolaryngologists. The reported incidence of postoperative hemorrhage is between 3% and

20%.[66] Peak incidence in postoperative bleeding occurs between days 5 and 7. Hemorrhage is classified as immediate bleeding, which occurs during surgery; early postoperative bleeding, which occurs in the first 24 hours after surgery; and delayed postoperative bleeding, which occurs more than 24 hours after surgery.[6,66–68] Postoperative bleeding is a serious emergency that warrants an immediate otolaryngology consult for evaluation and possible surgical management.

Patients with delayed posttonsillectomy bleeding are the ones who are usually seen at the ER. They are classified in 2 groups: those who are actively bleeding and those who have a blood clot in the tonsillar fossa. There is another group of patients who have had episodes of bleeding but at initial presentation at ER have no evidence of previous episodes of bleeding or active bleeding.

Patients who are not actively bleeding are evaluated for the presence of a clot in the tonsillar fossa. If no blood clot is present, then hemoglobin and hematocrit, as well as coagulation parameters, are drawn to assess the patients blood volume. These patients are usually admitted for observation. Posttonsillectomy patients are often dehydrated. When IV fluid resuscitation occurs and circulating volume is restored, collapsed arterial vessels expand and rebleeding occurs. For this reason, patients are admitted and observed for 24 hours after an episode of posttonsillectomy hemorrhage.

Patients who are not actively bleeding and have a clot in the tonsillar fossa should be managed by an otolaryngologist. If no otolaryngologist is available, then the patient is transferred to a tertiary center with available subspecialists. There is some debate in the otolaryngology community as to whether blood clots in the tonsillar fossa should be evacuated or not. Some advocate avoiding evacuating the clot and 24-hour hospital admission and observation, whereas others advocate removing the clot, especially, in patients in whom there is a suspicion of active bleeding but the oropharynx cannot adequately be assessed because of the presence of a large blood clot. Evacuation of the blood clot leads to active bleeding. Hence, one must be prepared to manage this. If this occurs, the probability that the patient needs surgical treatment is high. In a retrospective review done in 2004 of 90 children with posttonsillectomy hemorrhage, 90% of the children evaluated at ER for signs of bleeding necessitated surgical treatment.[67]

Patients who arrive at the ER with active bleeding from the tonsillar fossa should be evaluated immediately and treated by an ER physician. The ABCs of emergency care are used if needed. Immediate vital signs are taken. Two large-bore needles are used for IV access. If massive bleeding is present, then the patient is intubated to protect the airway. This situation rarely occurs but must be taken into consideration if necessary. If the patient is actively bleeding but the airway is stable, then treatment in the ER should aim at hemostasis. There are various techniques that are used to achieve this.

McGill forceps or a large sponge holder, several gauzes, and 1:10,000 diluted adrenaline solution are used to achieve temporary hemostasis. The gauzes are soaked in the solution, folded, and mounted on the tip of the McGill forceps. Then, the area of active bleeding is identified. A headlamp with tongue depressors is used to evaluate the oral cavity and the oropharynx for adequate visualization. If no headlamp is available, then any light source will suffice. The tongue is gently depressed with the nondominant hand, and the folded gauzes are applied with the dominant hand against the tonsillar fossa with significant pressure. This method has a twofold purpose. One is to exert pressure on the arterial bleeding to collapse the blood vessels. The second purpose is to impregnate the tonsillar vault with adrenaline. In patients who have limited bleeding, the tonsillar pillar is injected with lidocaine/epinephrine 1% 1:100,000. A 3-mL syringe is recommended for this purpose, and a long 25- or 27-gauge needle is used. The site of bleeding and the surrounding tissue is injected. Otolaryngology consult is highly advisable for all cases of postoperative bleeding because of the large number of patients who need surgical treatment. If no otolaryngologist is available, then the patient is transferred to a facility with otolaryngology services.

SUMMARY

EPs must be proficient in the short-term management of otorrhinolaringologic (ENT) conditions, especially those that require performing procedures. Most ENT conditions, injuries, and postoperative complications are initially evaluated in the ED. Several disorders can be evaluated in an outpatient setting; however, a subset of conditions such as complex auricular lacerations, moderate to severe epistaxis, peritonsillar abscess aspiration, and posttonsillectomy bleeding require immediate identification, expedite intervention, and proficiency in the execution of otolaringologic procedures. It is of utmost importance for the emergency practitioner to be proficient while performing these procedural skills.

REFERENCES

1. Murphy MF. Regional anesthesia in the emergency department. Emerg Med Clin North Am 1988;6:783–810.
2. Roberts JR. Otolaryngologic procedures. In: Roberts JR, Hedges JR, editors. Clinical procedures in emergency medicine. 5th edition. Philadelphia: Saunders Elsevier; 2010. p. 1197–215.
3. Salam GA. Regional anesthesia for office procedures: part I. Head and neck surgeries. Am Fam Physician 2004;69(3):585–90.
4. Avina R. Primary care local and regional anesthesia in the management of trauma. Clin Fam Pract 2000;2:533–50.
5. Labat G, Adriani J. 4th edition. Labat's regional anesthesia: techniques and clinical applications, vol. 107–30. St. Louis (MO): W.H. Green; 1985. p. 193–235.
6. Cummings CW, Flint PW, Haughey BH, et al, editors. Cummings otolaryngology – head and neck surgery. 5th edition. Philadelphia: Elsevier; 2010.
7. Mudry A, Pirsig W. Auricular hematoma and cauliflower deformation of the ear from art to medicine. Otol Neurotol 2009;30(1):116–20.
8. Ghanem T. Rethinking auricular trauma. Laryngoscope 2005;115(7):1251–5.
9. Jones SE, Mahendran S. Interventions for acute auricular hematoma. Cochrane Database Syst Rev 2004;(2):CD004166.
10. McCarter DF, Courtney AU, Pollart SM. Cerumen impaction. Am Fam Physician 2007;75(10):1523–8.
11. Roeser RJ, Ballachanda BB. Physiology, pathophysiology, and anthropology/ epidemiology of human ear canal secretions. J Am Acad Audiol 1997;8:391–400.
12. Roland PS, Smith TL, Schwartz SR, et al. Clinical practice guideline: cerumen impaction. Otolaryngol Head Neck Surg 2008;139(3 Suppl 2):S1–21.
13. Raman R. Impacted earwax—a cause for unexplained cough? Arch Otolaryngol Head Neck Surg 1986;112:679.
14. Grossan M. Cerumen removal—current challenges. Ear Nose Throat J 1998;77: 541–6, 548.
15. Dinsdale RC, Roland PS, Manning SC, et al. Catastrophic otologic injury from oral jet irrigation of the external auditory canal. Laryngoscope 1991;101(1 Pt 1):75–8.
16. Ansley JF, Cunningham MJ. Treatment of aural foreign bodies in children. Pediatrics 1998;101(4 Pt 1):638–41.

17. Davies PH, Benger JR. Foreign bodies in the nose and ear: a review of techniques for removal in the emergency department. J Accid Emerg Med 2000; 17:91–4.
18. Marin JR, Trainor JL. Foreign body removal from the external auditory canal in a pediatric emergency department. Pediatr Emerg Care 2006;22(9):630–4.
19. Schulze S, Kerschner J, Beste D. Pediatric external auditory canal foreign bodies: a review of 698 cases. Otolaryngol Head Neck Surg 2002;127:73–8.
20. Heim SW, Maughan KL. Foreign bodies in the ear, nose, and throat. Am Fam Physician 2007;76(8):1185–9.
21. Balbani AP, Sanchez TG, Butugan O, et al. Ear and nose foreign body removal in children. Int J Pediatr Otorhinolaryngol 1998;46:37–42.
22. DiMuzio J Jr, Deschler DG. Emergency department management of foreign bodies of the external ear canal in children. Otol Neurotol 2002;23:473–5.
23. Thompson SK, Wein RO, Dutcher PO. External auditory canal foreign body removal: management practices and outcomes. Laryngoscope 2003;113:1912–5.
24. Bressler K, Shelton C. Ear foreign body removal: a review of 98 consecutive cases. Laryngoscope 1993;103:367–70.
25. Votey S, Dudley JP. Emergency ear, nose and throat procedures. Emerg Med Clin North Am 1989;7:117–54.
26. D'Cruz O, Lakshman R. A solution for the foreign body in the nose problem. Pediatrics 1998;81:174.
27. Kadish HA, Corneli HM. Removal of nasal foreign bodies in the pediatric population. Am J Emerg Med 1997;15:54–6.
28. Zeinulabdeen M. New touch and pull method to remove foreign bodies from the ear. J Indian Med Assoc 1977;68:97–8.
29. Hanson RM, Stephens M. Cyanoacrylate assisted foreign body removal from the ear and nose in children. J Paediatr Child Health 1994;30:77–8.
30. Pride H, Schwab R. A new technique for removing foreign bodies of the external auditory canal. Pediatr Emerg Care 1989;5:135–6.
31. Henry LN, Chamberlin JW. Removal of foreign bodies from oesophagus and nose with the use of a Foley catheter. Surgery 1972;71:918–21.
32. Nandapalan V, McIlwain JC. Removal of nasal foreign bodies with a Fogarty biliary balloon catheter. J Laryngol Otol 1994;108:758–60.
33. Leffler S, Cheney P, Tandberg D. Chemical immobilization and killing of intra-aural roaches: an in vitro comparative study. Ann Emerg Med 1993;22(12):1795–8.
34. Tong MC, Van Hasselt CA, Woo JK. The hazards of button batteries in the nose. J Otolaryngol 1992;21:458–60.
35. Douglas R, Wormald PJ. Update on epistaxis. Curr Opin Otolaryngol Head Neck Surg 2007;15:180–3.
36. Hornung DE. Nasal anatomy and the sense of smell. Adv Otorhinolaryngol 2006; 63:1–22.
37. Cummings CW. Epistaxis. In: Cummings otolaryngology: head and neck surgery, vol. 40, 4th edition. Philadelphia: Elsevier, Mosby; 2005. p. 942–61.
38. Kucik C. Management of epistaxis. Am Fam Physician 2005;71(2):305–11.
39. Mayo Clinic First Aid. Available at: http://www.mayoclinic.com/health/first-aid-nosebleeds/HQ00105. Accessed December 11, 2011.
40. Dalens BJ. Regional anesthesia in children. In: Miller RD, editor. Miller's anesthesia. 7th edition. Churchill Livingstone, Philadelphia: Elsevier; 2009. p. 2527.
41. Hafner HM, Rocken M, Breuninger H. Epinephrine-supplemented local anesthetics for ear and nose surgery: clinical use without complications in more than 10,000 surgical procedures. J Dtsch Dermatol Ges 2005;3(3):195–9.

42. Fulling PD, Roberts JT. Fiberoptic intubation. Int Anesthesiol Clin 2000;38(3): 189–217.
43. Brown RS, Rhodus NL. Epinephrine and local anesthesia revisited. Oral Surg Oral Med Oral Pathol Oral Radiol Endod 2005;100(4):401–8.
44. Taleghani K, Sternbach G. Infraorbital nerve block. In: Rosen P, Chan T, Vilke G, et al, editors. Atlas of emergency procedures. St Louis (MO): Mosby; 2001. p. 160–1.
45. Kezirian GM, Hill FD, Hill FJ. Peribulbar anesthesia for repair of orbital floor fractures. Ophthalmic Surg 1991;22(10):601–5. Available at: http://www.ncbi.nlm.nih.gov/pubmed/1961618. Accessed December 11, 2011.
46. Simion C, Corcoran J, Iyer A, et al. Postoperative pain control for primary cleft lip repair in infants: is there an advantage in performing peripheral nerve blocks? Paediatr Anaesth 2008;18(11):1060–5.
47. Lynch MT, Syverud SA, Schwab RA, et al. Comparison of intraoral and percutaneous approaches for infraorbital nerve block. Acad Emerg Med 1994;1:514.
48. Roberts JR. Infraorbital nerve block. In: Roberts JR, Hedges JR, editors. Clinical procedures in emergency medicine. 5th edition. Philadelphia: Saunders Elsevier; 2010. p. 500–12.
49. Matsuba HM, Thawley SE. Nasal septal abscess: unusual causes, complications, treatment, and sequelae. Ann Plast Surg 1986;16(2):161–6.
50. Chukuezi AB. Nasal septal haematoma in Nigeria. J Laryngol Otol 1992;106(5): 396–8.
51. Wexner S, Armstrong L, French A, et al. Images in emergency medicine. Male with facial trauma. Septal hematoma. Ann Emerg Med 2011;57:541.
52. Kim YS, Kim YH, Kim NH, et al. A prospective, randomized, single-blinded controlled trial on biodegradable synthetic polyurethane foam as a packing material after septoplasty. Am J Rhinol Allergy 2011;25(2):e77–9.
53. Naghibzadeh B, Peyvandi AA, Naghibzadeh G. Does post septoplasty nasal packing reduce complications? Acta Med Iran 2011;49(1):9–12.
54. Günaydin RÖ, Aygenc E, Karakullukcu S, et al. Nasal packing and transseptal suturing techniques: surgical and anaesthetic perspectives. Eur Arch Otorhinolaryngol 2011;268(8):1151–6.
55. Last RJ, editor. Anatomy: regional and applied. 6th edition. Edinburgh (United Kingdom): Churchill Livingstone; 1978. p. 424–35.
56. Ursic C, Curtis K. Thoracic and neck trauma. Int Emerg Nurs 2010;18(4):177–80.
57. Galioto NJ. Peritonsillar abscess. Am Fam Physician 2008;77(2):199–202.
58. Rana RS, Moonis G. Head and neck infection and inflammation. Radiol Clin North Am 2011;49(1):165–82.
59. Strong EB, Woodward PJ, Johnson LP. Intraoral ultrasound evaluation of peritonsillar abscess. Laryngoscope 1995;105:779–82.
60. Buckley AR, Moss EH, Blokmanis A. Diagnosis of peritonsillar abscess: value of intraoral sonography. AJR Am J Roentgenol 1994;162:961–4.
61. Larawin V, Naipao J, Dubey SP. Head and neck space infections. Otolaryngol Head Neck Surg 2006;135:889–93.
62. Blaivas M, Theodoro D, Duggal S. Ultrasound-guided drainage of peritonsillar abscess by the emergency physician. Am J Emerg Med 2003;21:155–8.
63. Lyon M, Blaivas M. Intraoral ultrasound in the diagnosis and treatment of suspected peritonsillar abscess in the emergency department. Acad Emerg Med 2005;12:85–8.
64. Dewitz A. Soft tissue applications. In: Ma OJ, Mateer J, editors. Emergency ultrasound. New York: McGraw-Hill; 2003. p. 385.

65. O'Brien JF, Meade JL, Falk JL. Dexamethasone as adjuvant therapy for severe acute pharyngitis. Ann Emerg Med 1993;22(2):212–5.
66. Levin B. Post-tonsillectomy bleeding. Otolaryngol Head Neck Surg 2007;136: S56–8.
67. Krishna K. Post-tonsillectomy bleeding: a meta-analysis. Laryngoscope 2001; 111(8):1358–61.
68. Peterson J. Post-tonsillectomy hemorrhage and pediatric emergency care. Clin Pediatr 2004;43(5):445.

Critical Skills and Procedures in Emergency Medicine
Vascular Access Skills and Procedures

Gemma C. Lewis, MD[a], Stephanie A. Crapo, MD[a],
Jefferson G. Williams, MD, MPH[a,b,c,*]

KEYWORDS

- Venous access • Peripheral venous access • Central venous access • Intraosseus
- Ultrasound-guided vascular access

KEY POINTS

- Access to the venous and arterial vascular systems can provide key diagnostic information to emergency medicine providers, as well as a rapid route for emergency therapy for many conditions.
- With practice, emergency medicine providers should become quickly competent with methods to access the vascular system. Bedside ultrasonography can be used to improve the ease, safety, and rapidity of access to both the arterial and venous systems.
- When traditional intravenous access is difficult or unobtainable and fluid or medication administration is time sensitive, intraosseous access may be rapidly and reliably obtained with minimum procedural preparation or operator experience.

INTRODUCTION AND GENERAL PRINCIPLES

The body's vasculature has intrigued humans since ancient civilizations practiced bloodletting as the earliest form of phlebotomy. More scientific attempts to access and use the vascular system can be traced to the Middle Ages and followed to modern times alongside the quest to transfuse blood from one person to another. Intravenous (IV) devices and setup have developed from quills and animal bladders, to metal needles and glass bottles, to modern plastics and ever-improving synthetics.[1]

Currently, veins and arteries are accessed to give fluids, medicines, or blood products; for laboratory testing and invasive hemodynamic monitoring; or for procedural

The authors have no conflicts of interest or relevant financial relationships to disclose.
[a] Department of Emergency Medicine, University of North Carolina, 170 Manning Drive, CB # 7594, Chapel Hill, NC 27599-7594, USA; [b] North Carolina State Highway Patrol, 3318 Garner Road, Raleigh, NC 27610, USA; [c] Wake County Emergency Medical Services, 331 South McDowell Street, Raleigh, NC 27601, USA
* Corresponding author. Wake County Department of Emergency Medical Services, 331 South McDowell Street, Raleigh, NC 27601.
E-mail address: Jeff.Williams@Wakegov.com

reasons, such as the implantation of cardiac pacemaker wires. This article reviews the relevant skills and procedures for the emergency medicine provider for peripheral, central venous, and arterial access. The authors also discuss adjuncts to vascular access such as the use of ultrasound guidance, and other forms of vascular access such as intraosseus and umbilical cannulation, and peripheral venous cut-down. Vascular access skills and procedures are some of the most common and important in emergency medicine, and their mastery is critical for the emergency medicine provider.

Vascular structures may be identified and accessed by using common landmarks, by direct visualization or by feel alone, and with the assistance of imaging technology such as bedside ultrasonography. General indications for arterial puncture or cannulation in the emergency setting essentially are limited to blood gas sampling and invasive blood pressure monitoring. Venous puncture or cannulation has a longer list of indications, including laboratory testing and medication and fluid and blood product administration. In the case of central veins, cannulation is indicated for hemodynamic monitoring (eg, central venous pressure) and the administration of vasoactive medications ("pressors") or medications that would otherwise be more caustic to smaller peripheral veins. The general contraindications for vascular access include vascular access attempted through infected skin, vascular access in an extremity with an arteriovenous fistula, or vascular access where an arteriovenous fistula is planned, unless absolutely necessary.[2,3] In the following sections, the indications, contraindications, techniques, and procedures for each type of vascular access will be discussed.

PERIPHERAL VENOUS ACCESS SKILLS AND PROCEDURES
Peripheral Venous Catheter Placement

Accessing the peripheral venous system by venipuncture or for catheter placement is the most common invasive procedure in the emergency department.[2] Laboratory testing is often facilitated via sampling of venous blood, and many medications work faster when given intravenously rather than when given orally. In most patients, the peripheral veins are easily accessed at multiple sites.

Anatomy and physiology

Peripheral veins are located at varying depths from the skin surface and are readily identified by feel if not by sight. They are thin walled, and their relative pressure (and therefore engorgement and ease of access) may be increased by dependent positioning or by the use of a proximal tourniquet.[2,4]

When attempting peripheral venous access, one must consider and follow the following advice:

- Peripheral veins may be most easily accessed at "branch points" where 2 smaller veins merge into a larger one or where a vein is otherwise anchored by subcutaneous tissue and is less likely to move or "roll.[2]"
- Distal veins should be attempted before proximal ones.[5]
- The upper extremity is preferred to the lower extremity.[6]
- The site chosen should not overlie a joint, for catheter security, to improve flow through the catheter, and for maximum patient comfort and mobility.[2]

Indications and contraindications

Peripheral IV cannulation is indicated for medication or IV contrast administration, laboratory testing of venous blood, and fluid resuscitation.[2,5] For situations (eg, trauma) in which rapid administration of a large volume of crystalloid or colloid is warranted, catheter diameter has the largest effect on flow rate, and flow rates are lower with longer catheters. Maximum flow rates are achieved from large-bore short catheters.[2,7,8]

Peripheral IV access should not be attempted through overlying infected skin, or in the same extremity as a significant traumatic injury, burn, or edema. Cannulation of an extremity with an arteriovenous fistula or other dialysis access should also be avoided.[3] Sclerosing or vasoactive medications or otherwise extraordinarily concentrated solutions should be infused via central venous access if possible.

Stepwise procedure
Despite the routine and common nature of the procedure, care should be taken to ensure sterility and patient comfort. The required supplies are listed in **Box 1**. First, locate an appropriate site for needle entry into the skin. Clean the site and apply topical anesthesia several minutes before the procedure. Clean the site again with an antiseptic and wipe immediately before skin puncture. Apply a proximal tourniquet, if desired. Stabilize the vein with your nondominant hand. Insert the catheter and needle device into the skin at a 30° to 45° angle and advance into the vein. Vein entry is confirmed with a flash of blood in the catheter hub. Drop the angle of the needle and advance another 2 to 3 mm to ensure that the catheter is in the vein. Hold the hub of the needle and advance the catheter over the needle and into the vein. Withdraw the needle and hold your nondominant hand over the skin overlying the catheter/vein, to prevent free bleeding from the catheter. Release the tourniquet, if present. Collect blood as needed. Connect the IV tubing to the catheter hub, ensuring that IV solution fills the tubing. Secure the catheter with dressing and tape. Begin an IV infusion if desired, or secure a "saline lock" to be used later.[2,5,7,9]

Special considerations, complications, and pearls and pitfalls
If superficial extremity veins cannot be accessed and peripheral rather than central venous access is desired, practitioners should consider accessing the external jugular (EJ) vein or a deep vein, commonly a deep brachial vein. Ultrasound guidance can assist with either procedure. On ultrasonography, veins in cross section are black (fluid-filled, hypoechoic) circular structures that are nonpulsatile and easily compressible.[10,11]

The procedure for EJ cannulation is similar to that described earlier. Make the patient lie supine and stand behind his head. Turn the patient's head to the opposite side; the Trendelenburg position can assist in distending the vein. If the patient is cooperative, have him hum or Valsalva to increase the intrathoracic pressure and distend the vein. Enter the vein and secure the catheter as mentioned earlier, also

---

Box 1
Equipment needed for peripheral venous access

Gloves

Topical local anesthetic (especially for pediatric patients)

Catheter and needle device

Gauze, tape, and transparent dressing

Antiseptic solution or wipe

Tourniquet

IV tubing, flushes, syringe

ensuring that you cover the open catheter hub with a finger to prevent an air embolism (**Fig. 1**).

Deep brachial cannulation via ultrasound guidance is also similar to the above-mentioned procedure. Use a longer catheter, as standard length catheters will not be well secured in deeper tissue. Once the vein has been located, enter the skin after noting the static ultrasonographic image, or, if necessary, advance the needle under direct ultrasound guidance. Once the catheter has entered the vein, drop the angle of the needle, advance slightly, and then advance the catheter over the needle, through the deep tissue, and into the vein. Sometimes this requires the use of 2 hands or an assistant given the depth and/or toughness of overlying tissue.

Complications of peripheral venous catheter placement include extravasation of IV fluid (watch for progressive swelling at the site), hematoma formation, peripheral nerve palsy, and superficial thrombophlebitis.[2,3,9] Pain and paresthesia may occur after the procedure and likely will be temporary.

Other considerations for peripheral IV cannulation include ensuring recalling the purpose of the catheter before placement and preparing supplies for placement based on the patient. For example, peripheral IVs are often placed for the purpose of infusing contrast for a computed tomography scan or other imaging studies. Ensure that you know your local radiology protocols regarding the necessary and/or allowable locations and sizes for those catheters. In addition, extravasation of automatically injected IV contrast into extremity tissues can cause local necrosis and possibly compartment syndrome.[12] Ensure that any extravasation of IV contrast is treated appropriately and observed to ensure resolution. Last, IV access can be a challenge in the pediatric population. Once a peripheral catheter is established in a pediatric patient, ensure that you splint and/or extensively secure the catheter so that it is not lost or pulled out.[2]

Peripheral Venous Cut-Down

Although the numbers of venous cut-down procedures have decreased,[13] largely because of the ease and rapidity of intraosseous access via automatic drill and improved central access via ultrasound, it remains an important skill when other techniques have failed or are unavailable. In addition, when access to a larger vein is required, direct visualization via cut-down may be more successful than indirect visualization of other peripheral or central sites.

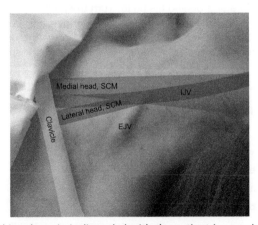

Fig. 1. The external jugular vein is distended with the patient in a supine position and the head turned toward the opposite side. Valsalva may assist in identifying the vein. EJV, external jugular vein; IJ, internal jugular vein; SCM, sternocleidomastoid.

The ideal vein for peripheral cut-down is the greater saphenous vein at the ankle.[13] It is the longest vein in the body and has a reliable and relatively superficial location. With an externally rotated lower extremity, the greater saphenous vein will be found 2.5 cm anterior and 2.5 cm superior to the medial malleolus.[2,13] Other access sites include the greater saphenous vein at the groin and the basilic vein at the elbow.

Indications and contraindications

Although venous cut-down may not be a frequently performed procedure, it is nonetheless indicated for resuscitation in any patient in whom easier and more rapid peripheral (or central) venous access has not or cannot be obtained. It may be useful for IV drug abusers with no peripheral veins, burn patients, and patients with extreme hypovolemia or hypotension. It is also a reliable technique in pediatric patients in whom other access cannot be gained.

However, venous cut-down is not without contraindications. The procedure should not be performed in patients who have a long bone fracture or vascular injury in the same extremity or in patients who have an infection overlying the proposed cut-down site. In addition, cut-down may be difficult and potentially harmful in patients with bleeding disorders and is unnecessary if peripheral access can be gained via another method.

Stepwise procedure

This procedure is often described in 2 separate phases: isolating the vein and then cannulating it.[2,13] **Box 2** lists the necessary equipment. These steps describe how to isolate and then cannulate the greater saphenous vein at the ankle. First, locate the vein near the medial malleolus as described previously. Stretch the skin over the incision site with the nondominant hand. Transversely incise the skin only superficially, using a No. 10 blade, from the anterior tibial border to the posterior tibial border to expose the subcutaneous tissue without incising the vein. Isolate the greater saphenous vein by inserting a curved hemostat along the posterior tibia and advancing, tip down, to the anterior tibia. Rotate the hemostat 180° so the tip is now pointing up. Open the hemostat to separate the saphenous vein from the surrounding tissue. Replace the curved hemostat with a straight hemostat, leaving the straight hemostat to elevate and control the vein.

Now that the vein is isolated, the operator can cannulate it. Using the Seldinger technique, insert a catheter and needle device (ie, a peripheral IV) into the isolated vein. Advance the catheter, and then remove the straight hemostat and needle. Insert a guidewire through the catheter, and then remove the catheter. Insert a dilator over the wire, dilate the vein, and then remove the dilator. Advance the large-bore fluid catheter over the guidewire, and then removed the guidewire. Begin infusing fluids through the catheter, place moist gauze over the incision, and wrap the site and extremity with a bulky gauze dressing.

Special considerations, complications, and pearls and pitfalls

Multiple methods exist to cannulate the vein once it has been identified. A surgical technique can be used, in which a small incision is made in the vein, and then IV tubing is sutured into place; the Seldinger technique can be used as described earlier, or, once the vein is isolated, the practitioner can simply insert a large-bore IV catheter into the vein.

As with any surgical procedure, complications of venous cut-down include bleeding and infection.[2,13] In addition, arterial injury or mistaken arterial cannulation can occur, as well as nerve injury, phlebitis, and thromboembolism. Also, cut-down can be complicated by surgical site infection or poor healing of the incision, which of course

| Box 2 |
| Equipment needed for peripheral venous cut-down (often as a premade kit) |

Sterile gloves, drapes, and gauze

Antiseptic solution

10- and 5-mL syringes

No. 10 and No. 11 scalpel blades

Local anesthetic

Curved Kelly hemostat

Small mosquito hemostat

Vein pick

Fine-toothed forceps

Iris scissors

Sharp tissue-cutting scissors

Sterile IV tubing and saline flushes

Central line kit (for Seldinger method)

Catheter and needle device, 16 or 18 gauge

Self-retaining skin retractors

Blood sampling equipment

Needle driver

Silk suture, 3-0 and 4-0

Roll gauze for bulky dressing

Transparent sterile dressing

Tape

would not occur with other methods of peripheral venous access, because there is no incision.

Last, the method chosen to cannulate the vein should be the one that the practitioner is able to perform most quickly and definitively, because the procedure may be life saving in this patient who otherwise does not have vascular access.

CENTRAL VENOUS ACCESS SKILLS AND PROCEDURES
Central Venous Catheter Placement

Should the critically ill patient require more invasive access, monitoring, or aggressive resuscitation, central venous access may be required instead of or in addition to peripheral venous access. Placing a central venous catheter allows one a stable, longer term access to large veins.[2,5,9,14,15] This access facilitates hemodynamic monitoring of the critically ill patient in the emergency department or in the intensive care unit and creates a route for the administration of multiple, sometimes caustic or vasoactive, medications that should not or cannot be given via peripheral veins.

Anatomy and physiology

The 3 most common sites to access the central venous system are the internal jugular (IJ) vein, the subclavian vein, and the femoral vein.[9] The anatomy of each site as well as the advantages, disadvantages, and special considerations for each are discussed.

Internal jugular anatomy The IJ vein exits the skull through the jugular foramen just anteromedial to the mastoid process and joins the subclavian vein at the sternoclavicular junction.[16] It increases in diameter as it descends, making it easier to cannulate below the cricoid cartilage. The carotid artery lies just medial and slightly deep. The right IJ vein is preferred because it takes a more direct route to the right atrium. The apex of the right lung is also lower than the apex of the left lung, slightly decreasing the risk of pneumothorax compared with the left side.[17]

The IJ vein is collapsible and compressible, which may make it a more preferred site to the subclavian, especially in anticoagulated patients.[2] It also distends; Trendelenburg or Valsalva enlarges the vein. Turning the neck to the contralateral side will straighten the vein (**Fig. 2**).

The IJ vein can be accessed by several different approaches: anterior, central, and posterior (see **Fig. 1**).[7,17]

- Anterior: Medial to the sternocleidomastoid (SCM) muscle at the level of the thyroid cartilage, 45° to the skin (30° in children), bevel up and direct the needle to the ipsilateral nipple. Stop if not entered by 5 cm and redirect, advancing in a more lateral direction.[7,17]

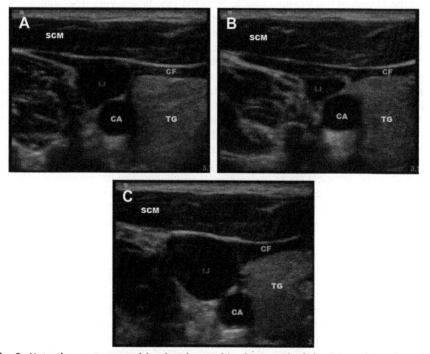

Fig. 2. Note the anatomy and landmarks on this ultrasound of the internal jugular vein, a common site of central access for the emergency provider. (*A*) The IJ is in a neutral position, somewhat amorphous, as the patient lies supine and breathes regularly. (*B*) The IJ is easily compressed by the ultrasound transducer as the operator ensures correct differentiation between the IJ and the carotid Artery. (*C*) The IJ is easily distended as the operator puts the patient in slight Trendelenburg position. CA, carotid artery; CF, cervical fascia; IJ, internal jugular; SCM, sternocleidomastoid; TG, thyroid gland.

- Posterior: 1 cm superior to where the EJ crosses the SCM lateral edge or one-third of the way from clavicle to mastoid process. Bevel at 3-o'clock position, 30° to 45° to the skin and direct the needle to the sternal notch.[7,17]
- Central: Superior apex of 2 heads of the SCM, bevel up 45°. Direct the needle to the ipsilateral nipple.[7,17]

Special considerations for the IJ The IJ venous access has several special considerations, advantages, and disadvantages. IJ cannulation should be avoided in cervical spine fractures and penetrating neck injury.[17] It should be considered carefully in left bundle branch block, because central venous catheter placement is a possible trigger for complete heart block.[18] Also, because the IJ vein courses alongside the carotid artery, carotid artery puncture is a possible complication. If arterial puncture is made via the guide needle, remove the needle and apply pressure for a minimum of 5 minutes (double if coagulopathy is present). Do not attempt IJ cannulation on the other side. If the catheter is placed in the carotid artery, do not remove the catheter—consult vascular surgery.[7] Advantages of the IJ vein include the direct course to right atrium for hemodialysis catheters and transvenous pacers.[7] Disadvantages include possible carotid artery puncture and patient preference.[7]

Subclavian anatomy At the lateral edge of the first rib, the axillary vein becomes the subclavian vein. It has a diameter of about 1 to 2 cm in adults. The subclavian vein joins the IJ vein at the thoracic inlet to form the innominate vein. The right and left innominate veins form the superior vena cava. The subclavian vein courses under the clavicle and is close to the apical pleura of lungs. The subclavian artery runs deep to the vein, separated by the anterior scalene muscle.

The subclavian vein is accessed by either an infraclavicular or supraclavicular approach. For the infraclavicular approach, find the junction of the medial and middle thirds of the clavicle. Insert the needle 1 cm inferior. The first rib acts as a protective barrier to the pleura and artery in this approach.[17] Entry can also be made at the deltopectoral groove, inferior to the clavicle. This is a longer approach, and the first rib cannot act as a protective barrier. For this approach, find the bend of the clavicle and insert the needle 1 cm inferior and 1 cm lateral.

The bevel of the needle should point caudally to guide the j-wire away from the IJ. Place your nondominant finger on the sternal notch, and aim for the sternal notch. If inserting the needle from the deltopectoral groove, the clavicle may be encountered. Walk the needle down the clavicle until the needle slips under the bone. Maintain the coronal plane in the needle. If the insertion point is more proximal, maintain a 10° angle to the skin.[9]

Consider that the supraclavicular approach[17,19–21] has been reported to have a higher success rate and less-frequent catheter malpositioning than the infraclavicular approach.[22] It also can be performed upright.[9] The needle insertion point is 1 cm lateral to the clavicular head of the SCM and 1 cm posterior/superior to the clavicle. Bisect the angle between the SCM and the clavicle and aim the needle toward the contralateral nipple. Direct the bevel medial, and angle the needle 10° to the horizontal. The subclavian vein is superficial in this approach, and the vein should be encountered within 2 to 3 cm. With an experienced operator, the supraclavicular approach has a similar if not superior complication rate to the infraclavicular approach.

Special considerations for the subclavian Subclavian venous cannulation has a low complication rate when done by an experienced provider.[7] To improve visualization of relevant landmarks and improve ease of catheter insertions with the infraclavicular approach, a bedside assistant can give caudal traction on arm. A rolled towel between scapulae helps to provide a better approach.[9] However, do not use this approach on the ipsilateral side of chest wall deformities, clavicle fractures, first or second rib fractures, or clavicle surgery. Advantages of subclavian venous access include a high degree of patient tolerance, a similarly low complication rate to the IJ, and the ease of insertion.[7] Disadvantages include risk of subclavian artery puncture (a noncompressible site) and an increased risk of pneumothorax.[7,9]

Femoral anatomy The location of the femoral vein makes it the largest, easiest, and possibly the most problematic site for central venous access.[7] It is encased in the femoral sheath with the femoral artery, nerve, and lymphatics. The femoral vein becomes the external iliac vein superior to the inguinal ligament. The anatomy of the vessels can be described with a simple mnemonic: NAVEL.[17] From lateral to medial, the structures in the sheath are femoral *n*erve, femoral *a*rtery, femoral *v*ein, *e*mpty space, *l*ymphatics.

Right-handed operators may find it easier to place right-sided femoral lines.[9] To find the vein, palpate the femoral artery. The vein lies about 1 cm medial to the arterial pulse in adults and about 0.5 cm in infants. The needle insertion site should be about 1 to 2 cm below the inguinal ligament to avoid retroperitoneal hematoma secondary to through-and-through puncture of the vein or artery. The bevel should be directed cephalad, and the needle should be at a 45° to 60° angle to the skin along the long axis of the thigh.[17]

Special considerations for the femoral vein Avoid ipsilateral placement of a femoral line if there is significant trauma to the lower extremity or deep venous thrombosis. Consider another site in case of abdominal trauma that may interrupt the inferior vena cava. Blood return below the diaphragm during cardiopulmonary resuscitation may be reduced, so consider placing the line at another site or placing the catheter tip near the diaphragm.[23] In pulseless arrest, when the femoral artery landmark is not available, the operator should place his thumb on pubic tubercle and his index finger on the anterior superior iliac spine. The femoral vein will be approximately at the "V" formed by the web space between the thumb and the index finger. The femoral vein is the largest and easiest central vein to access; however, there is a higher rate of venous thrombosis and line infection at this site.[24]

Indications and contraindications
Central venous access is indicated for patients who require hemodynamic monitoring, such as central venous pressure or a pulmonary artery catheter, for procedures such as hemodialysis or transvenous pacing or for the administration of medications such as vasopressors, sclerosing medications, and cytotoxic and chemotherapeutic agents. Given these indications, in the emergency setting, central access may be obtained during active resuscitation of critically ill patients.[14,15,17,22,25] In some cases, central access is used for patients in whom peripheral access cannot be gained. Nonetheless, depending on the catheter used, central access is not better than peripheral access for the purpose of rapid infusion of fluid during resuscitation. With the exception of an introducer sheath or a specifically made large-bore catheter ("trauma line"), large-bore peripheral IV access can provide more rapid infusion of fluids than most commonly used central lines.[7] Flow through a catheter is described by the Hagen–Poiseuille equation, which shows that flow is directly proportional to the pressure gradient and to the fourth power of the radius of the catheter.[8] It is inversely proportional to the length of the catheter. Thus, large-bore short catheters best achieve rapid fluid infusion.

$$Q = \Delta P(\pi r^4 / 8 \mu L)$$

where Q = flow, ΔP = pressure gradient, r = radius of internal catheter, L = length, μ = viscosity of fluid.

Many contraindications for central venous access are relative and depend on the patient's status and the urgency of the procedure. Site-specific contraindications and considerations have already been discussed. General contraindications include anatomic distortion, indwelling vascular hardware, injury proximal to the insertion site, and coagulopathy or thrombolysis.[7,17,26]

Stepwise procedure

The equipment required for placing a central venous catheter is listed in **Box 3**. There are several types of central lines, depending on the catheter's intended use. Selection of a line should be made with consideration of the current indication for the line and the patient's projected future course. Common central venous lines include[7]

- Single lumen: 16, 18, or 20 gauge; 8, 12, or 15 cm
- Double lumen: 18/18 gauge, 7.5 F; 15, 20, 25 cm
- Triple lumen: 18/18/16 gauge; 7 F; 15, 20, 25 cm
- Introducer sheath (Cordis): 9 F (11 gauge); 10, 13 cm

To insert a central venous catheter, first identify the optimal site using physical landmarks or ultrasound with the patient in the proper position based on the intended site. Prepare a sterile field that includes the necessary equipment. Always gown, prep, and drape in a sterile manner. Open the central venous catheter kit in a sterile manner, or have an assistant prepare the equipment in a sterile manner. Prepare the central venous catheter by flushing all ports and lumens with sterile saline. Administer topical anesthetic to all patients. Use a finder needle to locate the intended vein unless you are placing the catheter with ultrasound guidance. Using the dominant hand, hold the introducer needle on a 10-mL syringe and align it to the target. Puncture the skin and advance slowly through the soft tissues maintaining constant negative

---

Box 3
Equipment needed for central venous access (often in a kit, except gloves)

Sterile gown and gloves and mask and hair cover

Local anesthetic, syringe, small gauge needle

Sterile antiseptic solution

Finder needle (22 gauge)

Introducer needle (16 or 18 gauge)

Guidewire

No. 11 blade scalpel

Vein dilator

Full sterile sheet and sterile towels

Sterile normal saline flushes, 10 mL each

IV tubing, flushes, syringe

Central venous catheter

3-0 Silk suture with needle and driver

Antibacterial patch

Sterile gauze pads and sterile dressing

pressure by pulling back the plunger until a flash of venous blood returns into the syringe. Stabilize the needle with the nondominant hand and remove the syringe from the needle. Immediately occlude the needle hub with a finger to avoid air embolus. Insert the guidewire through the needle with the J-hook tip in front. Always hold the wire; do not release it. Remove the needle, maintaining control of the wire. Incise the skin with the No. 11 blade scalpel to accommodate the dilator and catheter. With a gentle twisting motion, insert the dilator over the guidewire and into the vessel. Remove the dilator. Advance the catheter over the guidewire. Remove the guidewire. Aspirate and flush all ports with sterile saline while holding the syringe upright to visualize and eliminate any remaining air. Suture the catheter in place and apply a transparent sterile dressing. Confirm placement of the subclavian and IJ lines with a chest radiograph.[9,17]

Special considerations, complications, and pearls and pitfalls

Ultrasound guidance for central venous catheter placement has gained in popularity and should be used if available and the operator is trained in its use.[9,10,27] Use of ultrasonography decreases the number of attempts and increases the first-attempt success rate of line placement. Ultrasonography is particularly useful when landmarks are obscured, such as in trauma or obesity. Both static and dynamic ultrasonography are used for central venous line placement. Static ultrasonography can be used to visualize the anatomy, after which the procedure is performed blind. Dynamic ultrasonography is used throughout the procedure. It is used for the IJ and femoral veins, and is also, but less commonly, used for the subclavian vein.[10]

To use ultrasonography for line placement, place a sterile sheath with transducer gel inside the sheath and sterile gel outside the sheath on the transducer. Using the linear probe in the transverse plane, locate the vein and corresponding artery. The vein will be compressible and thin walled compared with the artery. Center the vein in the image and estimate the depth.

Insert the needle distal to the transducer at approximately 45°. Aim the needle at the center of your transducer perpendicular to the long axis of the probe. Observe the image for the tip of the needle or for tissue movement. Angle the image distally to find the tip of the needle and then follow it until the vein is accessed.

A longitudinal technique for ultrasound-guided central line placement can also be used. Align the transducer with the long axis of the vein. Insert the needle at the distal end of the vein and direct it along the long axis, again watching for the needle tip and/or tissue movement. Once the flash of blood is obtained, continue catheter placement as described previously.

Complications of central venous catheter placement include pneumothorax (except femoral lines), arterial puncture, chylothorax, bleeding, vessel injury, arrhythmia, venous air embolism, cardiac tamponade, infection, airway compromise, thrombosis, and nerve damage.[7,9,17,28] To avoid these and increase the chances of success with central venous catheter placement, consider the following suggestions:

- When attempting a subclavian or IJ line, prep the entire ipsilateral part of the neck and anterior part of the chest to facilitate changing sites if there is failure at one site.
- If you discover no flow after removing the syringe, replace the syringe lightly and withdraw or advance slightly while aspirating.
- Use the guidewire with the J-tip pointing forward; do not reverse the wire because this can puncture vessels.
- There should be minimal resistance when advancing the guidewire. Do not force the wire. If it does not advance easily, reattach the syringe and aspirate to verify location inside the vessel. Reposition the needle if needed or turn the bevel.

- Always maintain control of the wire not only to avoid contamination but also to avoid losing the wire in the central circulation.
- After placing a subclavian or IJ line, the catheter tip should be in the superior vena cava. The right atrium is thin walled, and the catheter tip can perforate the right atrium.

Accessing and Using Indwelling Central Venous Catheters

Many patients present to the emergency department with indwelling central venous catheters. Unfortunately, patients who are being treated for cancer or who require hemodialysis, and therefore have previously implanted central venous access catheters, may develop illness or injury and require emergency medical care. Both partially implanted lines and fully implanted lines can provide convenient access to the vascular space, and the ability to troubleshoot malfunctions is key for the emergency practitioner.

Anatomy and physiology

For both fully and partially implanted central lines, the indwelling catheter tip lies either in the superior vena cava or in the right atrium. With partially implanted lines, the outside end of the catheter is tunneled subcutaneously and exits from the skin in a small incision.[29] The subcutaneous tunnel helps to prevent contamination of the line with skin flora. Often, a Dacron cuff is used to anchor the line subcutaneously.[14] With fully implanted lines, the outside end of the catheter is connected to a reservoir that is implanted subcutaneously.[14] No part of the line exits the skin. Many partially implanted lines are fully subcutaneous and connected to a reservoir, therefore converting them to a fully implanted line.[30]

Indications and contraindications for accessing indwelling central venous catheters

While indwelling central catheters are often convenient and preestablished sites for venous access, therefore omitting the need for painful attempts at other venous access, these lines are sensitive, often fragile, and a direct route to the patient's bloodstream. Care should be taken to only access them as necessary and always with the utmost attention to sterile technique. Indications to access an indwelling line include medication administration, phlebotomy, and simply a desire to use central access instead of new peripheral access (eg, to prevent needle sticks in a chronically ill patient). Indwelling lines may also be accessed in truly emergent situations to prevent death, ie, the use of a hemodialysis catheter in a patient during cardiac arrest. Dialysis catheters should only be accessed for reasons other than dialysis in a true emergency. Other contraindications for accessing indwelling central venous catheters include infection of the skin overlying the catheter or port, infection of the catheter, and suspected thrombophlebitis or obstruction of the line.[14,15,30,31]

Stepwise procedure

Sterile procedure must always be maintained during access of indwelling lines. **Box 4** lists the equipment necessary for indwelling line access. To access a partially implanted line, first ensure that the catheter clamp is closed. Then remove the covering from the end of the catheter. Clean both the catheter end and the luer adapter and allow to dry. Attach the luer adapter to the catheter end. If access is for blood sampling only, insert a 20-ga needle into luer adapter, open the catheter clamp, withdraw and discard 5 mL blood, discard needle and syringe, withdraw blood samples with a new 20-ga needle and syringe, and flush with appropriate solution for the line (normal saline or heparin solution). To follow blood sampling with an infusion, after

---

Box 4
Equipment needed to access an indwelling central venous catheter

Sterile gloves, mask, and hair cover

Local anesthetic, syringe, small-gauge needle

Sterile antiseptic solution

Sterile alcohol prep pads

Needle (20 gauge for partially implanted)

Noncoring type needle with right angle or straight angle, for fully implanted

Sterile drapes

Appropriate flush (saline or heparin) per type

IV tubing, syringes

Luer lock caps

Blood collection equipment

Sterile gauze pads

Sterile transparent dressing

---

the blood sample is drawn, attach IV tubing to the catheter end and infuse. Always close the catheter clamp between steps when no syringe is attached. When discontinuing the infusion, flush the catheter with appropriate solution, place luer cap on catheter end, and secure to the patient's chest wall. To avoid air embolism, do not use needleless caps.[30]

To access fully implanted catheters, use a noncoring needle to avoid damaging the catheter diaphragm and the skin over the reservoir. First, apply a topical anesthetic to the skin overlying the access site/reservoir. Clean the skin over the reservoir with iodine or chlorhexidine. Wipe off the solution with sterile alcohol prep pad. Flush the needle and tubing with normal saline and leave the syringe attached. Stabilize the reservoir with the nondominant hand, and insert the needle into the device until the needle reaches the opposite end. Flush with 2 to 3 mL normal saline; then withdraw 5 to 10 mL blood and discard. As with partially implanted catheters, close the catheter clamp when a syringe is not attached. Attach a new syringe to withdraw blood samples. If starting an infusion, clamp tubing and attach primed IV tubing. When discontinuing access, close clamp, attach appropriate flush, open clamp, and flush. Remove the noncoring needle and apply direct pressure to control bleeding. Apply a sterile dressing.[30]

Special considerations, complications, and pearls and pitfalls
It is important to know how to troubleshoot the nonfunctioning indwelling venous catheter. Common problems include malposition of the catheter tip against a vessel wall, wax buildup from infused lipids, and precipitated medications such as calcium and phosphate[31] or phenytoin or diazepam through a silicone line.[32] Intraluminal blood clot may also obstruct the line, and extraluminal clot may cause a one-way valve with retention of the ability to flush but not to aspirate. In this situation the indwelling line may be used, but with extreme caution.[31] An indwelling line should not be used or manipulated in the following situations:

- Central venous thrombus
- Sepsis or infection of the line or site of insertion

- Catheter dislodged from central venous system
- Mechanically obstructed line, because the obstruction can be released into circulation as an embolus.[33]
- Accessing hemodialysis catheters except in true emergency. Compromise of the dialysis catheter can lead to significant morbidity or mortality.

Complications may also occur when trying to restore line patency. These include catheter rupture, disconnection of the catheter from the implanted reservoir, hemorrhage, and contamination or infection.[31] If a line does not flush easily, do not increase force and pressure in a further attempt to flush the line. Separate peripheral access should be sought. The risks and benefits of manipulation of the indwelling line must be weighed before troubleshooting. Suggestions for troubleshooting indwelling lines include getting a chest radiograph to verify the catheter position, changing the patient's position (ie, Trendelenburg or reverse Trendelenburg), or having the patient perform a Valsalva. If the line is being used for parenteral nutrition and/or lipid infusion, consider waxy buildup. In this case, an injection of 70% ethanol in water, 0.1 N hydrochloric acid, or tissue plasminogen activator or urokinase may help. In the case of a medication precipitant, also consider injection of 0.1 N hydrochloric acid or 70% ethanol in water. For suspected thrombus, consider urokinase or tissue plasminogen activator injection, consider attempting to aspirate the thrombus with a syringe connected directly to the hub, or get a radiograph using contrast dye to evaluate the location of the obstruction. If these measures fail to restore patency to the line, the line may need to be replaced.[31]

OTHER VASCULAR ACCESS SKILLS AND PROCEDURES
Intraosseous Access

When peripheral IV access is unobtainable and fluid administration is time sensitive, intraosseous access may be rapidly and reliably obtained with a minimum of procedural preparation or operator experience. Initially introduced in 1922 by Drinker and Doan, this route of access was used extensively during World War II and then lost favor with the advent of plastic peripheral IV catheters. Since the 1980s, however, the intraosseous route has regained favor as a second-line venous access site[34] because it marries rapidity and reliability (**Table 1**).[35] Intraosseous access is recommended by the Advanced Cardiovascular Life Support (ACLS), Pediatric Advanced Life Support (PALS), and Advanced Trauma Life Support (ATLS) guidelines as the second-line access site of choice in resuscitation situations with class IIA evidence.[34] In military or tactical situations, it has replaced venous cut-down as the vascular access alternative when peripheral access cannot be obtained,[36] and it is becoming more frequently used in the prehospital arena.

Table 1 Rapidity and reliability of forms of vascular access in pediatric patients		
Access Type	**Average Time (min)**	**Success Rate (%)**
Peripheral	3.0	17
Central	8.4	77
Cut-down	12.7	82
Intraosseus	4.7	83

Data from Brunette DD, Fisher R. Intravascular access in pediatric cardiac arrest. Am J Emerg Med 1988;6(6):577–9.

Anatomy and physiology

Long bones have a rich and reliable blood supply from nutrient vessels. The medullary cavity, a space located deep to the bony cortices of the diaphysis, contains blood-rich venous sinusoids at either ends. These sinusoids drain into a central venous channel and provide an easily accessed route by which fluids and medications can be introduced into the venous system.[9]

The best site for intraosseous access in children is the flat medial plane of the proximal tibia, 2 cm below the tibial tuberosity. In adults, several other sites may be used because it is often difficult to obtain access via the tibia. Sites to be considered as alternates include the sternum, the humerus, the ileum, the distal femur, the medial malleolus,[9] the distal radius and ulna, and the clavicle.[34] In tactical or military environments, the sternum is generally protected by body armor and is therefore is favored.[36]

Indications and contraindications

Intraosseous access is contraindicated when there is an ipsilateral fracture or ipsilateral vascular injury proximal to the access site,[9] if there is an overlying burn or skin infection[34] or if the patient has severe osteoporosis or osteogenesis imperfecta.[9] Situations in which intraosseous access should be considered and used early include shock, sepsis, cardiac or respiratory arrest, multitrauma, high total body surface area burns, and status epilepticus.[34] However, in the absence of contraindications, intraosseous access is appropriate whenever there is impending cardiovascular collapse and peripheral vascular access cannot be obtained.[9]

Stepwise procedure

Unless performed in a situation in which time is of utmost and paramount importance, intraosseous access should be placed under sterile conditions. The equipment needed is listed in **Box 5**. Risks, benefits, and complications should be discussed with the patient if the clinical scenario allows. Appropriately prepare and drape the site desired for needle placement. If the patient is conscious or able to feel pain, use local anesthetic to anesthetize the site of placement paying particular attention to infiltration of the periosteum and the dermis. Stabilize the extremity. Using the dominant hand, place the needle against the skin and direct it perpendicular to the bone and, in children, away from the nearest physis. Apply constant pressure and begin to twist the needle clockwise. When the bony cortex is breached and the medullary cavity is entered, there will be a sudden decrease in resistance. At this point, the stylet should be removed and the needle stabilized with a bulky dressing (**Fig. 4**). In children who are expected to regain consciousness, a leg board to immobilize the extremity

---

Box 5
Equipment needed for interosseous access

Sterile drapes

Local anesthetic

Automatic intraosseous needle drill[a]

Gauze and tape

Antiseptic solution

Intraosseous needle

IV tubing, flushes, syringe

[a] *If available; see* **Fig. 3.**

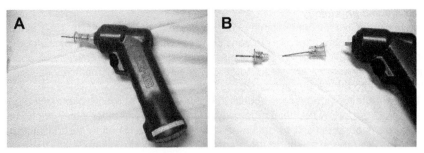

Fig. 3. An automatic drill can drastically increase the speed and ease of IO placement. (*A*) The drill is shown loaded with an intraosseus stylet/catheter. (*B*) The same drill/catheter/stylet is separated to show the component parts.

may be used. After stylet removal, a syringe may be applied to aspirate. Return of marrow confirms placement. Alternatively, successful administration of a continuous fluid infusion also confirms placement. As with any venous access site, the area should be observed for extravasation of fluids. A subsequent plain radiograph should be obtained once the patient is stabilized to confirm placement and rule out iatrogenic fracture.[9]

If available, a specialized drill may be used to insert the intraosseous needle (see **Fig. 3**). If such a device is used, follow the same procedure and angle of entry as described. Instead of manually twisting the device, squeeze the trigger of the drill. The abrupt decrease in resistance expected when the bony cortex is breached may

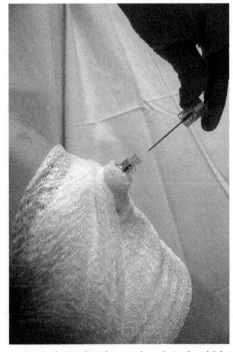

Fig. 4. Once the intraosseus catheter has been placed, it should be secured with a bulky dressing and the sharp stylet should be removed.

be dampened by use of the drill, so increased vigilance should be used to prevent through-and-through placement of the needle and subsequent infiltration into the deep tissues.[9]

Special considerations, complications, and pearls and pitfalls
Conditions that may contribute to unsuccessful intraosseous access placement include pathologically weak bone, clogging of the needle with bony fragments or marrow, penetration through the posterior cortex, or operator error in identifying landmarks.[34] In a successful placement of intraosseous access, complications are rare, on the order of less than 1%; however, the risk of complications increases with duration of needle placement, and the current recommendations are to replace intraosseous access with central venous access within 24 hours.[34] These include the rare occurrence of fat embolism, penetration of the physis in children, introduction of infection and subsequent development of osteomyelitis (0.6%)[37] or cellulitis (0.7%),[34] and iatrogenic fracture.[9] Extravasation of infusion contents into the surrounding soft tissues may result in compartment syndrome.[34] Placement of an intraosseous needle in the sternum carries additional risks, including pneumothorax, mediastinal injury, injury to the great vessels, and even death.[38]

Infusions and medications
Many types of resuscitation fluid are appropriate for intraosseous administration, including saline and dextrose solutions, lactated Ringer's solution, blood products, and plasma (**Fig. 5**). Rates of infusion are generally lower than those attained by peripheral lines.[39] Under experimental conditions, gravity infusion rates of 10 to 20 mL/min and pressure-driven rates of 40 mL/min have been attained.[40,41]

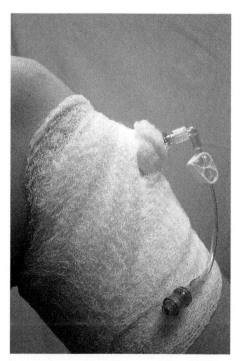

Fig. 5. An intraosseus line can be used just like a peripheral IV line.

Medication dosing is unchanged from the peripheral IV route.[42] Medications that have been safely given via intraosseous access are listed in **Box 6**.

Although many resuscitation medications can be given via endotracheal tube, intraosseous administration of medication is preferred according to the 2005 American Heart Association (AHA) guidelines for cardiopulmonary resuscitation and emergency

Box 6 Medications safely given via intraosseus access
Adenosine
Antibiotics
Antitoxins
Anesthetics
Atracurium
Atropine
Calcium gluconate
Calcium chloride
Contrast media
Dexamethasone
Diazepam
Digoxin
Dobutamine
Dopamine
Ephedrine
Epinephrine
Heparin
Insulin
Isoproterenol
Levarterenol
Lidocaine
Lorazepam
Mannitol
Morphine
Naloxone
Pancuronium
Phenobarbital
Phenytoin
Propanolol
Sodium bicarbonate
Succinylcholine
Thiopental
Vecuronium

and cardiovascular care. Given the ease with which intraosseous access can be obtained, there is almost no circumstance in which the endotracheal route should be used for medication administration.[9]

Umbilical Vessel Access

In the first week of life, a unique opportunity exists for rapid vascular access. Particularly in the setting of severe dehydration of a neonate, umbilical vessels may in fact be the only route of access available to the clinician.[43] Although the umbilical artery is a preferred site of access in a stable patient because of the added benefits of ease of arterial blood gas sampling and invasive hemodynamic monitoring, umbilical venous access is faster, easier, and is the recommended procedure for access in a neonate in need of rapid resuscitation in whom attempts at peripheral access have failed.[44]

Anatomy and physiology

The normal umbilical stump houses paired umbilical arteries that arise from the iliac arteries, and a single large umbilical vein that is contiguous with the portal vein[43] and returns blood via the ductus venosus into the inferior vena cava. Occasionally, there is a single umbilical artery, which can then be distinguished from the vein by its thick muscularis and smaller caliber.[44] The umbilical vein is typically accessible up to 2 weeks after birth. The umbilical arteries, in contrast, may close as early as 24 hours after birth and are almost always inaccessible after 7 days.[45] In nonemergent situations, the ideal placement is with the catheter tip at the junction of the inferior vena cava and the right atrium. However, in successful emergency cannulation, the umbilical venous catheter should extend only 2 to 3 cm beyond the abdominal wall to avoid entry into the portal system.[44]

Indications and contraindications

Umbilical venous cannulation is the preferred procedure in any neonate less than 2 weeks of age who require rapid fluid or medication resuscitation and in whom peripheral IV access attempts have failed. In a stable patient, umbilical arterial cannulation may be preferable.[44] Umbilical venous catheterization should not be performed if there are signs of infection in or around the umbilical stump, if the infant is greater than 2 weeks of age, or if an obvious abdominal abnormality or congenital defect is noted.[45]

Stepwise procedure

As with any form of vascular access, this procedure should be performed under sterile conditions. The required equipment is listed in **Box 7**. Risks, benefits, and complications should be discussed with the guardian. Clean and drape the entire lower abdomen, paying special attention to the umbilical stump. Place a purse-string suture in the umbilical stump leaving the ends free, and loosely wrap an umbilical tie around the base of the stump for tying should the need for rapid hemostasis arise. Flush the catheter with a heparinized solution and attach it to a regular syringe via a stopcock. For a premature neonate a 3.5F catheter is required, whereas for a term neonate a 5.0F catheter is appropriate. Incise the cord stump through and through at approximately 2 cm above the abdominal wall. Identify the single thin-walled vein. Remove any visualized clot within the vein lumen with forceps. Insert the catheter gently into the umbilical vein and aspirating frequently until good blood return is seen.[44] In emergent situations, the catheter need only be inserted 1 to 2 cm beyond the point of good blood return and radiographic confirmation of placement is not needed.[43] Once the catheter is advanced to the appropriate depth, tie the purse-string suture to secure the catheter. The umbilical tie may then be removed.[44]

Box 7
Equipment needed for umbilical venous cannulation

Sterile drapes

Antiseptic solution

Small-diameter nonabsorbable suture

Umbilical tape/tie

Umbilical vascular catheter

Scalpel

Forceps

Needle driver

Gauze

Special considerations, complications, and pearls and pitfalls
Proper technique is paramount for the successful placement of an umbilical venous catheter and to minimize complications. In emergent situations, the catheter need only be inserted 1 to 2 cm beyond the point of good blood return and radiographic confirmation of placement is not needed.[43] Care must be taken to prevent injury to the walls of the vessels, and to prevent any air from entering the central circulation.[44] Historical complication rates for umbilical venous access are higher than those for arterial access, at 20% and 10%, respectively.[46]

Complications that have been reported include thrombosis, air or thromboembolism, perforation of the vessels or bowel, local or systemic infection, organ or limb infarcts, hydrothorax, cardiac arrhythmias, pericardial effusion, tamponade, or erosion of the cardiac musculature.[43] Placement of the catheter in the portal system may result in hepatic necrosis, pulmonary embolism, or portal hypertension. A patent urachus may be mistaken for the umbilical vein and cannulated. This results in the return of urine rather than blood and should be easily recognized and remedied.[44]

Arterial Access and Catheterization

A critical component of the emergency management of many patients includes the acquisition of an arterial blood gas panel. Patients in extremis or those on mechanical ventilation may require continuous monitoring of arterial blood pressure and repeated blood gas measurements and therefore may benefit from arterial cannulation.[47] Since the first arterial catheterization was performed using a brass pipe in the carotid artery of a horse, techniques and devices have improved significantly.[48]

Anatomy and physiology
Common sites used for arterial access include the radial, brachial, and femoral arteries (**Table 2**). Frequently, these arteries run in neurovascular bundles, so care must be taken to avoid damage to nerves or cannulation of nearby veins.[47] Other possible sites of arterial puncture and catheterization include the dorsalis pedis and the posterior tibial, axillary, and temporal arteries.[49]

Indications and contraindications
Arterial blood sampling is indicated in any patient for whom determination of acid/base status and blood concentrations of oxygen and carbon dioxide (CO_2) is necessary for clinical decision making. It is also indicated for the determination of carboxyhemoglobin and methemoglobin levels when there is suspicion that these may be present.[50]

Table 2
Sites for arterial access and cannulation

Artery	Anatomy	Advantages	Disadvantages	Considerations
Radial	Volar wrist, radial side Enter at proximal wrist flexor crease	Superficial Easily palpated Collateral circulation via ulnar artery and palmar arcades	Small vessel	Allen's test
Femoral	Between ASIS and pubic symphysis Just below inguinal ligament Vein/nerve superficial and medial to artery	Largest vessel	Deep to nerve and vein Requires longer needle	Second choice for cannulation when radial artery is not an option
Brachial	Medial upper arm Between biceps brachii muscle and medial epicondyle Enter at antecubitum	Larger vessel	Patient must keep arm in extension while cannulated	Splits into radial and ulnar arteries so do not attempt distally Avoid median nerve, which is just medial to artery

Abbreviation: ASIS, Anterior Superior Iliac Spine.
Data from Stroud S, Rodriguez R. Chapter 46: Arterial puncture and cannulation. In: Reichman EF, Simon RR, editors. Emergency medicine procedures. New York: McGraw-Hill; 2004.

Arterial cannulation is indicated when there is need for repeated measurements of arterial blood gases, or when continuous blood pressure monitoring is required.

In patients in extremis, noninvasive methods of hemodynamic monitoring can markedly underestimate systolic pressures.[51] Arterial hemodynamic monitoring is recommended by the International Consensus Conference for Hemodynamic Monitoring in Shock whenever a patient is hypotensive despite the administration of vasoactive agents[25] and by the AHA for the management of acute myocardial infarction.[52] Continuous measurement of arterial blood pressure via arterial cannulation is second only to continuous aortic pressure measurements for accurate and precise hemodynamic monitoring and is superior to both oscillometric and auscultated peripheral blood pressure monitoring.[53] Synthetic vascular grafts should not be used for arterial sampling or cannulation.[47]

Contraindications for arterial puncture and cannulation include infection, trauma, burns, or skin irritation overlying the access site; severe peripheral arterial disease; inability of the physician to palpate the arterial pulsation at the intended access site; and the presence of bleeding disorders, current coagulopathy, or recent thrombolytic therapy. Synthetic vascular grafts should not be used for arterial sampling or cannulation.[47]

Stepwise procedure

This procedure should, like all vascular access procedures, be performed under sterile conditions, and risks and benefits of the procedure should be explained to the patient. Equipment required for the procedure is listed in **Box 8**. For this procedure, the patient should be positioned to maximize the skin exposure overlying the puncture site and to minimize the depth of the target artery. For the radial artery, this includes dorsiflexion of the wrist to approximately 60°. For the brachial and femoral arteries, this involves complete extension of the elbow and hip, respectively. Clean and drape the site of access, and then infiltrate the overlying skin with local anesthetic. Prepare the needle with an attached heparinized syringe by pulling back on the plunger to allow entry of a small amount of air. Locate the arterial pulsation with the nondominant hand or with the vascular probe of a portable ultrasonography machine. Advance the needle into the skin at a 30° to 45° angle with the bevel facing proximally until good blood return is seen in the syringe. Aspiration with the syringe plunger should not be necessary to obtain good blood return into the syringe. If no blood flow is encountered, withdraw

---

Box 8
Equipment needed for arterial cannulation

Sterile drapes

Antiseptic solution

Arm board

Gauze

Local anesthetic

Needles

Syringe

Arterial sampling needle and syringe or device

Arterial line manometer

Blood sampling equipment

the needle as far as the surface of the skin and then redirect before reentry to avoid arterial or venous damage.

If only one arterial blood sample is desired, collect 1 to 2 mL of blood and withdraw the needle. Hold pressure over the puncture site for 3 to 5 minutes to prevent hematoma formation, apply a pressure dressing the site. Remove any air in the blood sample, apply the cap, and send the sample to the laboratory on ice for immediate processing.[47]

If cannulation of the artery is desired, access of the artery is obtained as described for arterial puncture. However, several different devices exist for the introduction of the arterial catheter. First, a catheter-over-the-needle approach requires the use of exactly that: a needle sheathed by a vascular catheter similar to that used for peripheral IV access. No syringe should be attached to the catheter while access is being obtained. Once blood return is visualized in the hub of the needle, advance the catheter fully over the needle into the artery. Remove the needle leaving the catheter in place, confirming placement by the flow of pulsatile bright red blood from the catheter. Once placement is confirmed, attach IV tubing to the catheter, suture the catheter to the skin, and dress the site.[47]

The Seldinger technique, or catheter-over-a-guide-wire technique, generally results in higher success rates than a catheter-over-the-needle technique.[47] For this method, prepackaged 1-unit devices are available. After preparation and draping, remove the device from the packaging and the protective cover from the needle. Then test the guidewire to ensure ease of movement. Insert the needle as described for arterial puncture. When blood return is confirmed, advance the guidewire. If resistance is met, retract the guidewire and remove the device. A second attempt may be performed with a new device at a more proximal site. If the guidewire is inserted easily, then cut a small incision at the base of the guidewire with a No. 11 blade and then advance the catheter over the guidewire until the hub is at the skin. Remove the rest of the device leaving the catheter in place. Confirm appropriate placement with good arterial blood flow as described earlier, and attach IV tubing before suturing the catheter in place and dressing the site. In markedly hypotensive patients, none of these techniques may be successful and the arterial cut-down procedure must be performed to cannulate the artery. All arterial punctures should be rechecked frequently following placement to look for hematoma formation or limb ischemia. If cannulation is being performed for hemodynamic monitoring, it may be necessary to immobilize the limb in the position optimal for measurements.[47]

Special considerations, complications, and pearls and pitfalls

Before accessing the radial artery, appropriate assessment of collateral circulation from the ulnar artery should be performed via a modified Allen's test (**Fig. 6**). Grasp the limb to be used and occlude both the radial and ulnar arteries. Ask the patient to close the hand tightly to empty the tissues of blood. Then ask the patient to open the hand while occlusion of the radial and ulnar arteries is maintained. Once the hand is opened, release pressure on the ulnar artery. With normal collateral circulation the hand should flush pink within 7 seconds; 8 to 14 seconds is considered equivocal and more than 14 seconds is abnormal. Although an abnormal Allen's test is not an absolute contraindication to radial artery puncture or cannulation, it should prompt the provider to perform the procedure with increased caution and to monitor the patient more closely after the procedure.[47]

The overall incidence of complications from arterial access is less than 5%.[53] Relatively common complications include arterial thrombosis, injury to the artery, infection, or bleeding. When an arterial catheter is in place, the risk of infection

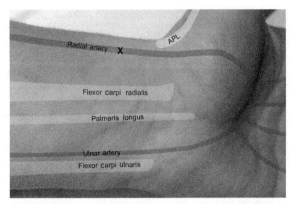

Fig. 6. Relevant wrist anatomy; an Allen's test should be performed before radial arterial line placement. APL, abductor pollicis longus tendon.

increases with the duration of catheterization.[54] There have been reports of neuropathic pain or direct nerve injury from hematoma formation after arterial puncture, particularly in patients with anticoagulaton.[55] Rare complications include arteriovenous fistula formation and limb ischemia.[47]

Accessing and cannulating the radial artery takes patience, a steady hand, and persistence, regardless of whether the operator is using a premade needle-catheter-guidewire device or catheter-over-needle approach (**Fig. 7**). Often, taking several minutes to palpate the patient's pulse in multiple locations throughout the wrist and forearm will give the operator a better sense of where the artery lies and runs. A slow gentle advance of the needle–catheter will minimize vasospasm and increase the operator's likelihood of success.

Alternative tests

Although now there are noninvasive methods of determining oxygenation and carbon dioxide levels, including pulse oximetry and end-tidal CO_2 monitoring, respectively, arterial blood gas sampling remains the definitive test for the true oxygen and CO_2 content of the blood. There is no replacement for the arterial blood gas for accurate acid/base status under most situations. Although venous blood gas may be an

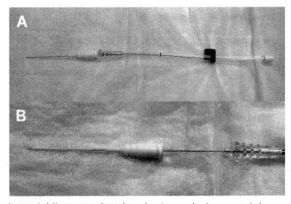

Fig. 7. Peripheral arterial lines may be placed using a device containing a guidewire (*A*) or by using a catheter-over-needle technique (*B*).

acceptable alternative to arterial blood gas for certain disease processes, such as diabetic ketoacidosis,[56] it is less accurate than blood gases from an arterial source in critically ill patients.[50]

SUMMARY

Accessing a patient's vascular system is critical to many facets of emergency care and is required for many diagnostic studies and therapeutic interventions. Peripheral, central, and alternate methods by which the vasculature may be accessed have reviewed in this article. The provider must be well versed in all these techniques and their nuances to appropriately apply the correct procedure to the correct patient at the correct time and setting. Mastery of the procedures reviewed is essential for the effective and complete practice of emergency medicine.

REFERENCES

1. Rivera AM, Strauss KW, Van Zundert A, et al. The history of peripheral intravenous catheters: how little plastic tubes revolutionized medicine. Acta Anaesthesiol Belg 2005;56:271–82.
2. Reichman EF, Oakes JL. Chapter 5: vascular access. In: Wolfson AB, editor. Harwood-Nuss' clinical practice of emergency medicine- fourth edition. Philadelphia: Lippincott Williams & Wilkins; 2005. p. 43–55.
3. Mulvey MA. Fluid and electrolytes: balance and disturbance. In: Smeltzer SC, Bare BG, Hinkle JL, editors. Brunner and Suddarth's textbook of medical-surgical nursing. 11th edition. Philadelphia: Lippincott Williams and Wilkins; 2008. p. 300.
4. Mbamalu D, Banerjee A. Methods of obtaining peripheral venous access in difficult situations. Postgrad Med 1999;75(886):459.
5. Feldman R. General principles of intravenous access. In: Reichman EF, Simon RR, editors. Emergency medicine procedures. New York: McGraw-Hill; 2004. p. 314–37.
6. Roseman JM. Deep, percutaneous antecubital venipuncture: an alternative to surgical cutdown. Am J Surg 1983;146(2):285.
7. Marino PL. Chapter 6: establishing venous access. In: Marino PL, Sutin KM, editors. The ICU book. 3rd Edition. Philadelphia: Lippincott, Williams & Wilkins; 2007. p. 107–28.
8. Pfitzner J. Poiseuille and his law. Anaesthesia 1976;31:273–5.
9. Wyatt CR. Chapter 33: venous and intraosseus access in adults. In: Tintinalli JE, editor. Tintinalli's emergency medicine: a comprehensive study guide. New York: McGraw-Hill; 2011. Available at: http://www.accessemergencymedicine.com. libproxy.lib.unc.edu/content.aspx?aID=6370085. Accessed June 25, 2012.
10. Sierzenski PR, Gukhool J, Leech SJ. Chapter 24: emergency ultrasound. In: Knoop KJ, editor. The atlas of emergency medicine. 3rd edition. New York: McGraw-Hill; 2010. Available at: http://www.accessemergencymedicine.com. libproxy.lib.unc.edu/content.aspx?aID=6008341. Accessed June 25, 2012.
11. Keyes LE, Frazee BW, Snoey ER, et al. Ultrasound-guided brachial and basilic vein cannulation in emergency department patients with difficult intravenous access. Ann Emerg Med 1999;34(6):711.
12. Wang CL, Cohan RH, Ellis JH, et al. Frequency, management, and outcome of extravasation of nonionic iodinated contrast medium in 69,657 intravenous injections. Radiology 2007;243(1):80–7.
13. Lanter PL, Williams J. Chapter 23- Venous cutdown. In: Roberts JR, Hedges JR, editors. Roberts and Hedges: clinical procedures in emergency medicine. 5th edition. Philadelphia: Saunders; 2009. p. 411–7.

14. Bothe A, Piccioni W, Ambrosino JJ, et al. Implantable central venous access system. Am J Surg 1984;147:565–9.
15. Dyer BJ, Weiman MG, Ludwig S. Central venous catheters in the emergency department: access, utilization, and problem solving. Pediatr Emerg Care 1995;11(2):112–7.
16. Denys BG, Uretsky BF. Anatomical variations of internal jugular vein location: impact on central venous access. Crit Care Med 1991;19:1516.
17. Feldman R. Chapter 38: central venous access. In: Reichman EF, Simon RR, editors. Emergency medicine procedures. New York: McGraw-Hill; 2004. p. 314–37.
18. Eissa NT, Kvetan V. Guide wire as a cause of complete heart block in patients with preexisting left bundle branch block. Anesthesiology 1990;73:772–4.
19. Nevarre DR, Domingo OH. Supraclavicular approach to subclavian catheterization: review of the literature and results of 178 attempts by the same operator. J Trauma 1997;42(2):305–9.
20. Sterner S, Plummer DW, Clinton J, et al. A comparison of the supraclavicular approach and the infraclavicular approach for subclavian vein catheterization. Ann Emerg Med 1986;15(4):421–3.
21. Yoffa D. Supraclavicular subclavian venipuncture and catheterization. Lancet 1965;2:614–7.
22. Dronen S, Thompson B, Nowak R, et al. Subclavian vein catheterization during cardiopulmonary resuscitation: a prospective comparison of the supraclavicular and infraclavicular percutaneous approaches. JAMA 1982;247:3227.
23. Cummins RO. Chapter Six. Advanced cardiac life support. Dallas (TX): American Heart Association; 1994. p. 1–13.
24. Deshpande KS, Hatem C, Ulrich H, et al. The incidence of infectious complications of central venous catheters at the subclavian, internal jugular, and femoral sites in an intensive care unit population. Crit Care Med 2005; 33(1):13–20.
25. Antonelli M, Levy M, Andrews PJ. Hemodynamic monitoring in shock and implications for management. Intensive Care Med 2007;33:575.
26. Graham AS, Ozment C, Tegtmeyer K, et al. Central venous catheterization. N Engl J Med 2007;356:e21.
27. Miller AH, Roth BA, Mills TJ, et al. Ultrasound guidance versus the landmark technique for the placement of central venous catheters in the emergency department. Acad Emerg Med 2002;9:800.
28. Eisen LA, Narasimhan M, Berger JS, et al. Mechanical complications of central venous catheters. J Intensive Care Med 2006;21:40.
29. Schanzer H, Kaplan S, Bosch J, et al. Double-lumen, silicone rubber, indwelling venous catheters. Arch Surg 1986;121:229–32.
30. Feldman R. Chapter 40: accessing indwelling central venous lines. In: Reichman EF, Simon RR, editors. Emergency medicine procedures. New York: McGraw-Hill; 2004. p. 342–8.
31. Feldman R. Chapter 39: troubleshooting indwelling central venous lines. In: Reichman EF, Simon RR, editors. Emergency medicine procedures. New York: McGraw-Hill; 2004. p. 338–41.
32. Taylor JP, Taylor JE. Vascular access devices: uses and aftercare. J Emerg Nurs 1987;13(3):160–7.
33. Rockoff MA, Gang DL, Vacanti JP. Fatal pulmonary embolism following removal of a central venous catheter. J Pediatr Surg 1984;19(3):307–9.
34. Luck RP, Haines C, Mull CC. Intraosseus access. J Emerg Med 2010;39(4): 468–75.

35. Brunette DD, Fisher R. Intravascular access in pediatric cardiac arrest. Am J Emerg Med 1988;6(6):577–9.
36. Ong RC, Mulvaney SW. Chapter e298: Military Medicine. In: Tintinalli JE, Kelen GD, Stapczynski JS, editors. Tintinalli's Emergency Medicine: A Comprehensive Study Guide. 7th ed. New York: McGraw-Hill; 2011. Avaiable at: http://www.accessemergencymedicine.com.libproxy.lib.unc.edu/content.aspx?aID=6394306. Accessed October 5, 2012.
37. Rosetti VA, Thompson BM, Miller J, et al. Intraosseus infusion: an alternative route of pediatric intravascular access. Ann Emerg Med 1985;14:885–8.
38. Fiser DH. Intraosseus infusion. N Engl J Med 1990;322:1579–81.
39. Ma OJ, Hoffman ME. Chapter 44: intraosseus infusion. In: Reichman EF, Simon RR, editors. Emergency medicine procedures. New York: McGraw-Hill; 2004. p. 383–9.
40. Hodge D, Delgado-Paredes C, Gleisher G. Intraosseus infusion flow rates in hypovolemic "pediatric" dogs. Ann Emerg Med 1987;16(3):305–7.
41. Schoffstall JM, Spivey WH, Davidheiser S, et al. Intraosseus crystalloid and blood infusion in a swine model. J Trauma 1989;29(3):384–7.
42. American College of Surgeons Committee on Trauma. ATLS: Advanced trauma life support for doctors, student manual. Chicago (IL): The American College of Surgeons; 2004.
43. Leacock BW, Milling TJ, Murphy AW, et al. Chapter 32: neonatal and pediatric intraosseus and central venous access. In: Tintinalli JE, editor. Tintinalli's emergency medicine: a comprehensive study guide. 7th edition. New York: McGraw-Hill; 2011. Available at: http://www.accessemergencymedicine.com.libproxy.lib.unc.edu/content.aspx?aID=6369974. Accessed June 26, 2012.
44. Reichman EF, Kang I. Chapter 45: umbilical vessel catheterization. In: Reichman EF, Simon RR, editors. Emergency medicine procedures. New York: McGraw-Hill; 2004. p. 390–7.
45. Lipton JD, Schafermeyer RW. Umbilical vessel catheterization. In: Henretig FM, King C, editors. Textbook of pediatric emergency medicine procedures. Baltimore (MD): Williams & Wilkins; 1997. p. 515–23.
46. Weber AL, DeLuca S, Shannon DC. Normal and abnormal position of the umbilical artery and venous catheter on the roentgenogram and review of complications. Am J Roentgenol 1974;120(2):361–7.
47. Stroud S, Rodriguez R. Chapter 46: arterial puncture and cannulation. In: Reichman EF, Simon RR, editors. Emergency medicine procedures. New York: McGraw-Hill; 2004. p. 398–410.
48. Hall WD. Stephen Hales: theologian, botanist, physiologist, discoverer of hemodynamics. Clin Cardiol 1987;10:487.
49. Nguyen HB, Huang DT, Pinsky MR. Chapter 34: hemodynamic monitoring. In: Tintinalli JE, editor. Tintinalli's emergency medicine: a comprehensive study guide. 7th edition. New York: McGraw-Hill; 2011. Available at: http://www.accessemergencymedicine.com.libproxy.lib.unc.edu/content.aspx?aID=6370270. Accessed June 26, 2012.
50. Markowitz DH, Irwin RS. Evaluating acid-base disorders: is venous blood gas testing sufficient? J Crit Illn 1999;14(7):403–6.
51. Cohn JN. Blood pressure measurement in shock: mechanism of inaccuracy in ausculatory and palpatory methods. JAMA 1967;13:972–6.
52. Antman EM, Anbe DT, Armstrong PW, et al. ACC/AHA guidelines for the management of patients with ST-elevation myocardial infarction. Circulation 2004;110:e82.

53. Lodato RF. Arterial pressure monitoring. In: Tobin MJ, editor. Principles and practice of intensive care monitoring. New York: McGraw-Hill; 1998. p. 733–47.
54. Schlichtig RI. Arterial catheterization: complications. In: Tobin MJ, editor. Principles and practice of intensive care monitoring. New York: McGraw-Hill; 1998. p. 751–6.
55. Nevasier RJ, Adams JP, May GI. Complications of arterial puncture in anticoagulated patients. J Bone Joint Surg Am 1976;35:1118–23.
56. Brandenburg MA, Dire DJ. Comparison of arterial and venous blood gas values in the initial emergency department evaluation of patients with diabetic ketoacidosis. Ann Emerg Med 1998;31:459–65.

Ultrasound-Guided Procedures in the Emergency Department— Needle Guidance and Localization

Alfredo Tirado, MD[a,*], Arun Nagdev, MD[b],
Charlotte Henningsen, MS[a,c], Pav Breckon, MD[d], Kris Chiles, MD[b]

KEYWORDS

- Ultrasound • Procedures • Central venous access • Nerve blocks
- Peripheral venous

KEY POINTS

- Probe selection is important, especially when considering the depth of the target structure. High-frequency linear probes should be used to visualize more superficial structures, whereas lower-frequency probes are useful when visualizing deeper tissues.
- Probe orientation is extremely important when performing ultrasound-guided procedures. Always keep the probe marker toward the left of the person performing the procedure, to line up the probe marker with the marker logo on the display screen to improve accuracy.
- Become familiarized with local anatomy and general layout of structures to be scanned, specifically when it comes to visualizing the target structures, whether vascular or nerve bundle.

INTRODUCTION TO PROCEDURAL ULTRASOUND
Background

Historically, medical ultrasound was born out of SONAR (Sound Navigation and Ranging) technology after World War II. As SONAR technology improved, it opened the door to diagnostic imaging, using high-frequency sound waves and the pulse-echo principle to display normal and abnormal anatomy. Its use in emergency medicine comes in response to an increasing need to rapidly diagnose life-threatening conditions at the bedside. As a result, ultrasound is being used in emergent procedures for difficult and challenging patients. Its use in this setting has improved efficiency and safety in patient care.

[a] EM Residency Program, FL Hospital, 7727 Lake Underhill Road, Orlando, FL 32822, USA;
[b] Department of Emergency Medicine, Highland General Hospital, University of California, 1411 East 31st Street, Oakland, CA 94602-1018, USA; [c] Sonography Department, Florida Hospital College, 7727 Lake Underhill Road, Orlando, FL 32822, USA; [d] Emergency Medicine Residency, Florida Hospital, Orlando, 7727 Lake Underhill Road, Orlando, FL 32822, USA
* Corresponding author. Department of Emergency Medicine, Florida Hospital-East Orlando, 7727 Lake Underhill Road, Orlando, FL.
E-mail address: tirado_alfredo@yahoo.com

Emerg Med Clin N Am 31 (2013) 87–115
http://dx.doi.org/10.1016/j.emc.2012.09.008
0733-8627/13/$ – see front matter © 2013 Elsevier Inc. All rights reserved.

emed.theclinics.com

To adequately perform these life-saving procedures using ultrasound guidance, knowledge of the machine functions is imperative. Familiarity of the instrumentation improves accuracy and efficiency. This article provides a brief introduction to the ultrasound physics and instrumentation necessary to perform procedural ultrasound, followed by a description of anatomic findings, techniques, and pitfalls that may be encountered.

Physics Principles and Instrumentation

The ultrasound image is generated as the transducer sends intermittent pulses into soft tissue. These pulses interact with the tissue through reflection and refraction at organ boundaries. Some of the echoes are reflected back to the transducer where they are processed by the ultrasound machine and presented on the display (**Fig. 1**).[1,2]

The ultrasound instrument processes each received echo and presents it as a visual dot corresponding to the anatomic location. The collection of these dots creates the gray-scale image, which is also known as brightness mode (or B-mode). The brightness of each dot corresponds to the strength of the reflection: the stronger the echogenicity, the brighter the dot; the weaker the echogenicity, the darker the dot (**Fig. 2**).

Probe Selection

Transducers operate under what is called the piezoelectric effect, which means pressure electricity. Certain materials (elements or crystals) have piezoelectric properties, which means that an applied voltage will deform the crystals, thus emitting a sound beam. The thickness of the transducer element determines the frequency of the transducer. High-frequency transducers range from 7 to 13 MHz, and low-frequency transducers range from 2 to 5 MHz.

Transducer frequency affects resolution and penetration. Higher frequencies yield better resolution or detail; however, they have poorer penetration. Lower-frequency transducers will yield poorer resolution, but will penetrate a greater distance. It is

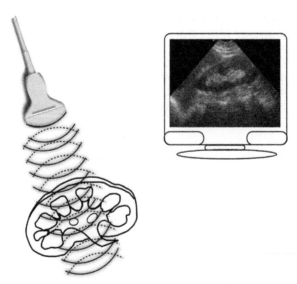

Fig. 1. Schematic representation of ultrasound waves traveling toward organ of interest being scanned.

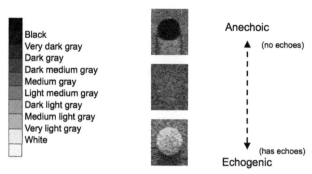

Fig. 2. Assignment of shades of gray related to the intensity of the received echo.

important to select the correct transducer frequency to obtain the penetration needed and still have the best resolution possible.

Transducer design also corresponds with anatomic structures to be imaged, and an appropriate match with frequency. A rectangular shape, known as a linear transducer, will have a high frequency and is excellent for imaging structures close to the skin's surface, such as vessels in the neck. Transducers that have a sector or convex shape are typically lower in frequency and are used to image deeper structures, such as the heart and gallbladder. **Fig. 3** shows different ultrasound transducers with their corresponding frequencies.

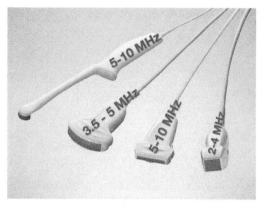

Fig. 3. Transducer selection with corresponding frequency.

Image Orientation

Orientation is imperative to understand, as are positioning and trajectory of the needle as it is being advanced. Each transducer has an orientation marker (**Fig. 4**) that correlates with a specific indicator on the display. For consistency, the orientation indicator on the display should be located toward the left of the person performing the procedure (**Fig. 5**).

The orientation of the transducer will depend on the object of interest being imaged. There are 2 basic axial planes that are primarily used in procedural guidance: longitudinal and transverse, noting that what may be transverse on a structure may not be exactly transverse to a body plane (**Fig. 6**).

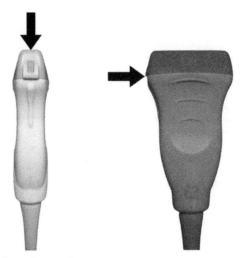

Fig. 4. Transducer orientation marker.

For consistency in procedural ultrasound, the indicator on the display should be aligned with the marker on the transducer. When imaging in the short axis or transverse plane, if the transducer marker is toward the left of the person performing procedure, then the transducer and display will be oriented correctly (**Fig. 7**).

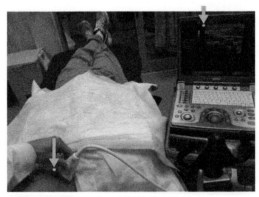

Fig. 5. Alignment of orientation marker with indicator on the display. (*Long arrow*) transducer marker, in reationship with (*short arrrow*) indicator in diplay.

Imaging Modalities

Most ultrasound imaging is performed using B-mode, which displays a 2-dimensional image. As previously mentioned, the reflected echoes appear as dots in which the brightness is proportional to the intensity of reflection.

Motion mode (also known as M-mode) is essentially B-mode stretched across a page. M-mode is primarily used in echocardiography of the adult and pediatric patient and for fetal heart imaging. It has also been used to evaluate for pneumothorax.

Doppler is another modality that is used to detect motion. The Doppler principle is based on a change in frequency attributable to motion, which is known as the Doppler

A   **B**

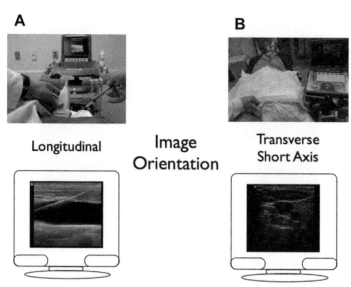

Longitudinal   **Image**   **Transverse**
                   Orientation   **Short Axis**

Fig. 6. Transducer orientation with basic axial views. (*A*) Demonstrates probe positioning to obtain a longitudinal or long-axis view of organ being scanned, in this case the IJ vein. (*B*) Demonstrates probe positioning to obtain a transverse or short-axis view.

effect. The Doppler shift is the difference in emitted frequency versus the received frequency. Doppler is primarily used to detect blood flow and can assess direction and velocity. Color Doppler also detects motion and is useful to identify the presence and direction of flow. In addition to identification of blood flow, Doppler has also been used in the detection of motion, such as urine jets in the bladder.

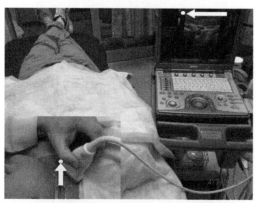

Fig. 7. Correct positioning of transducer with respect to marker in the display. If placed correctly, when moving the needle toward the transducer (*vertical arrow*), the marker will move the needle toward the display marker (*horizontal arrow*).

Artifacts

Artifacts represent deletions from or additions to an image that do not directly correlate with actual tissue. They are commonly seen and may be useful in diagnostic and

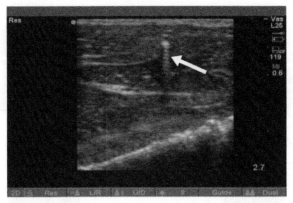

Fig. 8. Reverberation artifact (arrow points to the repeating reflections).

procedural ultrasound. Recognition of certain artifacts can help determine needle localization. The 3 major artifacts frequently identified in ultrasound-guided procedures are reverberation, refraction, and acoustic shadowing.

A reverberation artifact appears as multiple reflections that progressively weaken over time. It is caused by 2 strong reflectors. A needle is highly reflective and reverberation artifacts known as ring-down artifacts are frequently seen posterior to needles during procedural guidance (**Fig. 8**).

Refraction is a change in direction of the sound beam and is usually seen at the curve of a rounded object, such as the transverse axis of a vessel. It presents as a decrease or deletion of information known as an edge shadow (**Fig. 9**).

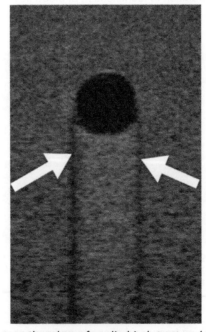

Fig. 9. Refraction artifacts at the edges of a cylindrical structure (*arrows* demonstrate edge artifact).

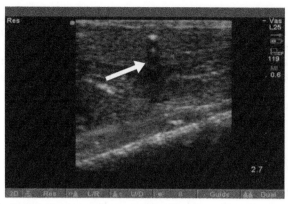

Fig. 10. Acoustic shadow (*arrow* points toward artifact).

An acoustic shadow occurs as the result of a highly attenuating structure, such as a calcification or metal. Posterior to a structure there will be a reduction in the amplitude of the sound beam. **Fig. 10** shows an example of this artifact.

Knobology

Ultrasound systems have similar functions, although the labeling may vary with different manufacturers. Knowledge of the locations and functions of basic controls ensures accuracy and efficiency when performing procedural guidance. Knobology is the study of the controls and their functions. The most important controls used for procedural guidance are image mode, transducer selection, gain, depth, calipers, and freeze.

ULTRASOUND-GUIDED CENTRAL VENOUS ACCESS
Background

Central venous access is an important procedure in the care of the critically ill patient in the emergency department (ED). Even with adequate training, the landmark technique approach carries complication rates that vary between 0.3% and 10.0%[3] and depend on multiple factors, including insertion site, host body habitus, and operator experience. Having adjuncts that can aid in these procedures is extremely valuable in our practice.

One such adjunct is ultrasound. Its use in central venous access has been described as early as 1978 for internal jugular vein localization,[4] with the first prospective randomized trial in 1990.[5] Since then, ultrasound has been used for central venous catheterization because of its ability to visualize target organs that otherwise would be impossible using landmark technique. Its use for central venous catheterization has demonstrated an increase in success rate, while reducing the number of attempts and complication rates for this procedure.[6–8]

In 2001, the Agency for Healthcare Research and Quality collected and reviewed data of common practices that could reduce the risk of adverse events related to exposure to medical care. They identified the 11 practices most highly rated in terms of strength of the evidence supporting more widespread implementation. Use of real-time ultrasound guidance during central line insertion to prevent complications was rated number 8 in this list, making it an essential component to our practice.[9]

Indications

Indications for ultrasound guidance are the essentially the same as for any central venous catheterization: intravascular depletion, hemodynamic monitoring, cardiopulmonary arrest, access for vasoactive medications, difficult peripheral intravenous (IV) access, total parenteral nutrition, and long-term IV access for medications, such as antibiotics.[3]

The added advantages obtained with ultrasound use are:

1. Localization of target vessels
2. Detection of anatomic variations
3. Real-time guidance
4. Detection of venous thrombosis

It can be extremely useful on high-risk patients, such as bariatric patients, end-stage renal disease, disorders of hemostasis, multiple prior catheter insertions, and intravenous drug users.[10–12]

Anatomy and Imaging

There are 3 major veins used for central venous access: the internal jugular (IJ), subclavian, and femoral veins. Although ultrasound guidance for the subclavian vein is possible, it can be challenging for novice users to perform, owing to anatomic barriers, such as the clavicle, that can make it a difficult procedure and a least-attractive site to perform. Femoral veins are also commonly used in the ED because of their low complication rate and ease of procedure; however, this location's inability to provide invasive hemodynamic monitoring information in a critically ill patient, the risks of thromboembolic events, and increased infection rate limits utility of the femoral veins. Therefore, in this article we focus on central venous access by the IJ vein.

The IJ vein originates from the jugular foramen at the skull base and courses inferiorly within the carotid sheath, accompanied by the internal carotid artery and vagus nerve. It descends posterior to the sternocleidomastoid muscle and lies laterally within the sheath. As it continues its trajectory, the inferior end of the vein passes deep between the sternal and clavicular heads of this muscle and then continues posterior to the sternal end of the clavicle, joining the subclavian vein to form the brachiocephalic vein (**Fig. 11**).[13,14]

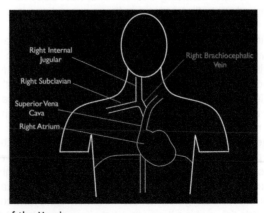

Fig. 11. Trajectory of the IJ vein.

There are 2 basic sonographic views used to obtain image of vessels: short axis or long axis. The short-axis view is a perpendicular view of the desired vessel. It is useful to evaluate structures surrounding the vein of interest. To obtain this image, simply follow the orientation rule discussed in earlier: probe marker toward the left of the person performing procedure, and align the marker from the probe with the indicator in the display (**Fig. 12**). **Fig. 13** shows an ultrasound image of the left IJ vein with all anatomic landmarks in view.

In contrast, the long-axis view is a parallel view of the vessel. This view has the advantage of allowing the user to assess the anterior and posterior walls of the vein being cannulated, helping to avoid double puncturing the vessel. To obtain this view, place the transducer in the long axis of the vessel with the probe marker away from the person performing the procedure (**Fig. 14**). **Fig. 15** demonstrates an ultrasound image of the long-axis view of the left IJ.

Once an image has been obtained, is important to differentiate between the vessels. Veins and arteries differ in 3 sonographic characteristics: compressibility, pulsatility, and respiratory variation. Veins are compressible, lack pulsatility, and have respiratory variation. Further confirmation could be accomplished by asking the patient to perform a Valsalva maneuver or placing the bed into a Trendelenburg position, in which case veins will increase diameter. Conversely, arteries are pulsatile, lacking both compressibility and respiratory variation.

As a note: The principles described for this procedure can be used in any of the different anatomic approaches for central venous access, but review of the anatomy is recommended to familiarize the user with sonographic findings.

Technique

This procedure requires a high-frequency transducer, sterile plastic cover kit (gel, probe cover, and securing elastic bands), a central venous catheter kit, and universal sterile precautions. The patient should be placed in a supine position, sterilized ,and draped in the usual fashion, including the sterile ultrasound probe with sterile gel in the sterile field. The ultrasound system should be placed parallel to the patient on the same side as the procedure to align anatomic landmarks with the image display.

Needle placement can be performed in either of the 2 views discussed earlier: short-axis or long-axis view. The short axis is also called the out-of-plane view, because the

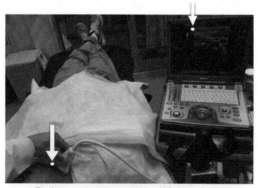

Probe marker toward *the left* of the person performing the procedure.

Fig. 12. Sonographic image of a short-axis view of the IJ vein with landmarks (*Long arrow* points toward transducer marker, *short arrow* marker in display).

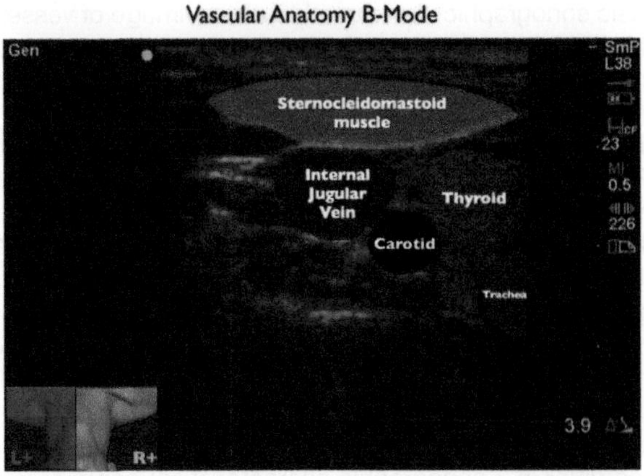

Vascular Anatomy B-Mode

Gen •

SmP
L38

Sternocleidomastoid
muscle

Internal
Jugular
Vein

Thyroid

Carotid

Trachea

.23

MI
0.5

226

3.9

Fig. 13. Positioning of transducer to obtain a short-axis view and align probe marker with indicator display.

transducer is placed perpendicular to the vessel and you see only a cross-sectional view of the needle. Care must be taken to avoid losing the tip of the needle. The long axis is called an in-plane view because the transducer is parallel to the vessel and the needle is kept entirely in the field of view. Studies have shown similar success rates for both approaches, slightly favoring the long-axis view; however, novice users seem to favor the short-axis view because it is the most common approach.[2,15] Selecting the correct approach will depend on level of comfort of the user and experience with the procedure.

Regardless of the approach, the next series of steps will be used for both techniques; to remember the technique we use the mnemonic: *EASE* (mnemonic created by Nagdev and Tirado). *EASE* stands for the following: *E*xamine for best location, *A*nesthetize early to reduce error, *S*tick with a 45° to 60° angle, and *E*valuate for placement.

*E*xamine. Place the patient in a supine position, with the ultrasound system at the patient's side. Place the transducer and assess for best location by comparing both anatomic sites (eg, right and left IJs). Care must be taken to examine for anatomic variations, width and depth of vessel, and sign of venous thrombosis (**Fig. 16**).

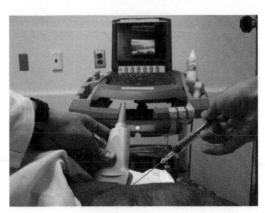

Fig. 14. Positioning of transducer to obtain a long-axis view of the IJ vein.

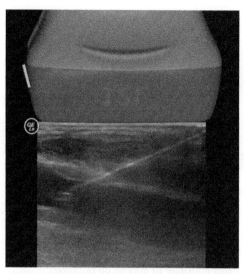

Fig. 15. Positioning of transducer to obtain a long-axis view of the IJ vein.

*A*nesthetize. Early anesthesia can reduce failure rate by controlling pain and movement of the patient while performing the procedure. Use lidocaine and inject around the trajectory of the needle, including muscles and subcutaneous tissue (**Fig. 17**).

*S*tick. The transducer with the probe cover is held in the nondominant hand resting on the patient's skin, and the 18-gauge needle is introduced with the dominant hand under real guidance, through the anterior wall of the vein and into the lumen.

In the short-axis approach, place the probe on top of the skin and center the vessel in the middle of the display (**Fig. 18**). To assess trajectory and distance of the needle to puncture the vessel, we use the principles of the Pythagorean Theorem for right-angled triangles (**Fig. 19**). If the vessel to cannulate is 1 cm deep, we need to

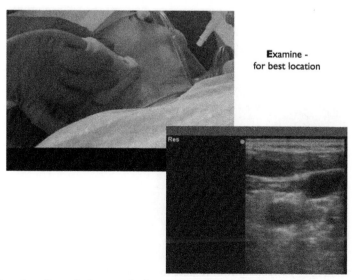

Examine -
for best location

Fig. 16. Examine. Correct placement of probe to examine for best location.

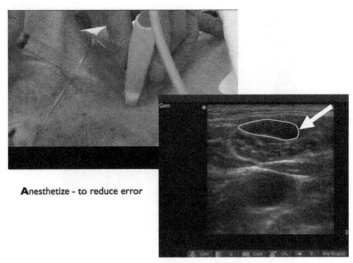

Anesthetize - to reduce error

Fig. 17. Anesthetize. Inject lidocaine to area to be canalized.

puncture the skin 1 cm away from the transducer at a 45° angle to create an isosceles triangle. In this case, the vessel should be punctured at 1.4 cm. The needle will tent on top of the vessel and as it goes through, a dot will appear in the field of view. Other artifacts might appear that can help to determine the needle tip, such as reverberation artifact and acoustic shadow.[2,15,16]

For the long-axis approach, is important to keep the hand stable to place the transducer parallel to the vessel. Note: If sliding of the transducer occurs, the incorrect vessel might be canalized. Thus, it is recommended to become familiar with the short-axis approach before the long axis. Once both the transducer and the vessel

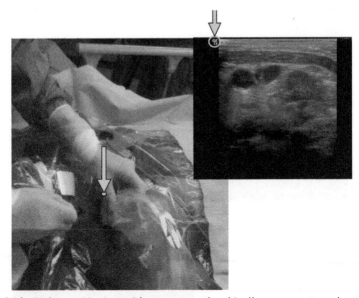

Fig. 18. Stick. Probe positioning with respect to the skin (*long arrow* transducer marker, *short arrow* display market).

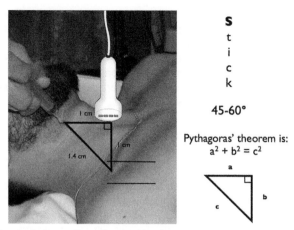

Fig. 19. Assessing trajectory of needle using Pythagorean Theorem.

are parallel, introduce the needle at a 45° to 60° angle aiming toward the probe marker, and follow the trajectory of the needle as it goes into the anterior wall of the vessel. If loss of trajectory occurs, gently withdraw the needle to the skin and reorient the needle toward the probe marker.

After the vein is punctured successfully, the ultrasound probe is removed and the procedure proceeds with the standard Seldinger technique.[2,15,16]

Evaluate. Ultrasound can be used to confirm the guide wire within the lumen before dilating the vessel.[17] The catheter appears as a linear "white" shadow that is best appreciated in the longitudinal ultrasound view (**Fig. 20**).

Pitfalls

- Probe orientation still is one of the most common pitfalls for the procedure. If performing a short-axis view, always keep the transducer probe marker toward the left of the person performing the procedure, and if in doubt on which side the marker is, place a fingertip on the skin until you can orient yourself to the display.

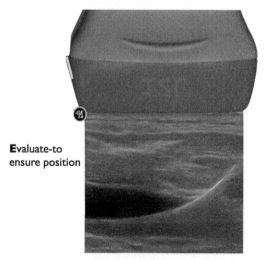

Evaluate-to ensure position

Fig. 20. Evaluate. Confirmation of intraluminal guidewire before dilating the vessel.

- Estimate the distance to the target vessel to avoid advancing the needle too deep and creating complications, such as carotid punctures or pneumothorax.
- Start at a 45° angle to keep the needle in the field of view.
- Always keep your eye on the needle and never advance the needle while looking at the screen because you might miss flashback.
- Last, always confirm wire placement before dilating the vessels, to avoid mechanical complications of the procedure.

ULTRASOUND-GUIDED PERIPHERAL VENOUS ACCESS
Background

Establishment of peripheral intravenous (PIV) access in the ED is a vital part of patient care both for analysis of blood samples and administration of fluids and medications. Traditional PIV access is attained by palpation and direct visualization using various combinations of needles and catheters (ie, angiocatheters). Although this method is successful during most attempts, it can be difficult in certain populations (eg, IV drug users, dialysis patients). Other options available to fulfill the urgent need for blood samples and fluid/medication administration include external jugular IVs, intraosseous lines, peripherally inserted central catheter (PICC) lines, and if necessary, central venous catheters. Although many of these options are available, they can be time-consuming and carry the risk of significant complications.

Ultrasound can aid in this process. As with central venous catheterization, it can detect deeper veins that are not apparent by palpation or direct visualization. By using the same technique as in ultrasound-guided central line placement, a care provider can access peripheral veins with excellent reliability and line stability.[18–21]

Indications

Indications are the same as for traditional PIV cannulation as a means to provide access to the patient's circulatory system. This access can be used for phlebotomy, delivery of medications and fluids in life-threatening conditions, and short-term nutrition administration. Ultrasound has been demonstrated to improve success rate in certain populations, such as bariatric patients, IV drug users, chemotherapy patients, patients with end-stage renal disease, nursing home patients with multiple IV scars, and recently hospitalized patients.[22,23]

Anatomy and Imaging

Although ultrasound can be used for any peripheral access approach, this section focuses on the 3 major vessels of the antecubital region: the basilic, cephalic, and brachial veins (**Fig. 21**). These veins are variable in location and are surrounded by nerves. Hence, ultrasound guidance is helpful when cannulating these veins.[14]

The basilic vein passes upward and anteromedially to the elbow, where it receives the medial cubital vein. Then it continues on the medial to the biceps brachii, deep to the fascia, until it joins the brachial vein and becomes the axillary vein at the border of the teres major. **Fig. 22A** demonstrates correct positioning of the transducer and **Fig. 22B** short-axis ultrasound view of the basilic vein.

The brachial vein forms the deep venous system, which can be isolated or paired to continue to the axillary vein. It is accompanied by the brachial artery and the nerves of the upper limb. **Fig. 23A** demonstrates correct positioning of the transducer and **Fig. 23B** short-axis ultrasound view of the brachial vein.

The cephalic vein lies laterally in the superficial fascia of the antecubital fossa and it ascends along the lateral side of the forearm and upper arm. **Fig. 24** demonstrates

Anatomy and Landmarks

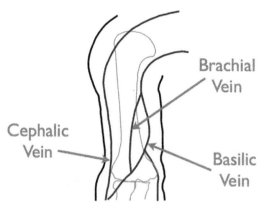

Fig. 21. Anatomic positioning of the major vessels of the antecubital region. the basilic, cephalic, and brachial veins.

correct positioning of the transducer and a short-axis ultrasound view of the cephalic vein.

As with central venous access, place the transducer in the short-axis view and scan the vessels in the antecubital fossa. Move the probe from lateral to medial to assess vessel location.

Technique

To perform this procedure requires all the equipment necessary for a traditional PIV approach: a high-frequency linear transducer, gel, and a long angiocatheter (at least 1.88 inch). Because this is a peripheral line, sterile sleeves or gel are not required, but if avoiding contact of blood products is a priority, the probe can be protected with Tegaderm after adding gel onto the surface of the transducer (**Fig. 25**).

Prepare the patient as shown in **Fig. 26**, with the patient in an upright and comfortable position, with tourniquet in place and the arm fully extended. Lay all materials on a flat surface within close reach of the anticipated IV site.

Anatomy and Landmarks

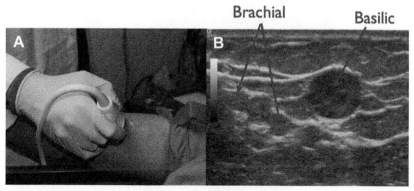

Fig. 22. (A) Transducer positioning to obtain basilic and brachial vein view. (B) Short-axis view of the basilic and brachial vein.

Anatomy and Landmarks
Cephalic Vein

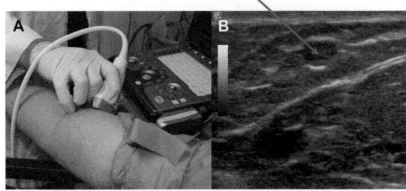

Fig. 23. (*A*) Transducer positioning to obtain cephalic vein view. (*B*) Short-axis view of the cephalic vein.

Examine the area for best location and evaluate the different veins of the antecubital fossa. Move the probe from lateral to medial and avoid applying excessive pressure to the surface of the skin, because this may cause veins to collapse. Hold the probe with the marker toward the left of the person performing the procedure to align the probe marker with the indicator in the screen display.

Using the short-axis approach, hold the angiocatheter, as shown in **Figs. 3–5**, and insert it at a 45-degree angle to the skin, centered in the middle of the probe. Remember to keep the probe perpendicular to the skin surface at all times. As soon as the needle is inserted in the skin, attempt to find the tip by sweeping distally with the probe. When the needle is located, determine if the trajectory needs to be adjusted by comparing its location with that of the target vein. Return the probe to its normal position (perpendicular to the skin), and advance the needle. Advance slowly and orient yourself with the screen to keep track of the needle tip. If the trajectory and alignment of the needle are appropriate, eventually the tip will begin to compress the wall of the target vein. When you observe this on the screen, very slowly advance the needle, while constantly

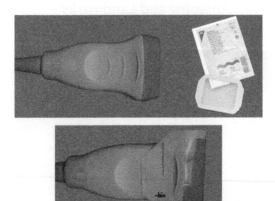

Fig. 24. Tegaderm to protect transducer from body fluids.

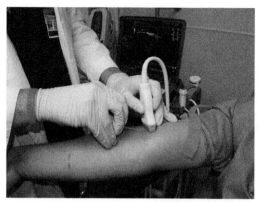

Fig. 25. Patient positioning for ultrasound-guided peripheral IV insertion.

watching for flash in the angiocatheter chamber. When flash is obtained, attempt to thread the catheter over the needle tip to cannulate the vein and secure the catheter.

When the catheter has been successfully inserted into the vein, you can evaluate for position by changing your plane of view to longitudinal. Determine if the tip of the catheter is inside the vascular space. Set the probe down and complete the IV process as usual.

Pitfalls

- One commonly encountered difficulty unique to ultrasound-guided peripheral access is the inability to determine if the catheter is in the vessel. The angiocatheter's flash chamber may fill up with blood, but between that instant and the attempt to pass the catheter over the needle, it may dislodge or puncture through

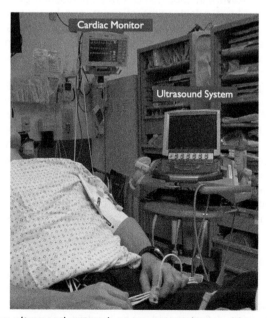

Fig. 26. Positioning ultrasound system in respect to patient position, placing ultrasound toward the head of the patient.

the vein. In addition, the catheter itself may accidentally dislodge the needle from the vessel lumen with the first attempted pass. If this is the case, you may meet resistance when trying to thread the catheter.

- Other complications of ultrasound-guided peripheral IV access are similar to any peripheral access procedures: venous infiltration, arterial puncture, nerve damage, pain, bleeding, and infection. Many of these adverse outcomes can be avoided with sterile technique, but most can be minimized by the use of ultrasound for real-time visualization.
- For a more reliable venous cannulation, a radial artery catheterization set may be used in place of the traditional angiocatheter. As soon as flash is seen in the plastic tubing, thread the guidewire past the tip of the needle, similar to the Seldinger technique.

ULTRASOUND-GUIDED NERVE BLOCKS
Background

EDs are the front line for painful injuries and conditions, with emergency physicians becoming the "de facto proprietor" of acute pain. Unfortunately, management of pain in the acutely injured patient is fraught with difficulty. The classically taught technique of IV opiate medication can lead to serious systemic side effects, including apnea, hypotension, and altered level of consciousness, leading clinicians to commonly underdose pain medications. Even at centers that specialize in treating acute pain, inadequate treatment of pain, oligoanalgesia, is a common phenomenon.[24,25]

Ultrasound-guided nerve blocks (UGNB) have recently become a mainstay in anesthesiology practice, demonstrating a high level of efficacy and safety. Ultrasound permits direct visualization of the needle, nerve, blood vessels, and associated structures and allows real-time imaging of anesthetic injection. Direct visualization has revolutionized regional anesthesia by making it safer for the more inexperienced practitioners. A Cochrane Review in 2009 demonstrated ultrasound-guided regional anesthesia to be quicker, have a faster time of onset, and be as efficacious as nerve stimulation.[26] Also, outside of the operating room, data from the US Army has shown early aggressive pain management, including ultrasound-guided regional anesthesia, not only reduces pain, but blocks the afferent neural pathways, a route thought to lead to chronic pain syndromes.[27]

Recently, emergency medicine providers have integrated UGNB into the clinical practice of the acutely injured patient as a part of the multimodal approach to pain management.[28–32] Along with pain reduction, UGNBs have been shown to be a useful adjunct in procedural sedations, specifically in patients who may be poor candidates for ED sedation. The goal of ED UGNB is different from that of our anesthesia colleagues. Whereas anesthesiologists measure success in terms of complete sensory and motor blockade, avoiding the need for general anesthesia, in the ED the goal is to effectively reduce pain in the acutely injured patient. We discuss 3 commonly performed ED nerve blocks that can be incorporated into clinical practice and aid in the pain reduction and clinical management of the acutely injured patient.

Patient Selection

Caution should be taken in patients judged to be at a high risk for compartment syndrome, and a discussion with consulting orthopedic surgical and/or pain services should occur before performing the procedure. Also, patients who are unable to cooperate with a neurologic examination because of intoxication, confusion, or dementia, or have an acute neurologic deficit, should not be blocked, because the operator will not be able to evaluate for neurologic complications following the procedure.

Positioning

Every patient, regardless of the block being performed, should have the same stepwise process undertaken to ensure safety and success. First, place the patient on a cardiac monitor, including pulse oximeter, and place the ultrasound system contralateral to the nerve being blocked (**Fig. 27**). The operator should be able to visualize both the ultrasound screen and the cardiac monitor in the same visual axis. The high-frequency linear probe is used for the blocks in this discussion, and should be cleaned in a standard manner (commonly a quaternary ammonia compound) between every use.

Supplies

Having a central location for all UGNB supplies, like a central line cart, allows the physician to efficiently gather the materials needed for a block. We recommend collecting a clear adhesive dressing that is large enough to cover the footprint of the transducer, a small-gauge syringe for the skin wheal, and a chlorhexidine skin prep. To perform the block, we recommend using a 3.5-inch 20-gauge to 22-gauge spinal needle attached to a 20-mL syringe (**Fig. 28**). Control syringes are ideal, but not required. For the novice provider, lidocaine with epinephrine is safer than bupivacaine because of the lower risk of LAST (local anesthetic associated systemic toxicity). We recommend always aspirating before injection to confirm lack of vasculature puncture, and halting the block if anechoic fluid is not seen on the ultrasound screen when anesthetic is deposited.

Individual Nerve Block Technique

Femoral nerve block

Indications The ultrasound-guided femoral nerve block is a basic and useful block for the emergency medicine provider. Classic indications include hip fractures (intertrochanteric and subtrochanteric), proximal and midshaft femur fractures, and patella injuries. The obturator and lateral femoral cutaneous nerves also innervate the proximal hip, but a well-performed femoral nerve block can still provide adequate analgesia to the area.

Anatomy The femoral nerve is one of the major branches of the lumbar plexus. It typically traverses inferior to the inguinal ligament lateral to the femoral vessels adjacent to the femoral artery. It lies beneath the fascia iliaca and superficial to the psoas muscle. A femoral block results in anesthesia to the entire anterior thigh and most of the femur and knee joint.

Survey scan Place the patient in a supine position. Attempt to externally rotate and abduct the hip, realizing that it is often not possible in the acutely injured patient and may not be needed. Place the linear probe with the probe marker facing the patient's right side just below and parallel to the inguinal crease. Locate the femoral artery and

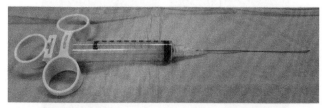

Fig. 27. Adequate needle. 3.5-inch 20-gauge to 22-gauge spinal needle attached to a 20-mL syringe.

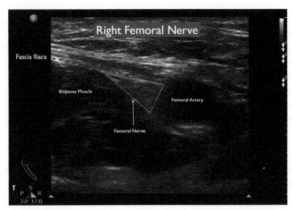

Fig. 28. Ultrasound of right femoral nerve with corresponding structures: fascia iliaca, iliopsoas muscle, femoral nerve, and femoral artery.

vein (similar to central venous cannulation). The operator should ensure that this is proximal to the take-off of the profunda femoris artery. Slowly move the probe lateral to identify the hyperechoic femoral nerve. The femoral nerve will have a triangle shape and a "honeycomb" appearance. Slightly fanning the probe in a caudal direction (from a perpendicular orientation) will often allow for better visualization of the nerve. The operator should also locate the fascia iliaca, which is the fascial covering that runs over the femoral artery and covers the femoral nerve (**Fig. 29**).

After cleaning the skin with an alcohol pad, place 2 to 3 mL of lidocaine with or without epinephrine about 0.5 to 1.0 cm lateral to the ultrasound probe. This will be the location of entry for the block needle, and adequate local anesthesia will allow for patient comfort during the block. Prep widely with a sterilizing solution, such as chlorhexidine. The ultrasound probe should be cleaned and covered with a sterile adhesive dressing across the contact surface (**Fig. 30**).

Technique We suggest a lateral to medial in-plane approach, aiming toward the corner of the femoral nerve (**Fig. 31**). After the femoral nerve and overlying fascia iliaca are identified, enter the skin with the needle bevel up about 0.5 to 1.0 cm lateral to the

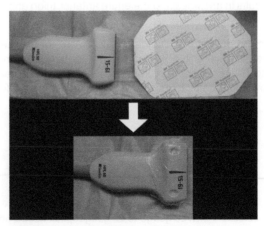

Fig. 29. Tegaderm technique as sterile adhesive dressing.

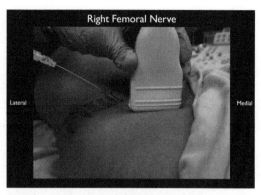

Fig. 30. In-plane approach, aiming toward the corner of the femoral nerve.

probe. The angle of entry will depend on the depth of the target depth of the fascia iliaca. More shallow angles of entry will improve needle visibility.

Advance the needle slowly, maintaining the shaft and tip in view at all times. Target the hyperechoic fascia iliaca overlying the iliopsoas muscle 1 to 3 cm lateral to the femoral nerve. Once beneath the fascia iliaca, aspirate to confirm the needle tip has not entered a vessel, and then slowly inject 3 to 5 mL of local anesthetic. With the needle tip in view, the spread of hypoechoic injectate should be visualized in real time with superficial movement of the fascia iliaca (**Fig. 32**). After confirming optimal needle tip location, proceed to inject a total of 10 to 20 mL of local anesthetic in 3-mL to 5-mL aliquots. If at any point the spread of local anesthetic is not visualized, intravascular injection should be suspected and the procedure halted. After injection, examine the patient for any signs of local anesthetic toxicity, such as perioral numbness, dizziness, or convulsions. Having your needle 1 cm lateral to the femoral nerve and vessels, yet under the fascia iliaca, reduces the risk of vascular puncture and intraneural injection.

Pitfall

- The most common pitfall of the UGNB of the femoral nerve is the failure to get under the fascia iliaca. Test doses of anesthetic should be visualized under the fascial plane with spread of anechoic fluid. Injecting anesthetic under the fascial plane and watching fluid track around the femoral nerve decreases the concern of intraneural and intravascular injection, while reducing patient discomfort.

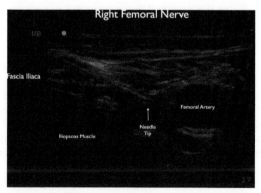

Fig. 31. Needle tip in view, with spread of injectate hypoechoic anesthesia with superficial movement of the fascia iliaca in femoral nerve block.

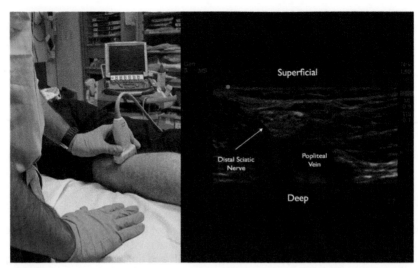

Fig. 32. Prone position for distal sciatic nerve block with sonographic images in screen display demonstrating distal sciatic nerve and popliteal vein.

Distal Sciatic Nerve Block at the Popliteal Fossa

Indications
The ultrasound-guided distal sciatic nerve block is an excellent block for distal tibia and/or fibula fractures, Achilles tendon rupture, pain control following ankle reduction, or other injuries to the lower extremity distal to the knee. Again, high-energy injuries to the distal tibia/fibula that are a concern for compartment syndrome should be blocked only in conjunction with the consulting service that will be managing the patient's inpatient course.

Anatomy
The lumbosacral plexus forms the sciatic nerve in the posterior aspect of the pelvis. As the nerve tracks down the posterior thigh, the nerve enters the popliteal fossa, bordered by the long head of biceps femoris superolaterally and by semimembranosus and semitendinosus superomedially. Just before entering the popliteal fossa, the distal sciatic nerve bifurcates into the common peroneal (medial) and tibial (lateral) nerves. A sciatic block at the popliteal fossa provides anesthesia to the distal leg, ankle, and foot.

Survey scan
We recommend prone positioning for the sciatic nerve bock. This enables the provider to place the probe on the patient without coming under the leg. Also, when performing the block in the prone position, needle movements will correlate with images on the screen (**Fig. 33**). If the patient's injuries do not allow for prone positioning (such as patients in cervical spine immobilization), the patient may be positioned supine with the lower leg supported in mild flexion at the knee, and the foot propped on enough pillows or blankets to allow for the probe to fit comfortably between the bed and the popliteal fossa (**Fig. 34**).

Place the linear probe with the probe marker facing the patient's right side at the popliteal crease. Locate the popliteal artery and vein (similar to a deep venous thrombosis scan). If performing the scan in the prone position, we recommend mild flexion at

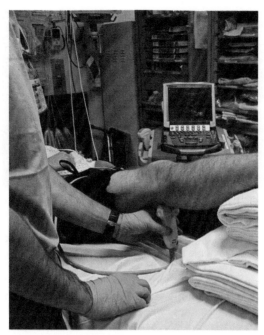

Fig. 33. Alternate supine position technique for distal sciatic nerve block.

the knee to prevent collapse of the popliteal vein. Once both the popliteal vein and artery are noted, locate the tibial nerve (superficial to the popliteal vein) and scan cephalad slowly. If you are unable to locate the neural bundle, fan the probe caudal (**Fig. 35**) to obtain the most perpendicular axis to the nerve, which allows for better visualization (an ultrasound phenomenon termed anisotropy). Slowly move the probe in a cephalad manner, following the tibial nerve until the common peroneal nerve is identified on the lateral aspect of the screen. As the probe is moved more cephalad, the 2 nerves will join together to form the distal sciatic nerve in the popliteal fossa (approximately 7–10 cm proximal to the popliteal crease).

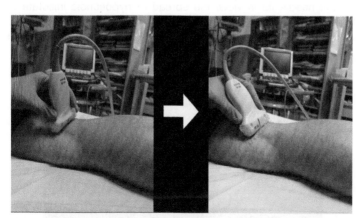

Fig. 34. Anisotropy phenomenon to obtain most perpendicular axis to the nerve, for better visualization.

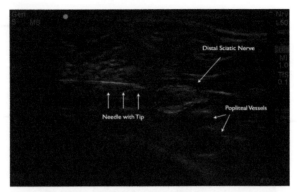

Fig. 35. Correct needle-tip positioning just above the sciatic nerve.

Unlike the femoral nerve block, in which the needle is placed just adjacent to the probe, for the distal sciatic nerve block, we recommend entering the skin much farther away from the probe. The distal sciatic nerve is often 2 to 4 cm deep to the skin surface, and a steep needle angle would prevent visualization of the needle tip on the ultrasound screen. We recommend measuring the depth of the nerve and entering the lateral knee/leg at a similar depth with a fairly flat angle. After cleaning the skin with an alcohol pad, place 1 to 2 mL of lidocaine with or without epinephrine in the specified location in the lateral knee/leg. This will be the location of entry for the block needle, and adequate local anesthesia will allow for patient comfort during the block. Prep widely with a sterilizing solution such as chlorhexidine. The ultrasound probe should be cleaned and covered with a sterile adhesive dressing across the contact surface.

Technique
Advance the needle slowly at a parallel angle to the probe with an in-plane technique, maintaining the shaft and tip in view at all times. Target the honeycomb appearance of the sciatic nerve without placing the needle directly into the nerve. We recommend placing the needle tip just above the nerve to reduce intraneural injection, while being close enough to get anesthetic deposited in an ideal location (**Fig. 36**). Aspirate to confirm there has been no vascular puncture, then slowly inject 3 to 5 mL of local anesthetic. With the needle tip in view, the spread of hypoechoic injectate should be visualized in real time (**Fig. 37**). Once a small bit of anechoic fluid has begun to encircle the nerve, the provider can reposition the needle tip and continue injecting in 3-mL to

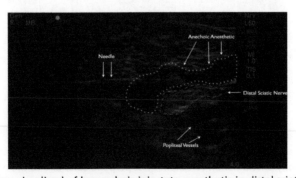

Fig. 36. Real-time visualized of hypoechoic injectate anesthetic in distal sciatic nerve block.

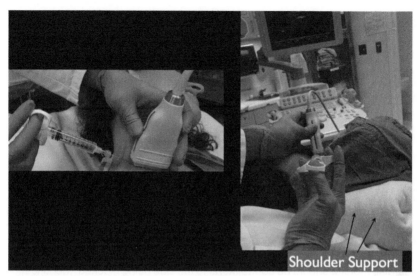

Shoulder Support

Fig. 37. Shoulder support with pillow or roll of sheets under the ipsilateral scapula to allow for more room for needle entry.

5-mL aliquots up to 20 mL of total anesthetic with a goal of forming a doughnut of hypoechoic fluid around the nerve. If at any point the spread of local anesthetic is not visualized, intravascular injection should be suspected and the procedure halted.

Pitfall

- The most common pitfall of the UGNB of the sciatic nerve at the popliteal fossa is not getting the anesthetic completely around the nerve. The popliteal fossa is filled with fat and local anesthetic is lipophilic. If the anesthetic is not placed in close proximity to the nerve, it will be easily absorbed by the adipose tissue and the block will not be effective. To obviate this pitfall, be sure to inject 3-mL to 5-mL aliquots with the needle positioned circumferentially around the nerve.

Interscalene Approach to the Brachial Plexus Block

Indications

The ultrasound-guided interscalene brachial plexus block is ideal for pain relief from arm abscesses, humeral fractures, elbow dislocations, and forearm injuries.

Anatomy

The brachial plexus originates from the C5-T1 ventral rami. The cords track between the anterior and middle scalene muscles (interscalene groove in the neck) and join the subclavian artery anterior to the first rib and posterior to the clavicle. This neurovascular bundle travels to the axilla and supplies both motor and sensory innervation to the entire upper extremity. A brachial plexus block provides anesthesia to the shoulder, arm, and elbow.

Survey scan

The patient should be positioned supine with the head of bed in approximately 30° reverse Trendelenberg and the patient's head turned to the contralateral side. We recommend placing a pillow or roll of sheets under the ipsilateral scapula to allow for more room for needle entry (**Fig. 38**). As previously stated, the ultrasound screen

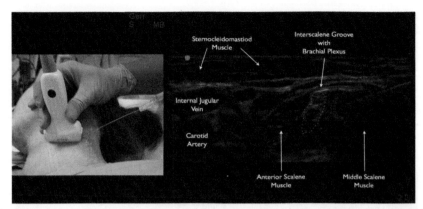

Fig. 38. Proper probe placement transverse on the neck (probe marker pointing to the patient's right), with corresponding sonographic findings: interscalene groove with brachial plexus, anterior scalene muscle, middle scalene muscle, and needle placement.

and cardiac monitor should be contralateral to the side being blocked. Identification of the interscalene location of the brachial plexus is often difficult and we recommend 2 techniques to improve success.

First, place the probe transverse on the neck (probe marker pointing to the patient's right), locating the carotid artery, IJ vein, and thyroid cartilage (**Fig. 39**). Identify the sternocleidomastoid muscle (SCM) and slowly move the probe laterally until the anterior and middle scalene muscles are noted. The cords of the brachial plexus will be found as large hypoechoic circular structures in the groove between the anterior and middle scalene muscles, commonly called the "stoplight" sign.

Alternately, place the high-frequency linear probe just proximal and parallel to the clavicle in the supraclavicular fossa with the probe oriented to the patient's right. The probe should be directed caudad and moved lateral to medial in a rocking fashion to identify the first rib and the subclavian artery traversing across the rib surface. The trunks of the brachial plexus should appear as hypoechoic oval structures posterolateral to the pulsatile subclavian artery and superficial to the first rib. From here, move the probe in a cephalad manner, following the plexus of nerves, until the probe is approximately at the level of the thyroid cartilage and in a transverse position on the neck. Here, you should recognize the bundle of hypoechoic nerve roots that rest between

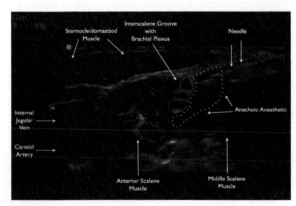

Fig. 39. Real-time visualized of hypoechoic injectate anesthetic in interscalene approach.

the anterior and medial scalene muscles deep to the SCM. If the anatomy is challenging to interpret, you can use color flow Doppler to confirm the vascular structures.

After cleaning the skin with an alcohol pad, place 2 to 3 mL of lidocaine with or without epinephrine about 0.5 to 1.0 cm lateral to the ultrasound probe. This will be the location of entry for the block needle, and adequate local anesthesia will allow for patient comfort during the block. Prep widely with a sterilizing solution such as chlorhexidine, and place a sterile drape. The ultrasound probe should be cleaned and covered with a sterile adhesive dressing across the contact surface.

Technique

We recommend a lateral to medial in-plane approach given this is a more advanced block. After the brachial plexus and surrounding structures are identified, enter the skin with the needle bevel up about 0.5 to 1.0 cm lateral to the probe. The external jugular vein may be in the path of your puncture; therefore, we recommend probe adjustment to be slightly medial or lateral to this easily located vein. Enter the skin at a shallow angle, which will improve needle visibility and improve safety.

Advance the needle slowly, maintaining the shaft and tip in view at all times. You will be entering through the middle scalene muscle and should try to get the needle tip into the interscalene groove. Aspirate to exclude vascular puncture and then slowly inject 3 to 5 mL of local anesthetic. With the needle tip in view, the spread of hypoechoic injectate should be visualized. After confirming optimal needle tip location, proceed to inject a total of 10 to 20 mL of local anesthetic in 3-mL to 5-mL aliquots. If at any point, the spread of local anesthetic is not visualized, intravascular injection should be suspected and the procedure halted. After injecting about 5 mL of anesthetic, the interscalene groove will be more noticeable, because the anechoic fluid should slowly separate the cords of the brachial plexus from the middle scalene muscle.

Pitfalls

- As mentioned, this is a more advanced block with a higher risk of complications because of the proximity of surrounding structures (pleura, subclavian vessels) and the complicated anatomy.
- Be sure to clearly delineate all structures before beginning your block and visualize your needle tip at all times, especially before injecting.
- This block is also associated with a risk of phrenic nerve involvement leading to hemidiaphragmatic paresis or paralysis. This should be assumed in all patients in whom the block will be performed. Very rarely does this affect patient breathing, but in patients with severe baseline respiratory pathology, the interscalene approach to the brachial plexus may not be ideal.
- Also, because of the inferior location of the of C8/T1 nerve root, the patient may get the least amount of sensory loss in the ulnar nerve distribution.

GENERAL NERVE BLOCK PITFALLS

From simple pain reduction to facilitating a procedure, the goal of a UGNB should depend on the patient. Common mistakes of novice providers include inadequate local anesthetic, poor visualization of the needle tip, and not visualizing the anechoic spread of anesthetic when injecting the recommended small aliquots. To reduce error, confirm the needle tip during the entire procedure, aspirate before all injections, and ensure deposition of anechoic fluid from the needle tip; this will ensure a high level of safety and success. And finally, the speed of the block is dependent on the proximity of the anesthetic deposition to the nerve epineurium. For less experienced providers, we recommend keeping a safe distance from the nerve, and therefore a moderate period of waiting (15–20 minutes) may be required before onset of the block.

REFERENCES

1. Kremkau FW. Diagnostic ultrasound: principles & instruments. 7th edition. St Louis (MO): Saunders; 2006.
2. Ma JO, Mateer JR, Bralivas M. Emergency ultrasound. 2nd edition. New York: McGraw-Hill; 2008.
3. Ernst A, Feller-Kopman D. Ultrasound-guided procedures and investigations: a manual for the clinician. 1st edition. New York: Taylor & Francis Group; 2006.
4. Ullman JI, Stoelting RK. Internal jugular vein location with the ultrasound Doppler blood flow detector. Anesth Analg 1978;57(1):118.
5. Mallory DL, McGee WT, Shawker TH, et al. Ultrasound guidance improves the success rate of internal jugular vein cannulation. A prospective, randomized trial. Chest 1990;98(1):157–60.
6. Turker G, Kaya FN, Gurbert A, et al. Internal jugular vein cannulation: an ultrasound-guided technique versus a landmark-guided technique. Clinics (Sao Paulo) 2009;64(10):989–92.
7. Karakitsos D, Labropoulos N, De Groot E, et al. Real-time ultrasound-guided catheterisation of the internal jugular vein: a prospective comparison with the landmark technique in critical care patients. Crit Care 2006;10(6):R162.
8. Leung J, Duffy M, Finckh A. Real-time ultrasonographically-guided internal jugular vein catheterization in the emergency department increases success rates and reduces complications: a randomized, prospective study. Ann Emerg Med 2006;48(5):540–7.
9. Shojania KG, Duncan BW, McDonald KM, et al. Making health care safer: a critical analysis of patient safety practices. Evidence Report/Technology Assessment No. 43. Rockville (MD): Agency for Healthcare Research and Quality; 2001. AHRQ Publication No. 01–E058, Summary.
10. Brusasco C, Corradi F, Zattoni PL, et al. Ultrasound-guided central venous cannulation in bariatric patients. Obes Surg 2009;19(10):1365–70.
11. Tercan F, Ozkan U, Oguzkurt L. US-guided placement of central vein catheters in patients with disorders of hemostasis. Eur J Radiol 2008;65(2):253–6.
12. Oguzkurt L, Tercan F, Kara G, et al. US-guided placement of temporary internal jugular vein catheters: immediate technical success and complications in normal and high-risk patients. Eur J Radiol 2005;55(1):125–9.
13. Moore KL. Clinically oriented anatomy. 5th edition. Philadelphia: Lippincott Williams & Wilkins; 2006.
14. Ahuja AT. Diagnostic and surgical imaging anatomy: ultrasound. 1st edition. Salt Lake City (UT): Lippincott Williams & Wilkins; 2007.
15. Cosby KS, Kendall JL. Practice guide to emergency ultrasound. 1st edition. Philadelphia: Lippincott Williams & Wilkins; 2006.
16. Noble VE, Nelson B, Nicholas Sutingo A. Manual of emergency and critical care ultrasound. 1st edition. New York: Cambridge University Press; 2007.
17. Stone MB, Nagdev A, Murphy MC, et al. Ultrasound detection of guidewire position during central venous catheterization. Am J Emerg Med 2010;28(1):82–4.
18. Keyes LE, Frazee BW, Snoey ER, et al. Ultrasound-guided brachial and basilic vein cannulation in emergency department patients with difficult intravenous access. Ann Emerg Med 1999;34(6):711–4.

19. Costantino TG, Parikh AK, Satz WA, et al. Ultrasonography-guided peripheral intravenous access versus traditional approaches in patients with difficult intravenous access. Ann Emerg Med 2005;46(5):456–61.
20. Brannam L, Blaivas M, Lyon M, et al. Emergency nurses' utilization of ultrasound guidance for placement of peripheral intravenous lines in difficult-access patients. Acad Emerg Med 2004;11(12):1361–3.
21. Schoenfeld E, Boniface K, Shokoohi H. ED technicians can successfully place ultrasound-guided intravenous catheters in patients with poor vascular access. Am J Emerg Med 2011;29(5):496–501.
22. Dargin JM, Rebholz CM, Lowenstein RA, et al. Ultrasonography-guided peripheral intravenous catheter survival in ED patients with difficult access. Am J Emerg Med 2010;28(1):1–7.
23. Stein J, George B, River G, et al. Ultrasonographically guided peripheral intravenous cannulation in emergency department patients with difficult intravenous access: a randomized trial. Ann Emerg Med 2009;54(1):33–40 [Epub 2008 Sep 27].
24. Wilson JE, Pendleton JM. Oligoanalgesia in the emergency department. Am J Emerg Med 1989;7(6):620–3.
25. Todd KH, Ducharme J, Choiniere M, et al. Pain in the emergency department: results of the pain and emergency medicine initiative (PEMI) multicenter study. J Pain 2007;8(6):460–6.
26. Walker KJ, McGrattan K, Aas-Eng K, et al. Ultrasound guidance for peripheral nerve blockade. Cochrane Database Syst Rev 2009;(4):CD006459.
27. Stojadinovic A, Auton A, Peoples GE, et al. Responding to challenges in modern combat casualty care: innovative use of advanced regional anesthesia. Pain Med 2006;7(4):330–8.
28. Blaivas M, Adhikari S, Lander L. A prospective comparison of procedural sedation and ultrasound-guided interscalene nerve block for shoulder reduction in the emergency department. Acad Emerg Med 2011;18(9):922–7.
29. Liebmann O, Price D, Mills C, et al. Feasibility of forearm ultrasonography-guided nerve blocks of the radial, ulnar, and median nerves for hand procedures in the emergency department. Ann Emerg Med 2006;48(5):558–62.
30. Beaudoin FL, Nagdev A, Merchant RC, et al. Ultrasound-guided femoral nerve blocks in elderly patients with hip fractures. Am J Emerg Med 2010;28(1):76–81.
31. Stone MB, Wang R, Price DD. Ultrasound-guided supraclavicular brachial plexus nerve block vs procedural sedation for the treatment of upper extremity emergencies. Am J Emerg Med 2008;26(6):706–10.
32. Herring AA, Stone MB, Fischer J, et al. Ultrasound-guided distal popliteal sciatic nerve block for ED anesthesia. Am J Emerg Med 2011;29(6):697.e3–5.

Ultrasound-Guided Procedures in the Emergency Department—Diagnostic and Therapeutic Asset

Alfredo Tirado, MD[a],*, Teresa Wu, MD[b], Vicki E. Noble, MD[c], Calvin Huang, MD, MPH[c], Resa E. Lewiss, MD[d], Jennifer A. Martin, MD[d], Michael C. Murphy, MD[e], Adam Sivitz, MD[f]

KEYWORDS

- Ultrasound • Procedures • Pericardiocentesis • Abscess • Lumbar puncture
- Paracentesis • Arthrocentesis • Thoracentesis

KEY POINTS

- Correct orientation of the probe is paramount for procedural ultrasound (ie, aligning the probe marker with the on-screen logo).
- Ultrasound is a diagnostic modality that can aid in the therapeutic intervention of some serious conditions such as pericardial tamponade, pleural effusions, and massive ascites.
- It is important for the user to pay close attention to the trajectory of the needle in all ultrasound-guided procedures. This ensures accuracy and reduces error.

ULTRASOUND-GUIDED PERICARDIOCENTESIS
Background

When patients are suspected of having a life-threatening pericardial effusion and cardiac tamponade, prompt diagnosis and treatment are imperative to improve chances of survival. Making the diagnosis of a pericardial effusion is often difficult based on

Disclosure: None.
[a] Department of Emergency Medicine, Florida Hospital-East Orlando, 7727 Lake Underhill Road, Orlando, FL 32822, USA; [b] EM Residency Program, Department of Emergency Medicine, Maricopa Medical Center, College of Medicine, University of Arizona, 2601 E. Roosevelt Street, Phoenix, AZ 85008, USA; [c] Emergency Ultrasound Division, Department of Emergency Medicine, Massachusetts General Hospital, Harvard University, 55 Fruit Street E00-3-B, Boston, MA 02114–2696, USA; [d] Emergency Ultrasound Division, Department of Emergency Medicine, St Luke's Roosevelt Hospital Center, 1111 Amsterdam Avenue, New York, NY 10025, USA; [e] Department of Emergency Medicine, Harvard Medical School, Mount Auburn Hospital, 330 Mount Auburn Street, Cambridge, MA 02138, USA; [f] Newark Beth Israel Medical Center and The Children's Hospital of New Jersey, Pediatric Emergency Medicine Fellowship, University of Medicine and Dentistry of New Jersey, 201 Lyons Avenue, Newark, NJ 07112, USA
* Corresponding author.
E-mail address: tirado_alfredo@yahoo.com

Emerg Med Clin N Am 31 (2013) 117–149
http://dx.doi.org/10.1016/j.emc.2012.09.009
0733-8627/13/$ – see front matter © 2013 Elsevier Inc. All rights reserved.

clinical findings alone. Bedside ultrasound can be used to determine if a pericardial effusion is present, to estimate the size of the fluid collection, to assess for cardiac tamponade, and to help guide an emergent pericardiocentesis.[1–7]

Indications and Contraindications

A bedside cardiac ultrasound should be performed when there is clinical suspicion for a pericardial effusion. If an effusion is noted on ultrasound, the heart should be assessed for any evidence of right atrial or right ventricular collapse. Diastolic collapse of the right atrium is the first sonographic sign encountered with increased pericardial pressures from a growing effusion. Once intrapericardial pressures exceed right ventricular pressures, end-diastolic right ventricular collapse is noted, and cardiac output is compromised. Right atrial and right ventricular collapses are best seen in the apical 4-chamber view of the heart.

Anatomy and Imaging

The pericardium is a thin, 2-layered structure that surrounds the heart. The outer layer is called the parietal pericardium. It is normally separated from the inner visceral pericardium by 25 to 50 mL of physiologic fluid. A pericardial effusion develops when infectious, serous, hemorrhagic, serosanguinous, or chylous fluid accumulates in between the parietal and visceral pericardium.

To determine if a pericardial effusion is present, 3 common cardiac views are used: the subxiphoid 4-chamber view, the parasternal long-axis view, and the apical 4-chamber view (**Fig. 1**). Although the parasternal short-axis view of the heart is typically obtained in most bedside cardiac ultrasound examinations, it is not one of the common views used during an ultrasound-guided pericardiocentesis.

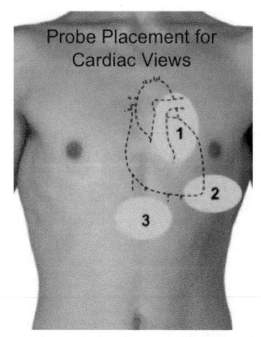

Fig. 1. Probe placement for standard cardiac views: (1) parasternal, (2) apical, and (3) subxiphoid.

Technique

Once the pericardial effusion has been localized on ultrasound, it is important to determine which approach will maximize chances of a successful pericardiocentesis, while minimizing the amount of damage inflicted on adjacent organs. If time permits, begin by prepping and draping the patient and the ultrasound transducer in a sterile fashion. Next, attempt to visualize the pericardial effusion with the subxiphoid, parasternal, or apical view of the heart (**Figs. 2–4**). Find an area where much pericardial fluid has accumulated close to the skin, and scan for a spot where there are no overlying organs obstructing the needle path to the heart.

In most situations, begin the scan with a low frequency (5–1 MHz) transducer to assess the heart and surrounding effusion. If the procedure is being performed with the needle entering the chest via the parasternal or apical approach, switching to a high-frequency transducer may provide better visualization of the needle and its trajectory into the pericardial sac (**Fig. 5**). With the apical or parasternal approach, the distance from the skin to the anterior pericardial sac is only a few centimeters, so using a high-frequency transducer enables better image resolution of the needle as it advances into the pericardial sac.

For the subxiphoid approach, place the probe just caudal to the xiphoid process and angle the face of the probe toward the patient's left shoulder. Insert the pericardiocentesis needle just cephalad to the transducer so that it bisects the ultrasound beams as it enters the pericardial space. The needle should be inserted at a 30° to 45° angle and directed toward the patient's left shoulder. Note that entering the thoracic cavity through the subxiphoid approach can put the patient at risk of liver or intestinal puncture.

During the parasternal approach, a long-axis view of the heart and pericardial effusion is obtained by placing the probe in the 3rd or 4th intercostal space, just left of the sternum. Insert the pericardiocentesis needle just lateral to the end of the transducer closest to the apex of the heart and direct the needle toward the patient's spine. Angle the ultrasound beams so that they bisect the needle as it enters the anterior pericardial sac (**Fig. 6**). With the anterior intercostal approach, there is a small risk of puncturing the internal mammary artery or accidentally lacerating the left anterior descending branch of the coronary artery.

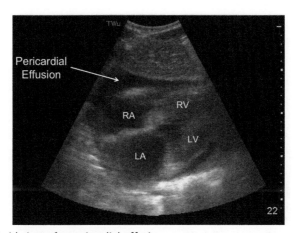

Fig. 2. Subxiphoid view of a pericardial effusion.

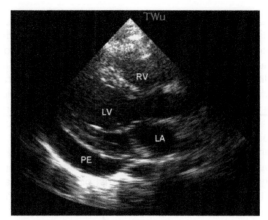

Fig. 3. Parasternal view of a pericardial effusion.

Under ultrasound guidance, the para-apical approach is becoming the most commonly used method for performing an emergent pericardiocentesis. In many patients, the largest collection of pericardial fluid is often seen collecting around the apex of the heart. Once an apical 4-chamber view of the heart is captured, the pericardiocentesis needle is inserted just lateral to the transducer (**Fig. 7**). The trajectory of the needle should be visualized as it enters the pericardial sac anterolaterally near the apex of the heart (**Fig. 8**). If lung is visualized overlying the apex of the heart (**Fig. 9**), movement of the probe in the medial and caudal direction may provide a more optimal needle entry site.

Once the pericardial sac has been entered, rapid injection of a few milliliters of saline will create bubbles in the pericardial sac that can be visualized on ultrasound. Agitated saline can help confirm needle placement before the Seldinger technique is used to introduce a catheter for serial drainage. If saline bubbles are noted in the cardiac chambers or in the subcutaneous tissues, reposition the needle under ultrasound guidance.

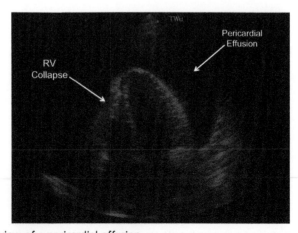

Fig. 4. Apical view of a pericardial effusion.

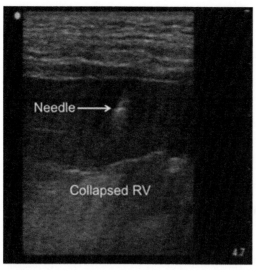

Fig. 5. Pericardiocentesis using ultrasound guidance with a high-frequency linear array transducer. RV, right ventricle.

Pitfalls

- Although there are no absolute contraindications for performing a bedside ultrasound-guided pericardiocentesis, it is important that hemodynamically stable patients with a large pericardial effusion should have their pericardiocentesis or pericardial window performed in the operating room by the most experienced personnel available.
- A pericardiocentesis performed using anatomic landmark guidance can put the patient at risk for inadvertent injury to the liver, cardiac chambers, coronary arteries, internal mammary artery, intercostal arteries, stomach, intestines, and lung. Knowledge of the surrounding anatomy and ultrasound guidance can help minimize these risks.

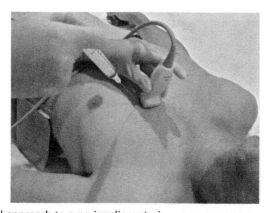

Fig. 6. Parasternal approach to a pericardiocentesis.

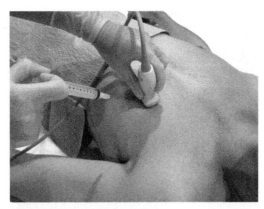

Fig. 7. Para-apical approach to a pericardiocentesis.

- Determine how deep the pericardial effusion is from the site of needle entry using the depth markers on the side of the ultrasound screen. Attempt the pericardiocentesis with a needle long enough to enter the pericardial effusion and permit wire insertion for a catheter placement in case serial drainage of the effusion is required.
- During the pericardiocentesis, it is important that the ultrasound beams are aimed to bisect the needle tip as it approaches the pericardial sac. You may need to fan or slide the probe away from the puncture site to maintain visualization of the needle tip as you advance the needle deeper into the patient.
- The optimal entry site may be some place between or around the 3 standard approaches noted in this article. Be flexible with your approach and scan around the heart to find the best for successful aspiration based on the patient in front of you.
- Do not be fooled by large anterior fat pads. Remember that most significant effusions will be seen circumferentially around the heart, and not just anteriorly. Additionally, fat pads tend to move in concert with the ventricular contractions and remain the same size, whereas pericardial effusions appear larger with each cardiac contraction as the ventricular wall constricts within the fluid.

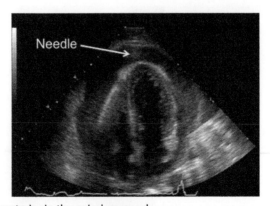

Fig. 8. Pericardiocentesis via the apical approach.

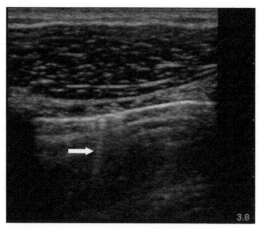

Fig. 9. White arrow demonstrates comet tail artifact between the 2 pleural surfaces.

- To maximize the collection of pericardial fluid available for aspiration, gently roll the patient over toward his or her left side. The pericardial fluid should settle near the apex of the heart for an ultrasound-guided para-apical pericardiocentesis attempt.

ULTRASOUND-GUIDED THORACENTESIS AND PARACENTESIS
Background

Thoracentesis and paracentesis are necessary for both diagnostic and therapeutic reasons. Both procedures are performed at the bedside by the clinician, traditionally using either physical examination findings or radiology-performed imaging to guide skin puncture. Point of care ultrasound not only can make the diagnosis of pleural effusions and ascites more accurately than physical examination and portable radiographs but also can help to guide the needle placement and can speak to the feasibility of the procedure in general. Indeed, there is ample evidence that ultrasound allows for real-time, accurate guidance and has the ability to decrease complications.[8,9]

Indications

Pleural effusions can be either unilateral or bilateral and can stem from multiple processes including heart failure, malignancy, infection, and hemorrhage. When an effusion accumulates enough volume, it can cause mass effect on the lung and diaphragm, leading to shortness of breath, pleurisy, and sometimes chest pain. Although chest radiography can demonstrate the presence of an effusion, it does not show the extent of diaphragm excursion or depth of the fluid pocket and cannot reveal lung/pleural adhesions—all of which can be seen with bedside ultrasound. In addition, chest radiography can be misleading if the patient is supine, whereas ultrasound is very accurate in supine patients. This can be particularly helpful in ventilated patients.[10] Thoracentesis can sample the pleural fluid for analysis, providing a diagnosis. Furthermore, removal of a volume of fluid will improve the patient's ventilatory mechanics and provide symptomatic relief.

Ascitic fluid is often the result of hepatic disease, which leads to portal hypertension and a hypoproteinemic state. Malignancy and hemorrhage are 2 other causes of abdominal free fluid. When much fluid accumulates, it can lead to a mass effect on the abdominal wall and on the diaphragm. This causes abdominal discomfort and can also lead to shortness of breath and decreased exercise tolerance. In rare cases, when abdominal pressures build high enough, right heart filling can be impaired as a result of compression of the inferior vena cava. Furthermore, ascitic fluid can become infected as a result of bowel flora translocation, thus leading to spontaneous bacterial peritonitis. Spontaneous bacterial peritonitis may be suspected when patients with known ascites present with signs of infection including, fever, leukocytosis, abdominal pain, and altered mental status. Diagnostic paracentesis and analysis of the fluid are essential to making this diagnosis. Large-volume paracentesis can provide symptomatic relief for patients. Bedside ultrasound can confirm the presence or absence of abdominal free fluid and can help to identify a fluid pocket of adequate depth for sampling. Furthermore, large vessels in the abdominal wall can be visualized and avoided. Finally, omental and bowel adhesions to the peritoneum can be identified.

Anatomy and Imaging

The pleural cavity is formed by a continuous membranous lining that surrounds and adheres to the lung parenchyma (visceral pleura) and the interior of the chest wall (parietal pleura). Normally, the pleural cavity has a scant lubricating layer of fluid that is too small to be visualized directly with ultrasound. As the visceral and parietal layers rub against one another with lung expansion, the surfaces slide against one another (ie, lung sliding). Furthermore, in normal lungs, there may be a "comet tail artifact," which is thought to represent reverberation artifact created by small microbubbles of fluid between the 2 pleural surfaces (**Fig. 10**). Pleural fluid can be seen above the liver or spleen in the mid-axillary line with the patient supine (**Fig. 11**) and is noted when there is a loss of the mirror image artifact (normally caused by the reflection of the diaphragm and the lack of sound reflection from the aerated lung) or when there is the continuation of the spinal shadow above the diaphragm when there is fluid in the thoracic cavity that can transmit ultrasound. It is also possible to see fluid in the posterior mid scapular line with the patient upright-seated position, and this is demonstrated as a black anechoic space separating the visceral and parietal pleura (**Fig. 12**). Below each rib runs the intercostal neurovascular bundle; because this is

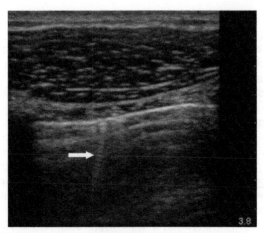

Fig. 10. Comet trail reverberation artifact artifact demonstrated by arrow.

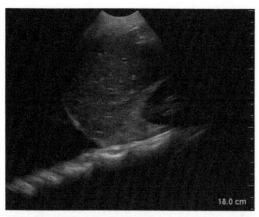

Fig. 11. Pleural fluid in mid-axillary line with patient in supine position.

hidden under the curvature of each rib, it will not normally be visualized sonographically.

The abdominal contents are covered by a membranous layer that adheres to the interior of the abdominal wall called the peritoneum. Running just above the peritoneal layer is the inferior epigastric artery—this should be identified and avoided when ultrasound is used to guide needle placement (**Fig. 13**). Free fluid in the abdomen is gravity dependent and will accumulate in the recesses between organs, specifically the hepatorenal (Morrison), splenorenal, and retrovesicular spaces. A minimum of about 250 mL of fluid can be sonographically visualized.[11] As the volume increases, the rest of the abdomen will fill with fluid and the peritoneum will be lifted off of the bowels.

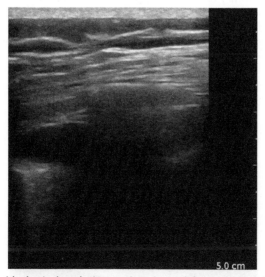

Fig. 12. Pleural fluid obtain by placing patient in upright position, with anechoic pace between visceral from parietal pleura.

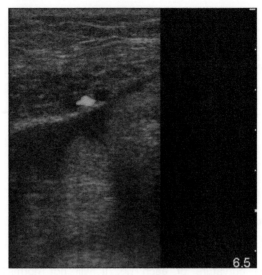

Fig. 13. Doppler image demonstrating inferior epigastric artery.

The fluid will appear as an anechoic region between the peritoneum and solid organs (**Fig. 14**).

Technique

Thoracentesis and paracentesis can be performed by aspirating fluid with a medium-gauge needle and syringe. More commonly, catheter-introducer kits are used; these kits will include either a plastic or a metal catheter sheathed over a longer introducer needle.

Both thoracentesis and paracentesis can be performed with ultrasound imaging, occurring preprocedurally or in real-time guidance. With either technique, the patient should be positioned with the ultrasound directly visible in the operator's line of sight (**Fig. 15**). It is important not to change the patient's position after marking the point of entry, because this can shift the pocket of fluid and move bowel into the path of the needle trajectory.

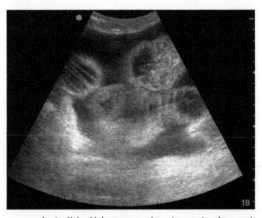

Fig. 14. Fluid appears anechoic (*black*) between the viscera in the peritoneal cavity.

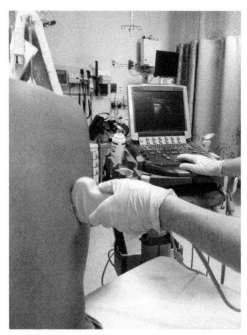

Fig. 15. Ultrasound system position, visible to the operator's line of sight.

When performing thoracentesis, first review relevant cell counts and coagulation factors and any prior imaging. The patient should ideally be placed in a seated position. This position will allow the gravity-dependent fluid to accumulate caudally and will also increase the distance between the pleural lining and the lung. Furthermore, large effusions tend to cause orthopnea, and as such, some patients may be unable to tolerate a supine or prone position. A high-frequency linear probe or a low-frequency curvilinear probe can be used for this procedure depending on operator preference and patient body habitus. As with any ultrasound application, the high-frequency linear probe will provide superior picture quality of the superficial structures but may be insufficient to visualize the lung parenchyma. The effusion and the diaphragm should be visualized and the skin marked. After sterile prep and drape, the skin should be anesthetized. The needle should be directed toward the rib, orthogonal to the skin surface, and the soft tissue should be infiltrated as the needle is passed. To ensure that the intercostal neurovascular bundle inferior to the rib is not injured, the tip of the needle should first touch the rib periosteum and then should be directed slightly cephalad until the rib is passed. This will ensure the track is immediately superior to the rib. After the pleural space is entered, the anesthetic needle can be withdrawn. A small skin incision is then made with a scalpel so that the larger introducer needle can be passed. While holding suction with the dominant hand, pass through the soft tissue along the same track. Once pleural fluid is expressed, advance the catheter off of the introducer needle, taking care to not advance the needle any farther into the body cavity. Once the catheter is within the effusion, the needle can be withdrawn completely and fluid can be removed. After the sampling is complete, the catheter can be withdrawn. Having the patient perform the Valsalva movement during this time will increase the intrathoracic pressure and reduce the chance of pneuomothorax.

When performing paracentesis, first review relevant laboratory data, including platelet count and coagulation factors. The patient can be placed in a right or left lateral decubitus position to maximize the fluid pocket. Begin by looking at the lower quadrants and identify the largest collection. The omentum and bowel loops should be visible in the far field. Next, scan the overlying abdominal wall for the epigastric vessels. Depending on body habitus, it may be helpful to switch to a high frequency (5–10 MHz) linear probe for vessel identification. The skin can then be marked for puncture, taking care to select an area away from the vessels. Sterilely prep and drape the skin. Perform soft tissue anesthesia with a smaller-gauge needle. Following this, a small skin incision can be made to help pass the larger introducer needle. In patients with tense ascites, it is often prudent to ensure that the puncture to the peritoneal cavity and the skin puncture not be in parallel, to prevent fistula formation. Holding suction with the dominant hand, pass the introducer needle through the soft tissue. Once fluid is expressed, thread the catheter into the peritoneum, taking care to not advance the needle any farther. Once the catheter is in place, the needle can be withdrawn and the fluid sampled.

Pitfalls

- When performing paracentesis, be sure to scan in multiple orientations when identifying the inferior epigastric arteries. If the probe axis is parallel to the vessel, the vessel may have similar appearance to a soft tissue plane. Additionally, if color Doppler is being used to identify vascular structures and if the probe is exactly perpendicular to the vessel, no color signal will be generated.
- When performing thoracentesis or paracentesis, the parietal pleura/peritoneal layer has the most innervation and may be the greatest source of discomfort when passing the catheter. When anesthetizing with the smaller-gauge needle after the fluid pocket is entered, consider withdrawing the needle slightly so that it is in close proximity to the membranous layer and depositing several milliliters of anesthetic agent.
- When performing skin puncture with the catheter-introducer needle for paracentesis, the nondominant hand can be used to hold skin tension orthogonal to the puncture site. This will create a "z-track," which will decrease postprocedural leaking.
- Both procedures have "traditional" landmarks and positioning, which do not necessarily apply when ultrasound is used. A large pleural effusion can be accessed with the patient recumbent if visualized in real-time. Abdominal free fluid can also be tapped with a patient supine as opposed to in a decubitus position.
- The lung and diaphragm are dynamic structures. Make sure you observe the full extent of excursion with the respiratory cycle.
- The intercostal neurovascular bundle is typically hidden inferior and proximal to the rib and usually cannot be visualized. The typical approach of needle insertion just cephalad to the rib will avoid vessel injury. However, anatomy can vary and thus it is important to examine the planned procedural site closely for anomalous vessels.
- Removal of large volumes may cause fluid shifts that can lead to patient instability. The traditional recommendation is to use caution when draining more than 1 L via thoracentesis, because this may lead to reexpansion pulmonary edema. However, there are recent studies that do not show an increased risk.[12,13] Removal of 8 L via paracentesis is considered large volume and this may lead to tachycardia and hypotension. Intravascular replacement with crystalloid and/or colloid is advisable.[14]

ULTRASOUND-GUIDED ARTHROCENTESIS
Background

When a patient presents with a painful and swollen joint, prompt diagnosis and evaluation are needed to distinguish a bursitis from a hemarthrosis, osteoarthritis, cellulitis, or a septic arthritis. A patient's history and physical examination may be limited in providing the information necessary to make an accurate diagnosis. Moreover, the physical examination alone may fail to suggest a joint effusion because of limited range of motion. Bedside ultrasound has proved to be superior to the physical examination in the detection of an effusion.[15]

When an effusion is identified, aspiration of synovial fluid may be necessary, such as when septic arthritis is a diagnostic concern.[16] Additionally, arthrocentesis may be of therapeutic benefit as occurs in the setting of hemarthrosis or inflammatory arthritis, allowing a decrease in the pressure within the synovial space and pain relief.[17] Bedside ultrasound can be used for assistance during diagnostic or therapeutic arthrocentesis.

Indications and Contraindications

A bedside ultrasound should be performed when a join effusion is suspected. Ultrasound has been found to be helpful in identifying effusions in smaller joints.[18] In larger joints, bedside ultrasound does not increase the likelihood of successful drainage, but it does result in more fluid drainage compared with the landmark technique.[19]

Bedside ultrasound by itself cannot distinguish the type of fluid present within the joint. Hemarthrosis, septic joint, and chronic inflammation may all have similar sonographic characteristics. An acute traumatic hemarthrosis appears hypoechoic but may be complicated by free-floating material (clot, fibrin, fat etc), making it appear more heterogeneous. Fluid within a septic joint may appear anechoic, often with internal echoes (providing a particulate appearance). Chronically inflamed joints as in degenerative arthritis may contain fluid that is hypoechoic or anechoic in appearance, making it difficult to distinguish from a septic effusion. Infectious arthritis is unique in that it classically presents with an increase in intra-articular fluid without an increase in synovial thickenss.[20]

There are no absolute contraindications to performing a bedside ultrasound to evaluate for the presence of an effusion. Once identified, bedside ultrasound may aid in dynamic arthrocentesis, thus decreasing potential complications.[21,22] This section will focus on ultrasound-assisted evaluation of the knee and elbow.

Anatomy and Imaging

Knee

A knee effusion may not be readily detectable on physical examination because of a patient's body habitus, the size of the effusion, or pain limiting knee flexion during the examination. Slight knee flexion will aid in beside ultrasound examination. This may be accomplished by placing a towel roll beneath the popliteal fossa.

The suprapatellar bursa extends approximately 6 cm superior to the patella, deep to the quadriceps tendon and in communication with the knee joint. A joint effusion is detected with increased distension of the suprapatellar recess with hypoechoic or anechoic fluid deep to the suprapatellar recess. To determine if a knee effusion is present, 6 common views may be used (**Fig. 16**A–D).

Technique

A high-frequency linear probe should be used with sterile water–based lubricant as a suggested conducting medium. A reference comparison view of the unaffected joint should be performed.

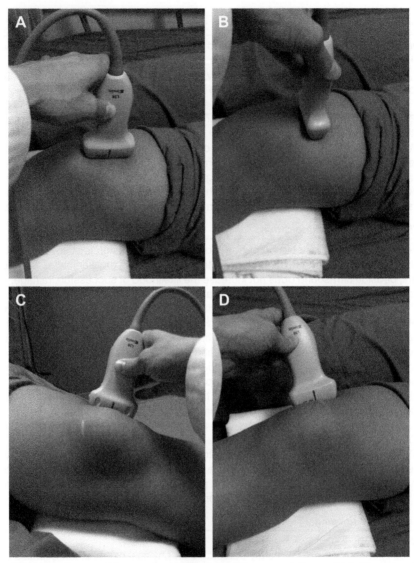

Fig. 16. Probe placement for standard knee views: (*A*) suprapatellar sagittal, (*B*) suprapatellar transverse, (*C*) lateral, and (*D*) medial.

As with all musculoskeletal bedside ultrasound applications, the sonographer should be sure to place and maintain the probe perpendicular to the anatomic structure of interest so as to avoid anisotropy and consequent misidentification of anatomic structures and misinterpretation of sonographic findings.[23]

The suprapatellar bursa should be imaged in the transverse and sagittal planes. With the patella serving as a landmark, take the image laterally for the lateral recess and medially for the medial recess (**Fig. 17**A–D).

In the static technique, identify the largest fluid pocket and mark to designate the optimal site for aspiration. Note the depth of the pocket and the optimal angle of approach. The ultrasound can be used to directly visualize and guide the needle

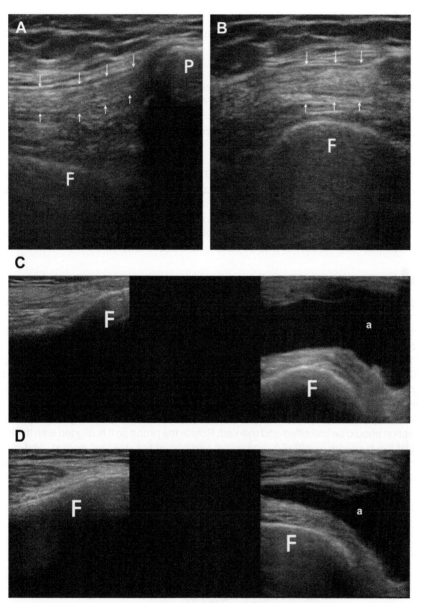

Fig. 17. (*A*) Normal knee. (*B*) Suprapatellar sagittal. (*C*) Suprapatellar transverse. (*D*) Coronal imaging at the lateral joint line or lateral recess (*left*) and (*right*) knee effusion seen as a hypoechoic collection of fluid in the suprapatellar bursa visualized along the lateral recess. Coronal imaging at the medial joint line or medial recess (*left*) and knee effusion (*right*) seen as a hypoechoic collection of fluid in the supra-patellar bursa visualized along the medial recess. F, femur; P, patella; arrows, quadriceps tendon. [a] Joint effusion.

into the fluid pocket. In the dynamic technique, sheath the probe in a sterile fashion and use sterile lubricant. Regardless of the approach used, maintain aseptic technique throughout the procedure.[23]

Elbow

An effusion in the elbow joint may be located in the anterior or posterior recess. The joint capsule, which lies between the radial head and capitellum (the anterior recess), distends anteriorly in the presence of effusion. A small amount of fluid (1- to 2-mm fluid stripe) visualized and measured sonographically within the anterior recess may be physiologic.[21]

The olecranon fossa, or posterior recess, is located distal to the medial and lateral epicondyles, where the posterior surface of the humerus flattens and then becomes depressed. In the sagittal plane, the triceps tendon will appear just below the epidermis and dermis as a hyperechoic fibrillar structure. The olecranon fossa is typically filled with adipose tissue and is known as the posterior fat pad. Sonographically, this appears as mid-gray echogenic material within the fossa. If an effusion is present, anechoic fluid pushes the fat pad superiorly and posteriorly.[21,23]

Technique

Place the patient's elbow in extension and hand in supination for imaging of the anterior recess in a sagittal plane (**Figs. 18** and **19**). The radial head and capitellum align with the joint capsule between them. This capsule will be anteriorly displaced in the presence of a pathologic effusion.[21]

Place the patient's elbow in 90° flexion when performing ultrasound assisted examination of the posterior recess.[24] When the posterior recess is located, the posterior fat pad will be observed within the olecranon fossa (**Figs. 20** and **21**A, B). In the presence of fluid, the fat pad will be superiorly displaced (**Fig. 22**A, B).

With the probe in the transverse plane in the posterior recess, the largest area of fluid collection should be identified and marked. Rotate the probe so it is aligned with the long axis of the humerus (sagittally), noting the location of the deepest pocket, and make a second mark that intersects with the first. This intersection would be the site of aspiration. The joint should be approached from the lateral aspect. A medial approach could

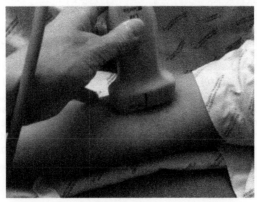

Fig. 18. Probe placement for standard visualization of the anterior recess of the elbow in sagittal view.

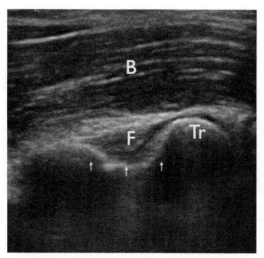

Fig. 19. Normal anterior elbow in sagittal view. B, brachialis muscle; F, anterior fat pad; Tr, trochlea; arrows, coronoid fossa.

result in triceps tendon, ulnar nerve, or superior ulnar collateral artery damage.[23,24] Direct the needle toward the patient's midline.[23] If real-time ultrasound guidance is performed, apply a sterile sheath to the probe and use sterile conducting medium.

Pearls and Pitfalls

- Comparison of the affected limb or joint with the unaffected side will aid in the identification of an effusion.
- Some pitfalls of ultrasound-assisted arthrocentesis are common to landmark-guided arthrocentesis. They pose the risk of iatrogenic infection.
- There is a risk of puncture of adjacent neurovascular structures. Ultrasound will aid in minimizing this risk, however, with the ability to distinguish vascular structures with color Doppler imaging.[23]
- Place the probe as perpendicular to the tendon or structure of interest as possible to avoid anisotropy.
- Gentle compression with the probe will aid in distinguishing a joint effusion from cartilage because fluid will compress and articular cartilage will not.[21]

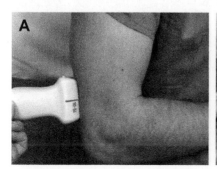
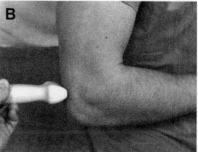

Fig. 20. Probe placement for standard posterior fossa elbow views: (A) sagittal and (B) transverse.

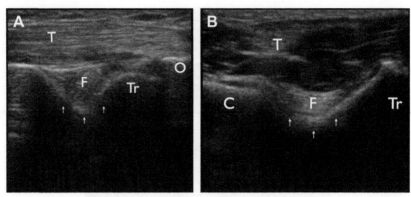

Fig. 21. Normal posterior elbow: (*A*) sagittal and (*B*) transverse. T, triceps; F, posterior fat pad; arrows, olecranon fossa; Tr, trochlea; O, olecranon; C, capitellum.

ULTRASOUND-GUIDED LUMBAR PUNCTURE
Background

Ultrasound-guided lumbar puncture was first described in the Russian literature in 1971.[25] Since then, multiple publications have reported on the utility of ultrasound to facilitate spinal anesthesia and lumbar puncture.[26–33] The literature has also documented that clinicians inaccurately identify lumbar interspaces with the standard palpation technique in 29% to 30% of cases.[34,35] Given this inaccuracy and given the increased risk of spinal cord injury, to access a lumbar interspace higher than the L3 vertebral body,[36] governing bodies in the anesthesia community recommend using assist devices such as ultrasound to select an accurate lumbar spinal access site.[37]

In addition to observational studies, there are a few small prospective, randomized controlled trials that compare ultrasound-guided lumbar puncture to landmark-guided lumbar puncture in the emergency department.[38,39] Although larger prospective cohort studies are needed to further define ultrasound's optimal use in lumbar

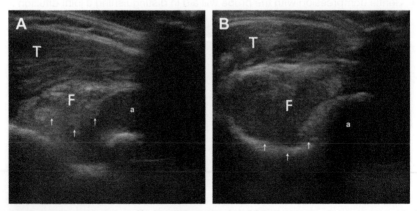

Fig. 22. Posterior recess joint effusion: (*A*). Sagittal and (*B*). Transverse. T, triceps; F, posterior fat pad; arrows, olecranon fossa; ª joint fluid.

puncture, these early studies suggest a trend toward improved success with ultrasound use, especially in obese patients (ie, body mass index $\geq$30 kg/m^2), whose surface lumbar landmarks are difficult to palpate.

Ultrasound indications

In clinical cases when lumbar puncture is indicated, the literature suggests that ultrasound use should be considered when certain patient characteristics and clinical scenarios exist (**Box 1**).[29,32,33,39,40]

Anatomy

In spinal ultrasound imaging, the identification of bony landmarks is imperative. Bone is a very dense tissue and reflects virtually all of the ultrasound waves that encounter its surface. Given the reflective properties of bone, the ultrasound monitor will display a bony surface as a hyperechoic (white) image with an area of anechoic (black) "shadowing" directly behind the structure (**Fig. 23**). The procedurally important lumbar anatomic structures that often are visualized with ultrasound assessment include (1) the lumbar spine with its associated spinous process and transverse processes; (2) the sacral spine; (3) the lumbar interspace; and (4) the ligamentum flavum. The following sections discuss the imaging and identification of these structures using ultrasound.

Technique

Patient positioning Recent observational trials in adult and pediatric populations support the positioning of patients in a sitting position with legs supported in a hip-flexed position. This position increases the interspinous distance and may favor an improved success rate for lumbar puncture. Although patient positioning is determined by patient tolerability and comfort, to the extent possible, this described positioning is recommended.[41,42]

Probe selection Linear (high-frequency) probes allow for higher resolution of superficial structures, making these the most commonly used transducers for imaging of spinal anatomy. However, in patients with an obese habitus and correspondingly deeper spinal structures, a low-frequency phased-array or curvilinear probe may provide better assessment of structures. If using a low-frequency probe, adjust and decrease the depth settings on the machine so to optimize assessment of spinal structures.

Probe orientation In lumbar ultrasound imaging, 2 main probe orientations are used: the transverse view and the longitudinal view. The goal of imaging in the transverse view is to determine the anatomic lumbar spinal *midline* by identifying the spinous

---

Box 1
Patient examination characteristics and clinical scenarios in which ultrasound use should be considered to guide lumbar puncture

- Obese patients with a body mass index $\geq$30 kg/m^2

- Pregnant patients

- Patients with lumbar edema

- Patients with a history of difficult prior lumbar punctures or difficult spinal access

- Patients with an examination demonstrating difficult-to-palpate or difficult-to-visualize spinal anatomy

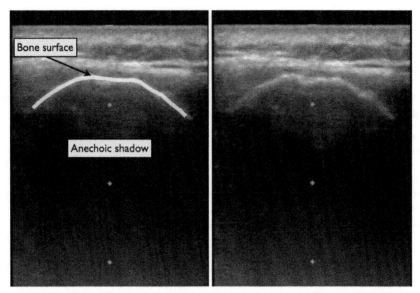

Fig. 23. On the left is a labeled bony spinous process, and on the right is an unlabeled structure. These images are obtained using ultrasound imaging in the longitudinal view.

processes. The goal of imaging in the longitudinal view is to locate the lumbar spinal *interspaces*.

Transverse view The transverse view is obtained by placing the probe perpendicular to the long axis of the spine (**Fig. 24**). The bony spinous process will often appear on the ultrasound monitor as a white hyperechoic convex rim with an associated anechoic shadow. Occasionally, the hyperechoic rim of the spinous process is not well visualized and only the anechoic shadow identifies the target structure. Often, paired hyperechoic structures may be visualized surrounding the spinous process, such as paired mammillary or transverse processes (**Fig. 25**). Identification of these symmetric structures surrounding the spinous process supports spinal midline

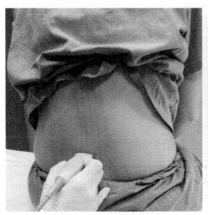
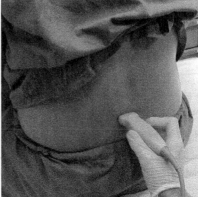

Fig. 24. Probe positioning in the transverse view.

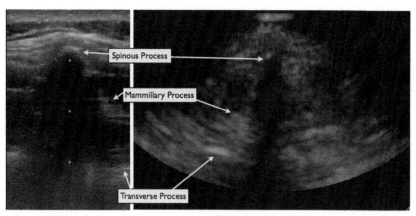

Fig. 25. The midline of the spine on ultrasound imaging in the transverse view. The left image is with use of a high-frequency probe, and the right image is with use of a low-frequency probe.

confirmation. Once identified, center the spinous process on the ultrasound display and then perform preprocedural labeling of the skin as directed in the following section.

Longitudinal View After the midline landmarks are identified with the transverse view, the longitudinal view should be performed with *continuous* reference to the marked and labeled midline. The longitudinal view is obtained by placing the probe's long axis parallel to the long axis of the spine (**Fig. 26**). Again, the key structure to identify is the spinous process. The spinous process should be the most superficial hyperechoic structure with an associated deep anechoic shadow. Care should be taken to confirm that the target structure is the spinous process and not a similar appearing deeper and lateral other bony structure. To confirm a structure is the spinous process, move the probe in a side-to-side direction away from and toward the identified spinal midline to confirm that the identified target structure is of the same general depth as the spinous processes identified on the transverse view. Once a spinous process is identified, move the probe cephalad and caudad to identify other contiguous spinous

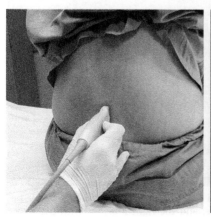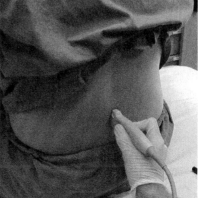

Fig. 26. Probe positioning in the longitudinal view.

processes. After another contiguous spinous process is identified, make fine adjustments with the probe to obtain an ultrasound image on the monitor that contains 2 contiguous spinous processes with a view between them into the spinal interspace. The goal with this view is to center the probe and image between the spinous processes and provide a direct ultrasonographic view into the hypoechoic (gray) interspace (**Fig. 27**). The spinal interspace is the optimal location for needle insertion during lumbar puncture; once it is identified, it should be marked and labeled as described in the following section.

Occasionally, deeper structures may be imaged within the spinal interspace, such as the ligamentum flavum. This structure typically appears as a hyperechoic linear structure within the depths of the interspace (**Fig. 28**). Unlike bone, this structure usually does not have an associated shadow. Sonographic depth assessment of this structure may provide a fairly accurate estimate of the spinal needle introduction depth needed to procure cerebrospinal fluid.

Exact lumbar interspace localization To perform the localization of an exact lumbar interspace, interrogate the midline spinal area of the lower back using the longitudinal view and attempt to localize the sacral bones. The sacral bones appear as fully continuous hyperechoic bony structures that do not have any associated interspaces. Once these bones are identified, move the probe cephalad until an interspace is identified (**Fig. 29**). The first visualized interspace should represent the L5-S1 interspace, with further cephalad movements of the probe allowing precise identification of additional interspaces.

Preprocedural labeling Preprocedural ultrasound guidance is only useful if accurate skin markings are made that clearly demarcate spinal anatomy and the access site. In the transverse view, the probe and monitor image should be centered over the midline spinous process. Once identified, use a surgical marking pen to make physical markings on the patient's skin adjacent to the midline of the probe (**Fig. 30**). For effective labeling and best adherence of ink to the skin, remove extraneous ultrasound gel from the skin with an alcohol wipe or towel before skin marking. In the longitudinal view, the probe and monitor image should be centered over the lumbar interspace

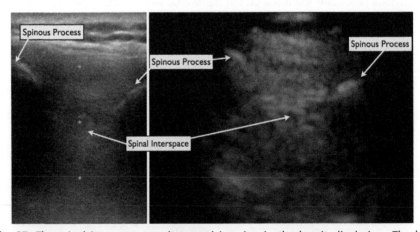

Fig. 27. The spinal interspace on ultrasound imaging in the longitudinal view. The left image is with use of a high-frequency probe, and the right image is with use of a low-frequency probe.

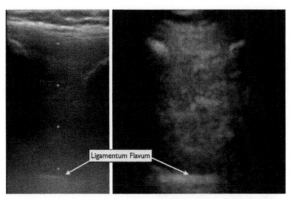

Fig. 28. Ultrasound appearance of the ligamentum flavum. The left image is with use of a high-frequency probe, and the right image is with use of a low-frequency probe.

with physical marks made adjacent to the midline of the probe (**Fig. 31**). Next, cross and connect the labeled markings made during the transverse and longitudinal views, which will effectively provide target "X" access points (**Fig. 32**). Once labeling is completed, standard aseptic site preparation may be performed and the spinal needle may be introduced at the identified "X" or a few millimeters below. Introduce the needle with a slight cephalad angulation so as to follow the contours of the spinous processes. Last, it is very important that patients maintain consistent positioning between the ultrasound-guided site labeling and the performance of the lumbar puncture. Even very small patient movements may change the correlation of the labeled skin surface marks and the underlying spinal structures.

Pitfalls

- The use of ultrasound to assess lumbar anatomy before lumbar puncture poses virtually no risk to patients. However, the inherent risk of the lumbar puncture procedure is the same as with the standard, landmark-guided procedure. Practitioners should also be mindful of the learning curve involved in becoming familiar with the technique and assessment of sonographic lumbar anatomy.

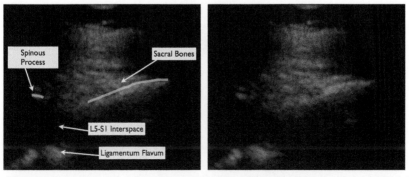

Fig. 29. When imaging with a low-frequency probe, the sacral bones and the L5-S1 interspace are identified. The left image is labeled, and the right image is not.

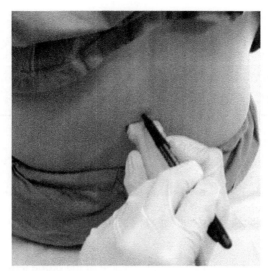

Fig. 30. Preprocedural labeling in the transverse view.

ULTRASOUND-GUIDED ABSCESS DRAINAGE
Background

Patients may present to the emergency department with a variety of infectious skin and soft tissue complaints ranging from simple cellulitis to purulent abscess. Making a clinical diagnosis about the nature and degree of a soft tissue infection may be difficult. This is reflected in the poor interrater agreement of the clinical examination findings and prediction of severity.[43,44] Bedside ultrasound has improved accuracy compared with physical examination findings alone in the detection of abscesses in adult and pediatric patient populations.[45–47] The information gained from soft tissue sonography can help determine not only whether a drainable subcutaneous fluid

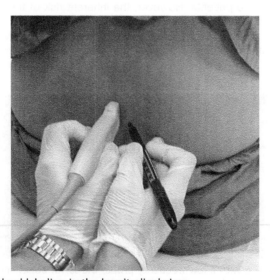

Fig. 31. Preprocedural labeling in the longitudinal view.

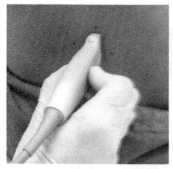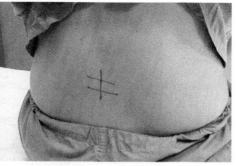

Fig. 32. After making physical markings on the patient's skin adjacent to the midline of the probe in both views, multiple access sites are mapped out by crossing and connecting the labeled markings.

collection exists but also the optimal drainage strategy and location, and it can be used to guide the eventual incision or aspiration.

Ultrasound Indications

A bedside soft tissue ultrasound should be performed on any soft tissue infection when there is a question of an underlying fluid collection. In cases when there is obvious abscess with fluctuance or drainage, the examination can help to delineate the extent of the underlying lesion and determine whether further invasive drainage is required. Low probability cases may reveal unexpected findings of an occult abscess. Once it is determined that drainage is required, the surrounding soft tissue should be assessed for structures such as local vasculature, nerves, or connective tissue that should be avoided during the incision and drainage.

Anatomy and Imaging

Normal soft tissue findings consist of a relatively thin layer of subcutaneous tissue with an organized echotexture. Deep to the subcutaneous tissue are hypoechoic muscle layers bordered by hyperechoic fascia. With cellulitis, the soft tissue appears diffusely thickened and echogenic, with a breakdown of the organized architecture (**Fig. 33**A). Eventually, with progressive edema, this creates a "cobblestone" appearance, with the presence of anechoic edema surrounding subcutaneous fat (see **Fig. 33**B). In contrast, an abscess appears as an ovoid collection of fluid (**Fig. 34**A). This collection may seem contiguous with surrounding cellulitic tissue or have a well-demarcated echogenic border (see **Fig. 34**B). Although a purulent collection often appears hypoechoic to anechoic, it may also appear isoechoic to hyperechoic compared with surrounding tissues.[48] Gentle downward pressure with the ultrasound transducer may reveal fluid moving within the collection.[49] The presence of posterior acoustic enhancement may also help to identify the liquid nature of an isoechoic or hyperechoic abscess cavity. Doppler may reveal hyperemia of the surrounding tissues and should reveal an absence of flow within the abscess cavity (**Fig. 35**).

Ultrasound Technique

Soft tissue ultrasonography is performed with a linear high-frequency transducer (≥7.5 MHz). Assessing the lesion depends on the location, with infections on the trunk and extremities providing minimal obstruction, whereas those on joints, in folds, or between creases may be technically challenging. The scan should start from an

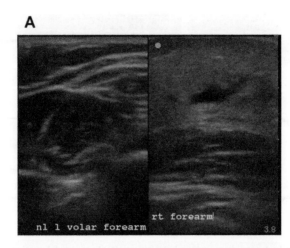

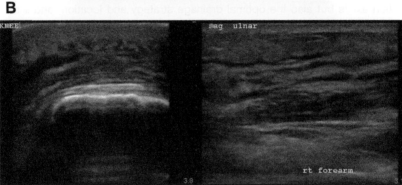

Fig. 33. (*A*) Comparison between normal soft tissue (*left*) and infected soft tissue with small fluid collection (*right*). Note the doubling of size of the subcutaneous tissue layer and the gray echogenicity. (*B*) Cobblestoning in cellulitis.

area of healthy tissue and pan across the lesion to the opposite side, repeating in an orthogonal plane. Measure the size and depth of the abscess, as well as the depth required for the incision. A sinus tract may extend to the surface, whereas the main abscess cavity lies not directly below but off at an angle.

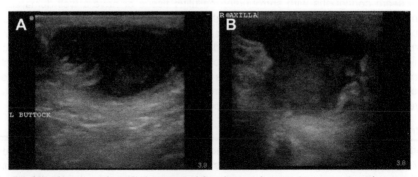

Fig. 34. (*A*) Abscess with well-demarcated borders and posterior acoustic enhancement, with some internal echoes. (*B*) Irregular shaped abscess with mixed echogenic contents.

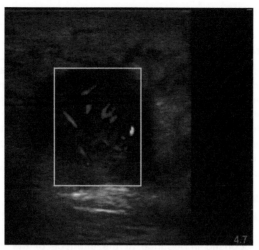

Fig. 35. Evaluated for an abscess, this shows a Doppler flow pattern consistent with adenitis. Also noted are the surrounding cellulitic changes (cobblestoning). An abscess should not have Doppler signal within the cavity.

Pitfalls

- There are no absolute contraindications for performing a soft tissue ultrasound, but care should be taken to ensure appropriate probe sterilization after performance on even a nonpurulent skin lesion.[50]
- Incomplete examination of the area may underestimate the extent of the abscess. Make sure the image has enough depth, and be sure to scan all the way through the lesion and not just in one area.
- Performing a blind incision and drainage procedure carries the inherent risks of injury to unseen adjacent structures, having an unsuccessful procedure because of inadequate localization, or having an unsuccessful procedure because of inadequate assessment of the abscess extent.

ULTRASOUND-GUIDED FOREIGN BODY REMOVAL
Background

Retained subcutaneous foreign bodies are of great concern to emergency physicians because of their ability to serve as a focus for wound infection. A focused evaluation including history and physical examination may not be adequate to rule out a foreign body. Anderson and colleagues[51] reported that 38% of foreign bodies were missed by the treating physician when imaging studies were not obtained.

Radiographs are most useful for detecting glass and metal larger than a few millimeters foreign bodies with sensitivities at greater than 95% when adequate penetration and multiple views are obtained. Radiographs are not useful for the detection of radiolucent objects such as rubber, plastic, and organic matter (wood, thorn, or cactus spines), with sensitivities ranging from 5% to 15%.[51]

The use of ultrasound for the detection of foreign bodies was introduced on 1978.[52] Detection of soft tissue foreign bodies has improved with faster scanners and processing applications. Studies have been performed in various tissue models such as cadavers and chicken thighs, with few small studies performed in humans.[53–55] Reported sensitivity ranges from 43% to 98%, and specificity ranges from 59% to

98%.[53–56] Ultrasound has been able to detect objects as small as 0.5 mm and as deep as 4 mm with improved sensitivity with increasing size of the foreign body.[55,57,58]

Ultrasound Indications

Ultrasound is recommended for the evaluation of radiolucent and radiopaque foreign bodies. Although metal and glass foreign bodies are visible on radiographs, ultrasound can give more precise information and the degree of soft tissue injuries. Ultrasound can determine not only the location of the foreign body but also the size, shape, and orientation. Real-time imaging allows the clinician to image nearby structures, such as blood vessels, that should be avoided during the removal. Surrounding muscle, tendons, ligaments, or neurovascular structures can also be evaluated for injury. Ultrasound reduces procedural time and surgical outcome.[59–61]

Anatomy and Imaging

Most foreign bodies appear echogenic on ultrasound with artifactual changes depending on the type of foreign body.[62] The degree of echogenicity is related to the differences in acoustic impedance at the interface of the foreign body and surrounding tissue. Metal and glass cause a comet tail or reverberation artifact (**Fig. 36**). Gravel has strong posterior shadowing similar to gallstones (**Fig. 37**A). Organic material such as wood, thorn, or plastic appears hyperechoic and may show posterior acoustic shadowing (see **Fig. 37**B). The artifact occurring depends primarily on the surface of the foreign body instead of the composition. Smooth and flat surfaces produce dirty shadowing or reverberation. Objects with irregular surfaces produce clean shadowing.[63] Additionally, organic materials may cause an inflammatory response with developing hemorrhage, edema, and hyperemia leading to a hypoechoic halo (**Fig. 38**). Presence of a hypoechoic halo and use of power Doppler to detect inflammatory changes can aid in foreign body detection.[57,64,65]

Technique

A high-frequency ($\geq$7.5 MHz) linear array transducer is used for evaluation of soft tissue. Very superficial structures may be difficult to visualize because they lie outside the focal zone of the transducer. A standoff pad or water bath can be used to optimize the image by aligning the focal zone of the transducer with the area of interest. Water

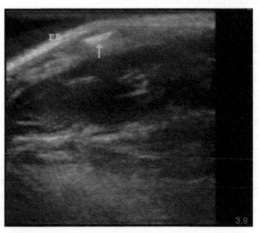

Fig. 36. Glass foreign body (*arrow*) with minimal reverberation artifact.

A

B

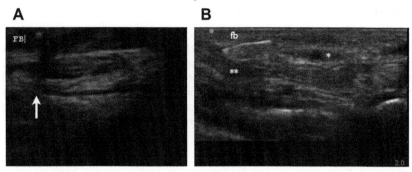

Fig. 37. (A) Foreign body (wood) with posterior acoustic shadowing (*arrow*). (B) Another wooden foreign body without shadowing. Note position adjacent to tendon (*double asterisk*) and artery (*asterisk*).

baths do not require the use of ultrasound gel and avoid compression of the soft tissue, which minimizes discomfort to the patient.[66]

It is important to scan slowly through that soft tissue as an object can be easily missed because of its similar appearance to the surrounding tissue and potential lack of shadowing. The area of interest should be scanned on both longitudinal and transverse planes. Objects are best viewed when the plane of the transducer beam is perpendicular to the surface of the foreign body. Rotating the transducer so the beam is oblique to the foreign body diminishes the echoes returning to the transducer.

Pitfalls

- Diagnostic pitfalls include misidentification of a structure. False-positive findings have been reported from the presence of calcifications, hematoma, scar tissue, trapped air, or sesamoid bone.[53,54,57] Careful scanning of the length of the object in multiple planes may differentiate a foreign body from artifact or bone.
- Limitations of ultrasound evaluation for soft tissue foreign body is primarily related to sonographer experience.
- Familiarity with ultrasound appearances of foreign bodies and their artifacts is essential.

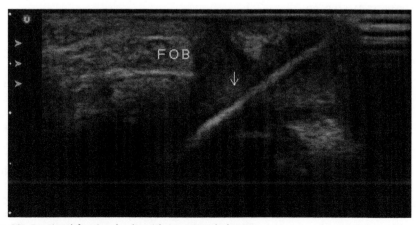

Fig. 38. Retained foreign body with associated abscess.

SUMMARY

Bedside ultrasound can be an effective tool for diagnosis of common conditions such as: ascities, joint, pleural and pericardial effusion. Prompt recognition and treatment of these conditions can be life saving in some cases, but it requires performing procedures that can be challenging. The use of this technology can help physicians identify best placement for needle insertion to improve success rates while decreasing complications. With adequate training and experience, physicians can incorporate this technology to their practice and help improve patient care.

REFERENCES

1. Tsang TS, Enriquez-Sarano M, Freeman WK, et al. Consecutive 1127 therapeutic echocardiographically guided pericardiocenteses: clinical profile, practice patterns, and outcomes spanning 21 years. Mayo Clin Proc 2002;77:429–36.
2. Lindenberger M, Kjellberg M, Karlsson E, et al. Pericardiocentesis guided by 2-D echocardiography: the method of choice for treatment of pericardial effusion. J Intern Med 2003;253:411–7.
3. Vayre F, Lardoux H, Pezzano M, et al. Subxiphoid pericardiocentesis guided by contrast two-dimensional echocardiography in cardiac tamponade: experience of 110 consecutive patients. Eur J Echocardiogr 2000;1:66–71.
4. Wu TS, Finlayson R. Advanced emergency ultrasound applications. EM Reports 2011;32(6):1–16.
5. Ainsworth CD, Salehian O. Echo-guided pericardiocentesis: let the bubbles show the way. Circulation 2011;123(4):e210–1.
6. Otto C. The practice of clinical echocardiography. 3rd edition. Philadelphia: Saunders, Elsevier; 2007.
7. Inglis R, King AJ, Gleave M, et al. Pericardiocentesis in contemporary practice. J Invasive Cardiol 2011;23(6):234–9.
8. Jones PW, Moyer JP, Rogers JT, et al. Ultrasound-guided thoracentesis: is it a safe method? Chest 2003;123(2):418–23.
9. Patel PA, Ernst FR, Gunnarsson CL. Evaluation of hospital complications and costs associated with using ultrasound guidance during abdominal paracentesis procedures. J Med Econ 2012;15(1):1–7.
10. Xirouchaki N, Magkanas E, Vaporidi K, et al. Lung ultrasound in critically ill patients: comparison with bedside chest radiography. Intensive Care Med 2011;37(9):1488–93.
11. Rose JS. Ultrasound in abdominal trauma. Emerg Med Clin North Am 2004;22(3): 581–99, vii.
12. Abunasser J, Brown R. Safety of large-volume thoracentesis. Conn Med 2010; 74(1):23–6.
13. Feller-Kopman D, Berkowitz D, Boiselle P, et al. Large-volume thoracentesis and the risk of reexpansion pulmonary edema. Ann Thorac Surg 2007;84(5):1656–61.
14. Nasr G, Hassan A, Ahmed S, et al. Predictors of large volume paracantesis induced circulatory dysfunction in patients with massive hepatic ascites. J Cardiovasc Dis Res 2010;1(3):136–44.
15. Kane D, Balint PV, Sturrock RD. Ultrasonography is superior to clinical examination in the detection and localization of knee joint effusion in rheumatoid arthritis. J Rheumatol 2003;30:966–71.
16. Rios CL, Zehtabchi S. Evidence-based emergency medicine/rational clinical examination abstract. Septic arthritis in emergency department patients with joint pain: searching for the optimal diagnostic tool. Ann Emerg Med 2008;52:567–9.

17. Courtney P, Doherty M. Joint aspiration and injection. Best Pract Res Clin Rheumatol 2005;19:345–69.
18. Dewitz RS, Paul AI. Ultrasound assisted ankle arthrocentesis. Am J Emerg Med 1999;17(3):300–1.
19. Wiler JL, Constantino TG, Filippone L, et al. Comparison of ultrasound-guided and standard landmark techniques for knee arthrocentesis. J Emerg Med 2010;39(1):76–82.
20. Adhikari S, Blaivas M. Utility of bedside sonography to distinguish soft tissue abnormalities from joint effusions in the emergency department. J Ultrasound Med 2010;29(4):519–26.
21. Valley VT, Stahmer SA. Targeted musculoskeletal sonography in the detection of joint effusions. Acad Emerg Med 2001;8(4):361–7.
22. Stahmer SA, Filippone LM. Ultrasound guided procedures. In: Roberts JR, Hedges JR, editors. Clinical procedures in emergency medicine. 5th edition. Philadelphia: Saunders; 2010. p. 1259–87.
23. Dewitz A, Jones R, Goldstein J. Additional ultrasound- guided procedures. In: Mateer MA, editor. Emergency ultrasound. 2nd edition. New York: McGraw-Hill; 2008. p. 507–37.
24. Parrillo SJ, Morrison DS, Panacek ES. Arthrocentesis. In: Roberts JR, Hedges JR, editors. Clinical procedures in emergency medicine. 5th edition. Philadelphia: Saunders; 2010. p. 971–85.
25. Bogin IN, Stulin ID. Application of the method of 2-dimensional echospondylography for determining landmarks in lumbar punctures. Zh Nevropatol Psikhiatr Im S S Korsakova 1971;71(12):1810–1 [in Russian].
26. Cork RC, Kryc JJ, Vaughan RW. Ultrasonic localization of the lumbar epidural space. Anesthesiology 1980;52(6):513–6.
27. Currie JM. Measurement of the depth to the extradural space using ultrasound. Br J Anaesth 1984;56(4):345–7.
28. Grau T, Leipold RW, Conradi R, et al. Ultrasound imaging facilitates localization of the epidural space during combine spinal and epidural anesthesia. Reg Anesth Pain Med 2001;26(1):64–7.
29. Grau T, Leipold RW, Conradi R, et al. Efficacy of ultrasound imaging in obstetric epidural anesthesia. J Clin Anesth 2002;14(3):169–75.
30. Grau T, Leipold RW, Fatehi S, et al. Real-time ultrasonic observation of combined spinal-epidural anaesthesia. Eur J Anaesthesiol 2004;21(1):25–31.
31. Peterson MA, Abele J. Bedside ultrasound for difficult lumbar puncture. J Emerg Med 2005;28(2):197–200.
32. Ferre RM, Sweeney TW. Emergency physicians can easily obtain ultrasound images of anatomical landmarks relevant to lumbar puncture. Am J Emerg Med 2007;25(3):291–6.
33. Stiffler KA, Jwayyed S, Wilber ST, et al. The use of ultrasound to identify pertinent landmarks for lumbar puncture. Am J Emerg Med 2007;25(3):331–4.
34. Broadbent CR, Maxwell WB, Ferrie R, et al. Ability of anaesthetists to identify marked lumbar interspace. Anaesthesia 2000;55(11):1122–6.
35. Furness G, Reilly MP, Kuchi S. An evaluation of ultrasound imaging for identification of lumbar intervertebral level. Anaesthesia 2002;57(3):277–80.
36. Boon JM, Abrahams PH, Meiring JH, et al. Lumbar puncture: anatomical review of a clinical skill. Clin Anat 2004;12:544–53.
37. Schaffartzik W, Hachenberg T, Rust J, et al. Anaesthics incidents - Injuries caused by regional anaesthesia - closed claims of the North German Arbitration

Board. Anasthesiol Intensivmed Notfallmed Schmerzther 2011;46(1):40–5 [in German].

38. Pisupati D, Heyming TW, Lewis RJ. Effect of ultrasonography localization of spinal landmarks on lumbar puncture in the emergency department. Ann Emerg Med 2004;44(4):S83.

39. Nomura JT, Leech SJ, Shenbagamurthi S, et al. A randomized controlled trial of ultrasound-assisted lumbar puncture. J Ultrasound Med 2007;26(10): 1341–8.

40. Shah KH, McGillicuddy D, Spear J, et al. Predicting difficult and traumatic lumbar punctures. Am J Emerg Med 2007;25(6):608–11.

41. Sandoval M, Shestak W, Sturmann K, et al. Optimal patient position for lumbar puncture, measured by ultrasonography. Emerg Radiol 2004;10(4):179–81.

42. Abo A, Chen L, Johnston P, et al. Positioning for lumbar puncture in children evaluated by bedside ultrasound. Pediatrics 2010;125(5):e1149–53.

43. Marin JR, Bilker W, Lautenbach E, et al. Reliability of clinical examinations for pediatric skin and soft-tissue infections. Pediatrics 2010;126(5):925–30.

44. Murray H, Stiell I, Wells G. Treatment failure in emergency department patients with cellulitis. CJEM 2005;7(4):228–34.

45. Sivitz AB, Lam SH, Ramirez-Schrempp D, et al. Effect of bedside ultrasound on management of pediatric soft-tissue infection. J Emerg Med 2010;39(5):637–43.

46. Squire BT, Fox JC, Anderson C. ABSCESS: applied bedside sonography for convenient evaluation of superficial soft tissue infections. Acad Emerg Med 2005;12(7):601–6.

47. Tayal VS, Hasan N, Norton HJ, et al. The effect of soft-tissue ultrasound on the management of cellulitis in the emergency department. Acad Emerg Med 2006;13(4):384–8.

48. vanSonnenberg E, Wittich GR, Casola G, et al. Sonography of thigh abscess: detection, diagnosis, and drainage. AJR Am J Roentgenol 1987;149(4):769–72.

49. Loyer EM, DuBrow RA, David CL, et al. Imaging of superficial soft-tissue infections: sonographic findings in cases of cellulitis and abscess. AJR Am J Roentgenol 1996;166(1):149–52.

50. Frazee BW, Fahimi J, Lambert L, et al. Emergency department ultrasonographic probe contamination and experimental model of probe disinfection. Ann Emerg Med 2011;58(1):56–63.

51. Anderson MA, Newmeyer WL 3rd, Kilgore ES Jr. Diagnosis and treatment of retained foreign bodies in the hand. Am J Surg 1982;144(1):63–7.

52. Hassani SN, Bard RL. Real time ophthalmic ultrasonography. Radiology 1978; 127(1):213–9.

53. Bray PW, Mahoney JL, Campbell JP. Sensitivity and specificity of ultrasound in the diagnosis of foreign bodies in the hand. J Hand Surg 1995;20(4):661–6.

54. Gilbert FJ, Campbell RS, Bayliss AP. The role of ultrasound in the detection of non-radiopaque foreign bodies. Clin Radiol 1990;41(2):109–12.

55. Banerjee B, Das RK. Sonographic detection of foreign bodies of the extremities. Br J Radiol 1991;64(758):107–12.

56. Turkcuer I, Atilla R, Topacoglu H, et al. Do we really need plain and soft-tissue radiographies to detect radiolucent foreign bodies in the ED? Am J Emerg Med 2006;24(7):763–8.

57. Jacobson JA, Powell A, Craig JG, et al. Wooden foreign bodies in soft tissue: detection at US. Radiology 1998;206(1):45–8.

58. Failla JM, van Holsbeeck M, Vanderschueren G. Detection of a 0.5-mm-thick thorn using ultrasound: a case report. J Hand Surg 1995;20(3):456–7.

59. Shiels WE 2nd, Babcock DS, Wilson JL, et al. Localization and guided removal of soft-tissue foreign bodies with sonography. AJR Am J Roentgenol 1990;155(6): 1277–81.
60. Rockett MS, Gentile SC, Gudas CJ, et al. The use of ultrasonography for the detection of retained wooden foreign bodies in the foot. J Foot Ankle Surg 1995;34(5): 478–84 [discussion: 510–1].
61. Eggers G, Haag C, Hassfeld S. Image-guided removal of foreign bodies. Br J Oral Maxillofac Surg 2005;43(5):404–9.
62. Schlager D. Ultrasound detection of foreign bodies and procedure guidance. Emerg Radiol 1997;15(4):895–912.
63. Rubin JM, Adler RS, Bude RO, et al. Clean and dirty shadowing at US: a reappraisal. Radiology 1991;181(1):231–6.
64. Fornage BD, Schernberg FL. Sonographic diagnosis of foreign bodies of the distal extremities. AJR Am J Roentgenol 1986;147(3):567–9.
65. Davae KC, Sofka CM, DiCarlo E, et al. Value of power Doppler imaging and the hypoechoic halo in the sonographic detection of foreign bodies: correlation with histopathologic findings. J Ultrasound Med 2003;22(12):1309–13 [Quiz: 1314–6].
66. Blaivas M, Lyon M, Brannam L, et al. Water bath evaluation technique for emergency ultrasound of painful superficial structures. Am J Emerg Med 2004; 22(7):589–93.

Critical Cardiovascular Skills and Procedures in the Emergency Department

Anita J. L'Italien, MD[a,b,*]

KEYWORDS

- Emergent pericardiocentesis • Cardiac pacing
- Implantable cardioverter-defibrillator • Cardioversion • Defibrillation
- Sudden cardiac arrest • Tachyarrhythmias • Induced hypothermia

KEY POINTS

- Emergent pericardiocentesis for cardiac tamponade can be lifesaving in a prearrest or arrest situation.
- Temporary emergent cardiac pacing is a way to ensure or restore myocardial depolarization and can be lifesaving.
- It is important for emergency physicians to have a basic understanding of pacemaker (PM) and implantable cardioverter-defibrillator (ICD) function and to be familiar with the possible complications of these devices.
- Prompt recognition and treatment of tachyarrhythmias can be lifesaving. It is of utmost importance for the emergency physician to know the indications, contraindications, and complications of cardioversion and defibrillation.

EMERGENT PERICARDIOCENTESIS

Pericardiocentesis, the aspiration of fluid from the pericardial sac, was first performed in 1840.[1] Cardiac tamponade occurs when the pericardial effusion causes hemodynamic compromise or circulatory collapse. Emergent pericardiocentesis for cardiac tamponade can be lifesaving in a prearrest or arrest situation. The pathophysiology clinical presentation, and detailed review of the procedure for emergent pericardiocentesis are discussed in this article.

The pericardial sac is inelastic. When fluid accumulates in the sac, it progressively increases the intracardiac pressure until it impairs filling of the right heart, which leads

[a] Department of Emergency Medicine, Wake Emergency Physicians, PA, 3000 New Bern Avenue, Medical Office Building, Raleigh, NC 27610, USA; [b] Department of Emergency Medicine, University of North Carolina, 170 Manning Drive, CB#7594, Chapel Hill, NC 27599-7594, USA
* Corresponding author. Department of Emergency Medicine, Wake Emergency Physicians, PA, 3000 New Bern Avenue, Medical Office Building, Raleigh, NC 27610.
E-mail address: l'italien@weppa.org

Emerg Med Clin N Am 31 (2013) 151–206
http://dx.doi.org/10.1016/j.emc.2012.09.011
0733-8627/13/$ – see front matter © 2013 Elsevier Inc. All rights reserved.
emed.theclinics.com

to a decrease in cardiac output. The degree to which this occurs depends more on how quickly the fluid accumulates rather than the absolute volume of the fluid. The pericardial sac is able to stretch and accommodate a much larger volume of fluid with a slow accumulation. In contrast, even 50 mL of rapid accumulation can lead to cardiovascular collapse.[2] Causes of pericardial effusions include trauma, post-cardiac surgery, myocardial rupture after infarction, aortic dissection, malignancy, infections, connective tissue disease, and volume overload states such as cirrhosis, congestive heart failure, nephritic syndrome, and liver failure.[3]

The diagnosis of cardiac tamponade is clinical. **Box 1** shows the most common signs and symptoms associated with cardiac tamponade. No single finding or a combination of findings is sensitive or specific for cardiac tamponade. Beck's triad, consisting of hypotension, muffled heart sounds, and jugular venous distention, is present in less than 30% of patients and is more likely to be seen with rapid accumulation of pericardial fluid.[4,5] Pulsus paradoxus is often difficult and time consuming to measure and is not specific to cardiac tamponade (**Box 2**).[5]

Direct visualization with the use of ultrasound is the best tool to confirm the presence of an effusion and should be used when available.[7] This method has sensitivities and specificities approaching 100% when performed by emergency physicians[6] and is rapid and noninvasive. The presence of tamponade is suggested by the collapse of the right ventricle during diastole, abnormal septal movement, and decreased respiratory variation of the inferior vena cava, which should collapse during inspiration.[2] Tamponade is also one of the causes of pulseless electrical activity (PEA) arrest and should be considered in this situation.[8]

Box 1
Symptoms and signs of cardiac tamponade

Symptoms

- Dyspnea
- Confusion
- Dizziness
- Fatigue
- Chest pain
- Palpitations

Signs

- Tachycardia
- Hypotension
- Jugular venous distention
- Muffled heart sounds
- Friction rub
- Pulsus paradoxus
- Low-voltage electrocardiogram (ECG)
- Electrical alternans on ECG
- Enlarged heart on radiograph
- Pulseless electrical activity (PEA)

Box 2
Pulsus paradoxus

Pulsus paradoxus is an exaggeration of the normal inspiratory decrease in blood pressure. It is a classic finding of cardiac tamponade but not pathognomonic. It is defined as a drop in systolic blood pressure greater than 10 mm Hg during inspiration. It is detected by feeling the pulse, which may disappear or diminish significantly during inspiration. However, if the patient is breathing deeply, it should be interpreted with caution. It can also be measured by sphygmo-manometry. The blood pressure cuff is inflated more than the patient's systolic pressure. During deflation, it should be identified when the first Korotkoff sound is audible during expiration, but disappears during inspiration. As the cuff pressure drops, another point is reached when the first blood pressure sound is audible throughout the respiratory cycle. The difference between these 2 points is the measure of pulsus paradoxus. It can also be seen with pulmonary emphysema, asthma, obesity, heart failure, constrictive pericarditis, cardiogenic shock, pulmonary embolus, and labored respirations.[6]

The only indication for pericardiocentesis in the emergency department (ED) is cardiac tamponade causing life-threatening hemodynamic instability or PEA arrest.[9] Ultrasound-guided pericardiocentesis has proved to be safe with a low complication rate in experienced hands.[10] Unfortunately, cardiac tamponade is an uncommon occurrence in the ED, and pericardiocentesis is not routinely performed.[11] It should therefore be reserved for life-threatening cardiac tamponade, when each minute counts.

There are no absolute contraindications to pericardiocentesis for life-threatening hemodynamic instability.[3] If collapse is not imminent, definitive treatment should first be sought. Pericardiocentesis in the setting of aortic dissection or myocardial rupture carries an increased risk of intensified bleeding and extension of the dissection or rupture when decompression occurs.[12–14] Sternotomy in the operating room or ED thoracotomy is preferred for traumatic cardiac tamponade, as there is a high rate of recurrence and this approach seems to improve survival.[15–18] However, pericardiocentesis may still be useful and lifesaving in the above-mentioned settings as a temporizing measure when the patient is in a prearrest (unconscious, hypotensive, or agonal) or arrest state.[19]

There are 2 approaches to emergent pericardiocentesis: blind and ultrasound-guided. The approach chosen should be the one most familiar to the provider. Intravenous (IV) fluids can often temporize the patient's hemodynamics and should be administered while preparing for the procedure and/or arranging for definitive care.[20] Vasopressors such as dopamine, norepinephrine, dobutamine, and isoproter-enol may also be used.[21–23] With either technique, placing a pigtail drainage catheter into the pericardium using the Seldinger technique should be considered, as reaccumulation can occur.[24,25]

The blind approach carries an increased risk of complications compared with the ultrasound-guided technique.[10,26,27] Attaching an electrocardiogram (ECG) lead to the puncture needle is thought to help identify the location of the needle during blind aspiration, as contact with the ventricular epicardium by the needle creates a "current of injury" or ST segment elevation on the ECG tracing.[3] This technique increases preparation time, makes the procedure more cumbersome, and creates a risk of fibrillation of the heart if proper electrical grounding is not optimal.[28] It also does not provide an adequate safeguard against myocardial injury. For these reasons, it is not routinely recommended.[29]

Ultrasound-guided pericardiocentesis, first described in 1979, is a safe and effective method of relieving pericardial tamponade.[10,30,31] It is also the preferred method.[2,28,32] It has the advantage of allowing the provider to visualize correct needle placement and choose the shortest route to the effusion, while having fewer complications than the blind technique.[10] A subxyphoid, parasternal, or apical approach can be used.[3]

To perform the blind procedure, assemble necessary equipment as recommended in **Box 3**. Use sterile techniques and universal safety measures to prepare the patient. Anesthetize the skin and subcutaneous tissues. If a subxyphoid approach is chosen, elevate the head of the bed so that the fluid accumulates inferiorly by gravity. Puncture the skin just below and to the left of the xyphoid process, as shown in **Fig. 1**. Aim the needle to the patient's left shoulder at a 30 to 45 degree angle from the skin. Once under the costal margin, decrease the angle of the needle to 15 to 30 degrees from the skin and advance with continuous aspiration until blood or fluid is obtained. The needle can be redirected to the right shoulder or directly cephalad if the initial attempt is unsuccessful.[33] For a parasternal approach, insert the needle in the fourth or fifth intercostal space, 3 to 5 cm lateral to the sternal border and just above the rib to avoid the neurovascular bundle that runs along the inferior margin of the rib.[34,35] Withdraw as much fluid as possible. The emergency physician may witness immediate improvement in the patient's hemodynamics after the procedure is done. A drainage catheter should be placed at this time if rapid reaccumulation is a concern.[29] Obtain a chest radiograph after the procedure to evaluate for complications such as pneumothorax or hemothorax.[3]

Equipment is the same for the ultrasound-guided technique except for the addition of the ultrasound machine. The provider needs a 3.5- to 5.0-MHz frequency probe (**Fig. 2**). If the ultrasound machine has a cardiac preset, use it. It orients the arrow

---

Box 3
Equipment for emergent pericardiocentesis

Skin antiseptic

Sterile drape

25-Gauge needle for local anesthetic infiltration

1% or 2% Lidocaine for local anesthesia

16- to 18-Gauge (5.1–8.3 cm) polytef-sheathed venous needle

60-mL Syringe

Specimen-collecting tubes

Plastic tubing (30 cm)

3-Way stopcock

No. 11 blade scalpel

4 × 4-in Gauze dressing

Topical antibiotic ointment

Optional for catheter placement

Sheath introducer set: floppy tipped guidewire, dilator, and introducer sheath 65 cm standard pigtail angiocatheter (6F–8F) with multiple side holes

Sterile saline

2- to 5-mL Syringes

3-Way stopcock

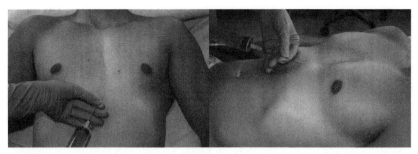

Fig. 1. Blind subxyphoid approach to pericardiocentesis. The skin is punctured between the xyphoid process and the left costal margin at a 30° to 45° angle to the skin.

on the monitor to the right side of the image, opposite to that of abdominal imaging. If not, the following descriptions still apply, but the operator will need to rotate the probe indicator to the opposite direction to obtain the same orientation on the screen.[3]

Identify the best location for needle insertion. This location is the place where the largest fluid accumulation is closest to the body surface without intervening vital structures.[29] Check the following cardiac views: subcostal 4 chambers or subxyphoid view, parasternal long axis view, and apical 4-chamber view (**Fig. 3**).

The normal pericardium appears as a single brightly echogenic stripe adjacent to the myocardium (**Fig. 4**).[3] An effusion appears as an anechoic (black) space between the pericardial and visceral pericardium (**Fig. 5**).[3] Less than 50 mL in the dependent part of the pericardial space is normal.[3] Effusions can be categorized as small (<10 mm), moderate (10–15 mm), or large (>15 mm); however, the size of the effusion is not as important as the pressure it exerts on the heart as discussed previously.[3,36]

Once the location of entry is chosen, the angle of the transducer is used to determine the trajectory of the needle, the entry site is marked, and sterile preparation is achieved. Needle insertion can be done blindly or under direct ultrasound visualization, although the latter is technically more difficult and requires sterile preparation of the ultrasound probe. Attach the catheter needle to the 60-mL syringe, and advance while aspirating until the needle enters the pericardial space. If using direct ultrasound guidance, the practitioner should notice tenting of the pericardium just before needle entry into the pericardial space. If confirmation of the needle location is needed, corroborate position by injecting 5 mL of agitated saline.[10] See **Box 4** for details. Fluid

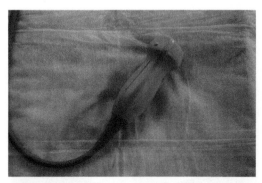

Fig. 2. Low-frequency phased array ultrasound probe. The small flat surface is good for scanning through intercostal spaces.

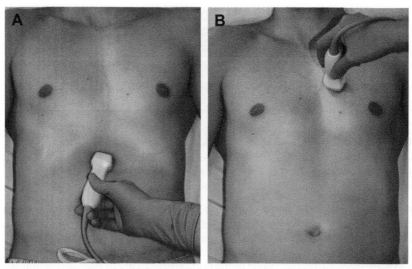

Fig. 3. (*A*) Subxyphoid view. Hold probe at a 15° angle to the chest wall, aim toward the left shoulder with probe indicator toward the patient's right. (*B*) Parasternal long axis view. The transducer is perpendicular to the third or fourth intercostal space to the left of the sternum with the indicator to the patient's right. The apical 4-chamber view is obtained by rotating the patient to their left side, placing the probe in the fifth intercostal space, aiming toward the right shoulder with indicator in the same direction.

can then be aspirated directly into the 60-mL syringe until hemodynamic stability is achieved. Place a drainage catheter at this time, if desired. Obtain a chest radiograph to evaluate for complications.

If a drainage catheter is to be placed, advance a guidewire through the needle sheath after the needle enters the pericardial space. Make a stab incision in the skin at the entry site, and use a dilator over the guidewire. Remove the dilator and guidewire, leaving the introducer sheath in place. Traditionally, the introducer sheath is removed and the guidewire left in place; the catheter is then passed over the guidewire. Either method can be done; however, experience at the Mayo Clinic has shown that occasionally the catheter tip pulls the guidewire out of the pericardial sac,

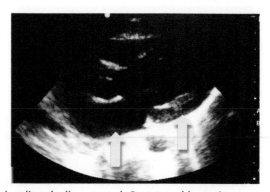

Fig. 4. Normal pericardium (*yellow arrows*). Parasternal long view.

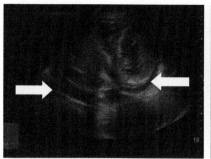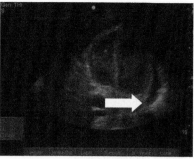

Fig. 5. Pericardial effusion appears as an anechoic/black space between the parietal and visceral pericardium (*white arrows*).

whereas this is less likely to occur using the introducer sheath.[29] A pigtail angiocatheter is inserted through the introducer sheath, and fluid is aspirated. The introducer sheath is then removed. Injection of agitated saline is repeated to confirm proper placement if necessary, as explained in **Box 4**. The catheter is then secured to the chest wall by suture, antibiotic ointment is applied, and an appropriate sterile, occlusive dressing is placed over the site.

The blind approach carries a 4% to 40% rate of complications.[26,27] Ultrasound-guided pericardiocentesis has a much lower rate of both major (1.2%–1.6%) and minor complications (3.5%) in experienced hands.[10] The most serious complication is laceration of the coronary arteries. Punctures of the myocardium do not usually cause any serious consequences. Vasovagal episodes are treated with atropine. **Box 5** provides details for possible complications of the procedure.

Pericardiocentesis is infrequently performed, and the risk of complications is greater because of less familiarity and experience with the procedure by the provider. **Box 6** provides advices on optimizing success and minimizing complications.

Pericardiocentesis has the potential to be a lifesaving procedure in the presence of cardiac tamponade and is an important skill in which emergency physicians must be proficient.

EMERGENT CARDIAC PACING

In the 1950s, Zoll and Leatham[42–44] demonstrated the effectiveness of transcutaneous (TC) pacing. The first implantable PMs were developed in the late 1950s followed by improved techniques in transvenous (TV) pacing.[45] Cardiac pacing is a way to ensure or restore myocardial depolarization and can be lifesaving.[46,47] It can be accomplished by either a TC or TV method. TC pacing delivers an electrical impulse across

---

Box 4
Agitated saline

Agitated saline can be used to confirm catheter placement within the pericardium. To create agitated saline, use two 5-mL syringes, one filled with air and the other with saline, each connected to a 3-way stopcock. Rapidly inject back and forth between the 2 syringes to aerate the saline, and then quickly inject it into the sheath while visualizing it directly with ultrasound. The contrast appears as dense opacification of the pericardial space.

Box 5
Complications of emergent pericardiocentesis

Laceration of coronary artery

Puncture of myocardium

Pneumothorax

Hemopneumothorax

Pneumopericardium

Tachydysrhythmias

Puncture of peritoneal cavity

Liver laceration

Acute pulmonary edema[37]

Right ventricular dilatation[38,a]

Vasovagal episodes

[a] Can occur when volumes greater than 1 L are removed.

---

the chest wall to stimulate the myocardium. TV pacing stimulates the ventricle directly using an intravenous electrode.

The approach chosen depends on the experience of the provider with each method, the comorbidities of the patient, and the time available to initiate the pacing. TC pacing

---

Box 6
Tips for emergent pericardiocentesis

- Apical aspiration—direct the needle parallel to the long axis of the left ventricle toward the aortic valve.

- The internal thoracic artery runs about 1 cm lateral to the sternal border; avoid this when using a parasternal approach by inserting the needle 3 to 5 cm lateral to the sternum.

- Neurovascular bundles run along the inferior margins of the ribs; insert the needle over the rib to avoid these structures.

- If using a subxyphoid approach, elevate the head of the bed up to 45° to allow the fluid to accumulate inferiorly.

- Decompress abdominal distention with a nasogastric tube before attempts at pericardiocentesis.

- If a catheter is placed for continued drainage, manual aspiration is preferred over vacuum suction, as it avoids collapse of the tubing. Intermittent drainage rather than continuous should be done to avoid clogging the drain.

- Hypovolemia can cause collapse of the right heart during diastole, mimicking cardiac tamponade.

- An intrapericardial blood clot can be echogenic and missed on ultrasound.[39]

- An epicardial fat pad can be seen anteriorly and should not be mistaken for an effusion.

- There is a high rate of false-negative results in pericardiocentesis in the setting of traumatic hemopericardium because of clotted blood and significant false-positive results.[40,41]

- An 18-gauge thin-walled needle is preferred over a larger-bore needle, which is more likely to lacerate the myocardium.

is the technique of choice in the ED because it can be initiated quickly and is noninvasive and less technically difficult.[48] It is generally used as a temporizing measure until TV pacing can be initiated. TV pacing is best reserved for urgent rather than emergent situations because of the time required to gain venous access and the skill required to float the electrodes successfully. However, it may be necessary if attempts at TC pacing are unsuccessful.

Box 7 summarizes the various clinical situations in which emergent cardiac pacing is indicated. The patient is typically symptomatic or hemodynamically unstable with hypotension, chest pain, pulmonary edema, syncope, or altered mental status. Pacing experience in the pediatric population has been limited but is used in similar conditions.[49,50]

Box 8 provides a list of contraindications to emergent cardiac pacing. This method is rarely successful in bradyasystolic arrest and is not standard practice: if used in this situation, it should be initiated within 10 minutes to provide maximum potential benefit.[51] Drug- or toxin-induced arrhythmias have not been shown to respond to pacing and specific antidotes, inotropic medications or vasopressors are more successful in restoring hemodynamic stability.[52–55] The hypothermic heart is easily prone to ventricular fibrillation (VF), which is difficult to revert and can be initiated by pacing. Rewarming should be attempted first. However, attempts at pacing can be supported as a last resort if other interventions fail.[56]

A list of equipment and supplies needed for TC and TV pacing is found in **Boxes 9** and **10**, respectively. It is important to be familiar with the equipment available at one's institution before the need to use it arises.

Pacing Generator

The generator typically has 3 control buttons (**Fig. 6**). The *output* knob controls the amount of electrical current that is delivered to the myocardium and usually ranges from 0.1 to 20 mA. The *sensitivity* knob allows for the generator to sense the patient's intrinsic cardiac activity and to function in a demand, or synchronized, mode. This mode is preferred, as it prevents a pacing stimulus from occurring during the relatively refractory period of ventricular repolarization, which can precipitate VF. To *increase*

Box 7
Indications for emergent cardiac pacing

- Symptomatic sinus bradycardia
- Sinus arrest
- Symptomatic[a] sick sinus syndrome
- Tachybrady syndrome
- Overdrive pacing of tachydysrhythmias refractory to pharmacologic treatment
- Acute myocardial infarction with new LBBB, RBBB, or bifasicular block[48]
- Malfunction of implanted PM if patient is PM-dependent
- Symptomatic type II second- and third-degree heart block
- Prevention or treatment of recurrent torsades de pointes

Abbreviations: LBBB, left bundle branch block; RBBB, right bundle branch block.
[a] Symptoms includes hypotension, altered mental status, respiratory distress, heart failure, and cardiac ischemia.

Box 8
Contraindications for emergent cardiac pacing

- Asymptomatic or relatively stable rhythm
- Asystole[57]
- Bradyasystole (relative)
- Prosthetic tricuspid valve specific to TV pacing[57]
- Hypothermia (relative)
- Interruption of cardiopulmonary resuscitation (CPR)[58]
- Drug- or toxin-induced dysrhythmias

---

the sensitivity, *decrease* the setting or millivolts. At high millivolt values, the generator functions in an asynchronized mode and paces continuously. The *rate* knob controls the number of discharges or beats per minute (bpm). It should be set at 60 to 80 bpm or 10 to 20 bpm more than the intrinsic rate for overdrive pacing.

Pacing Catheter

Temporary TV catheters may be unipolar or bipolar. Bipolar catheters have a cathode (+) or stimulating electrode at the tip of the catheter, whereas the anode (−) is 1 to 2 cm proximal to the tip. Unipolar catheters have the cathode at the tip, and the anode is located in the pacing generator, proximally on the catheter, or on the patient's chest. Regardless of the catheter type, all stimulation is bipolar. A flexible balloon catheter is frequently used in the emergency setting. The balloon near the tip helps guide, or float, the catheter into the right ventricle (**Fig. 7**).

Introducer Sheath

This sheath may be prepackaged with the pacing catheter or in a separate set. It contains a pacer port whose opening is covered by a perforated elastic seal that allows manipulation of the catheter. A side port allows for central venous access. The sheath must be larger than the pacing catheter. The size of the catheter refers to the outside diameter, whereas the size of the introducer sheath refers to the inside diameter. Therefore, a 6F catheter fits in a 6F sheath.

Procedure for TC and TV Pacing

Connect the patient to a continuous cardiopulmonary monitor with peripheral IV access established. Apply the 2 electrode pads to the patient's chest (**Fig. 8**). Turn on the portable pulse generator (**Fig. 9**). Provide sedation and pain medication as needed

---

Box 9
Equipment for TC pacing

- Pacing generator (defibrillator)
- Adhesive pacing pads
- Sedation/analgesia
- Airway equipment and intubating drugs
- Resuscitation equipment and drugs

Box 10
Equipment for TV pacing

- Insulated connecting wire with alligator clamps at each end or a male-to-male adaptor
- Fresh battery and a spare
- Pacing generator
- Flexible TV cardiac pacing catheter
- 12-lead ECG machine or cardiac monitor, well grounded
- 10-mL syringe
- 1% lidocaine
- 19- and 26-gauge needles
- Skin antiseptic
- Sterile drapes
- Sterile gloves and gown
- Central catheter kit—introducer sheath must be one size larger than the pacing catheter (sheath, guidewire, dilator, and introducer needle)
- No. 11 blade scalpel
- Needle holder
- 3-0 or 4-0 silk sutures on needles
- Tegaderm

Some or all of these may be found in prepackaged kits.

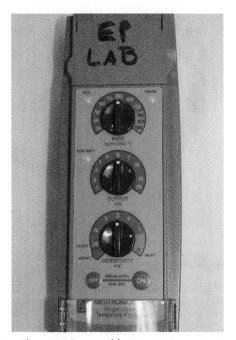

Fig. 6. Pacing generator. There are 3 control buttons: rate, output, and sensitivity.

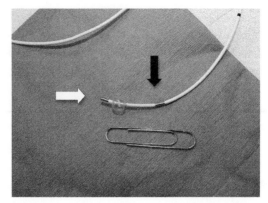

Fig. 7. Balloon-tipped pacing catheter. White arrow indicates the cathode (+) and back arrow indicates the anode (−).

A

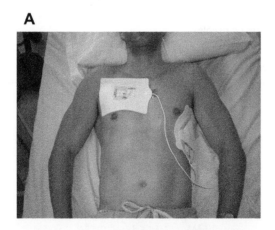

B

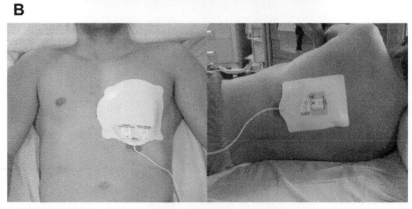

Fig. 8. (A) Pad placement for transcutaneous pacing. (B) Alternate anteroposterior placement.

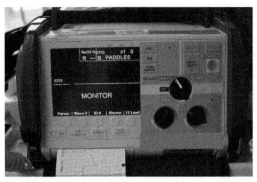

Fig. 9. Portable pulse generator/defibrillator.

with agents such as fentanyl, morphine, Versed, and Ativan. Attempt to pace. **Box 11** provides the detailed steps. Only asynchronous pacing can be done with this method.

Should the patient require TV pacing, obtain consent if possible. The patient should be connected to a continuous electrocardiographic monitor with peripheral IV access established and the venous access site chosen. The left subclavian vein and the right internal jugular vein are the preferred sites, as they have the straightest anatomic path to the right ventricle.[59–61] The choice depends on the provider's experience with these access sites and the patient's comorbidities and body habitus. Ultrasound should be used to guide access of the internal jugular vein when available, as it has been shown to decrease complications.[62–64]

Box 12 lists the steps for emergent TV pacing. The pacing catheter balloon should be checked for leaks by inflating with 1.5 mL of air and submerging in sterile saline.

Box 11
Steps for TC pacing

1. Secure IV access.

2. Have airway and resuscitation equipment drugs readily available.

3. Place pacing pads on patient (see **Fig. 8**).

4. Connect to pacing generator/defibrillator machine (see **Fig. 4**).

5. Connect ECG leads to the patient and to the pacing generator.

6. Provide sedation and/or analgesia.

7. Turn on machine.

8. Set the beats per minute at 10 to 20 beats higher than the patient's intrinsic rhythm for overdrive pacing or 60 to 80 bpm for bradycardias.

9. Set the milliamperes to lowest current.

10. Set the machine to pacing mode. Slowly increase the current (milliamperes) until capture is achieved.

11. Confirm electrical and mechanical capture.[a]

12. After capture is established, decrease the milliamperes as much as possible while maintaining capture.

[a] Mechanical capture is confirmed by the presence of a pulse corresponding to the paced electrical activity on the monitor.

The ECG recording helps to localize the tip of the catheter during placement because the PQRS complex morphology changes depending on where it is located. When contact is made with the right ventricular wall, ST segment elevations are seen. See **Table 1** for corresponding positions and patterns. If ultrasound is available, obtain

---

Box 12
Steps for ECG-guided TV pacing

1. Assemble all equipment.

2. Check the integrity of the catheter balloon.

3. Insert a new battery into the generator.

4. Connect the positive lead of the pacing catheter to the positive connector terminal on the generator cable (**Fig. 10**).

5. Connect the negative lead to any V lead of a well-grounded ECG machine using a male-to-male connector or an insulated wire with alligator clips at each end.

6. Set the rate, sensitivity, and output on the generator.

   a. Rate: 80 or 10 bpm faster than the intrinsic rate

   b. Sensitivity: set low for asynchronized mode

   c. Output: lowest voltage

7. Choose the site of IV access.

8. Use sterile technique to gain venous access.

9. Place the introducer sheath in the vein.

10. Place catheter into the introducer sheath.

11. Advance catheter until it is in the superior vena cava, about 10 to 12 cm for internal jugular and subclavian approach.

12. Inflate the balloon with 1.5 mL of air and lock the inflation port.

13. Advance the catheter until it makes contact with the right ventricle (see **Table 1**).

14. Deflate the balloon by releasing the inflation port.

15. Remove the negative lead from V and insert it into the negative connector terminal on the generator cable (see **Fig. 6**).

16. Turn on the generator (see **Fig. 6**).

17. Increase the output until capture is achieved.

18. Confirm electrical and mechanical capture.[a]

19. Determine the sensing threshold and set it (see text).

20. Tighten the valve on the sheath to prevent the catheter from moving.

21. Extend the sheath to its full length.

22. Secure the catheter to the skin.

23. Cover with appropriate sterile occlusive dressing.

24. Continue to monitor the patient closely.

25. Obtain a chest radiograph.

Abbreviations: IJ, internal jugular; SC, subclavian.
[a] Mechanical capture is confirmed by the presence of a pulse corresponding to the paced electrical activity on the monitor.

Table 1
PQRS morphologies seen during ECG-guided transvenous pacing catheter placement

Location	ECG Pattern	Apperance
Above atrium	P and QRS are negative	
High right atrium	Large negative P & QRS, P wave much larger than QRS	
Mid right atrium	Isoelectric (biphasic) P waves	
Low right atrium	Smaller, upright P wave	
Right ventricle	Small and upright P wave, large negative QRS	
Right ventricular wall[a]	Large negative QRS, ST elevation	
Inferior vena cava	Decreased amplitude of P and QRS complexes, P wave morphology changes	
Pulmonary artery	P wave becomes negative, QRS complex decreases	

[a] Desired location for pacing.

a subxyphoid view of the heart. The catheter is seen longitudinally as it enters the right atrium and then the right ventricle. A pacing spike followed by a QRS complex on the cardiac monitor indicates electrical capture.[48] Mechanical capture is confirmed by palpating a corresponding pulse.

After capture is achieved, adjust the output and sensitivity settings. The threshold is the minimum current necessary to maintain capture. It is usually less than 1.0 mA.[48] To determine the threshold, reduce the current slowly until capture is lost. Repeat this several times for an accurate value. The output should be set approximately 2 times the threshold to ensure ongoing capture. If synchronous pacing is desired, set the rate to 10 bpm greater than the intrinsic rate and the sensitivity to asynchronous

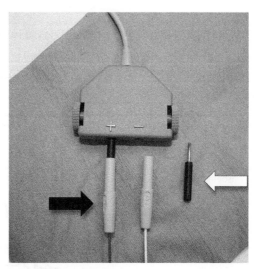

Fig. 10. Reusable adaptors (*white arrow*) are necessary to connect the electrodes (*black arrow*) to the generator cable (*seen in blue*).

mode (low millivolts). Be sure capture is taking place; then, adjust the sensitivity mode to midposition and gradually decrease the rate until pacing is suppressed by the intrinsic rhythm. If this does not work, increase the sensitivity setting. If pacing is triggered by P or T waves or artifact, decrease the sensitivity. Set the millivolts to about half the sensitivity threshold.

Most complications are associated with the TV approach and involve central venous access or the leads and generator (**Box 13**). An ECG machine that is not well grounded can induce VF,[65] which is suggested by the presence of artifact on the tracing.

Box 13
Complications of emergent cardiac pacing

- Development of VF or acceleration of the rhythm with overdrive pacing
- Failure to recognize underlying VF
- Complications specific to TV pacing
  - Cardiac perforation
  - Arrhythmias
  - Fracture of the wire with embolization
  - Phrenic nerve injury
  - Cardiac tamponade
  - Dislodgement of lead
- Central-venous-access-associated complications
  - Pneumothorax, hemothorax
  - Infection, thrombosis
  - Vessel laceration
  - Arterial puncture
  - Air embolus

Box 14 provides suggestions to optimize success and minimize complications. It is especially important to ensure that there is mechanical capture in the presence of electrical capture. During attempts at TV pacing, a chest radiograph is helpful in determining the cause for failure to pace. Defibrillation and cardioversion are safe in the presence of a TV pacing catheter. The patient should be frequently reassessed, as loss of capture can occur. **Box 15** provides tips for troubleshooting failure to capture. If TC pacing is successful, immediate plans should be made for insertion of a TV pacing catheter, either in the ED or by a cardiologist.

MANAGEMENT OF PMS AND ICDS IN THE ED

An implantable PM is a device that uses electrical impulses to regulate the heart's intrinsic rhythm or to reproduce that rhythm. An ICD is a programmable device able to detect potentially fatal cardiac rhythms and generate large electrical impulses to abolish those rhythms. The use of these devices has increased dramatically during the past few decades and will continue to do so as technology advances and the US population ages. Emergency physicians must have a basic understanding of PM and ICD function and be familiar with the possible complications of these devices. The indications for PM and ICD placement are found in **Boxes 16** and **17**, respectively.[66]

A PM is composed of 3 basic components: the leads or wires, the electrodes, and the pulse generator. The leads communicate between the electrodes and the pulse generator. The electrodes have sensing and pacing abilities and may be TV or epicardial. They are connected to a hermetically sealed box, commonly of 1 to 2 in diameter, which houses the pulse generator (**Fig. 11**). The pulse generator contains a battery and a circuit board. The circuit board is a minicomputer that processes information from the heart and responds to that information. The pulse generator is typically embedded into a pocket created in the anterior chest wall just beneath the clavicle, although it may be found in other locations on the torso. The PM may be programmed to pace continuously or only as needed, termed "on demand" (**Fig. 12**).

Similar to PMs, ICDs are composed of a pulse generator and electrodes capable of sensing and pacing. In addition, ICDs have electrodes that are capable of defibrillation. Technology has advanced such that one lead is capable of housing all sensing, pacing, and defibrillation functions, although there are many models with multiple leads that are still in use. There is also one or more larger coils that dissipate heat during high-voltage impulses. Electrodes sense the intrinsic rhythm and have preset thresholds for pacer and defibrillation functions. Modern ICDs incorporate multiple algorithmic programs that allow for different ICD responses according to the rhythms sensed, such as low-energy cardioversion or high-energy defibrillation.

PM Modes

There are numerous PM modes; the North American Society of Pacing and Electrophysiology and the British Pacing and Electrophysiology Group[67] classify them using a 5-position lettering system. Most PMs use only the first 3 positions. It is important to understand the basics of PM classification to better troubleshoot potential device complications (**Table 2**). Here is an illustrative example: In AAI mode, the intrinsic heart rate is sensed in the atrial chamber (position II = A). The response to the sensed event is to inhibit PM pacing (position III = I). If there is no intrinsic heart rate sensed, the atrial chamber is paced at a prespecified rate (position I = A). The most common modes are DDD, DDDR, VVIR, and AAIR.

Box 14
Tips and troubleshooting

TC pacing

- In women, place the pads under the breast tissue rather than over it.
- Place the pads as far from an implanted device as possible, at least 8 cm.

TV insertion

- If the balloon inflation syringe does not spontaneously fill with air when the inflation port is released, remove the catheter and check the integrity of the balloon.
- Do not attempt to aspirate air from the balloon, as it can cause it to rupture.
- If the catheter advances past the right ventricle, withdraw it into the right atrium, give it a twist, and readvance it.
- If ectopy develops during catheter advancement, withdraw the catheter until the ectopy stops and readvance it.
- Lidocaine can help desensitize the myocardium if ectopy persists.
- Contact with the right ventricle is shown by an ST elevation pattern, or "current of injury," on the ECG tracing.

Confirming capture

- The ECG tracing should demonstrate an LBBB pattern.
- If an RBBB pattern is seen, the catheter is probably in the coronary sinus or left ventricle because of perforation of the septum.
- Electrical capture does not equal mechanical capture. Check the patient for a corresponding pulse.
- Auscultation of the heart may reveal a small murmur secondary to tricuspid insufficiency from the catheter presence, a clicking sound, or paradoxic splitting of S2.

CPR

- VT and VF secondary to the PM are rare. Another cause should be sought.
- Defibrillation and cardioversion are safe with temporary PMs.
- Chest compressions can be performed over the pads. There is no danger of electrical injury due to insulation of the electrodes, but minor shocks may be felt by health care personnel in contact with the pads.

Chest radiograph

- A properly placed catheter will appear on the AP view of a chest radiograph as pointing slightly inferior and near the lateral border of the heart. The tip points anteriorly on the lateral view.
- If the catheter is pointing away from the chest wall on the lateral view of the radiograph, it is probably in the coronary sinus.
- Catheter tip outside the cardiac silhouette suggests myocardial perforation.

In the presence of a permanent PM

- Severe bradycardia or asystole may occur if the temporary PM fails to capture and the permanent PM senses the signals and inhibits pacing.

Abbreviations: AP, anteroposterior; VT, ventricular tachycardia.

Box 15
Failure to capture—troubleshooting

- Check generator battery.
- Obtain chest radiograph to evaluate lead placement.
- Reposition adhesive pads on chest wall.
- Check electrical contacts and connections.
- Increase output current.
- Decrease sensitivity setting to induce asynchronous pacing.
- Evaluate for pneumothorax, pericardial effusion, or tamponade.
- Evaluate for hypoxia, acidosis, and electrolyte abnormalities.
- Obtain ECG to assess rhythm and presence of myocardial ischemia.

Approach to the Patient with Potential PM or ICD Complications

Patients with device complications may present with a variety of symptoms, which are usually nonspecific (**Box 18**). The standard approach includes assessing hemodynamic stability, obtaining device information, and performing a 12-leadECG. PMs and ICDs record a large amount of information. The device manufacturer typically has an electrophysiology technician who comes to the ED and interrogates the device to determine if it functions properly, if shocks are delivered appropriately, or if an arrhythmia is present. Adjustments in the preset values and thresholds can be

---

Box 16
Indications for PM placement

- Symptomatic second- and third-degree heart block[a]
- Asymptomatic second- and third-degree heart block with
  - Greater than 3-s periods of asystole
  - Escape rate less than 40 bpm
  - Presence of neuromuscular disorders
- Bifascicular or trifascicular block
  - Intermittent third-degree heart block
  - Type II second-degree heart block with alternating bundle branch block
- Post-ST-segment elevation myocardial infarction with
  - Third-degree heart block
  - Second-degree infranodal block with alternating bundle branch block
- Also recommended for
  - Symptomatic bradycardia or sinus pauses[a]
  - Recurrent syncope caused by carotid sinus hypersensitivity
  - Hypertrophic cardiomyopathy with sinus node or atrioventricular dysfunction
  - Prevention or termination of some types of tachyarrhythmias

[a] Symptoms include syncope or presyncope, fatigue, seizures, congestive heart failure, or confusion.

> **Box 17**
> **Indications for ICD placement**
>
> - SCA or unstable sustained VT without an identifiable cause that is completely reversible
> - Structural heart disease with stable or unstable sustained VT
> - Syncope of undetermined origin with hemodynamically significant sustained VT or VF induced at electrophysiologic study
> - LVEF 35% or less secondary to myocardial infarction at greater than 40 days post–myocardial infarction in those with NYHA functional class II or III
> - LVEF 30% or less secondary to myocardial infarction at greater than 40 days post–myocardial infarction in those with NYHA functional class I
> - LVEF 35% or less with nonischemic dilated cardiomyopathy in those with NYHA functional class II or III
> - Nonsustained VT due to prior myocardial infarction, LVEF 40% or less, and inducible VF or sustained VT at electrophysiologic study
> - Also consider for
>   - Hypertrophic cardiomyopathy
>   - Unexplained syncope with a history of LV dysfunction
>   - Cardiomyopathy
>   - Brugada syndrome
>   - Long QT syndrome
>
> *Abbreviations:* LV, left ventricular; LVEF, left ventricular ejection fraction; NYHA, New York Heart Association; SCA, sudden cardiac arrest.

made to optimize device function. Battery depletion and lead fractures can also be detected. If interrogation is not available, an attempt can be made to assess the function of the device through careful examination of the ECG and magnet application. If the underlying problem cannot be determined, the patient may require consultation with a cardiologist and/or admission to the hospital. **Box 19** provides a general approach to the patient with potential PM or ICD complications. Unstable patients require prompt treatment following advanced cardiac life support (ACLS) algorithms, with the addition of application of a magnet in the case of PMs.

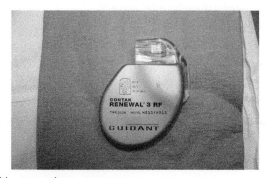

Fig. 11. Implantable pacemaker.

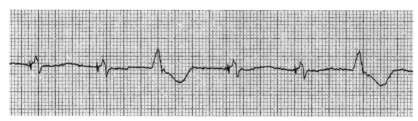

Fig. 12. Demand pacing. First 2 ventricular beats are initiated by the pacemaker. The third beat is the patient's native ventricular beat, which occurs before it is time for a pacer spike to be generated.

Electrocardiographic Interpretation of Paced Rhythms

One should be able to interpret the ECG of paced rhythms to make an assessment regarding the functioning of the PM. Atrial pacing is present if there is a pacer spike followed by a P wave and the patient's intrinsic QRS complex (**Fig. 13**). If there is a pacer spike before every P wave, there is 100% pacing. If there are pacer spikes before only some P waves, then demand pacing is occurring, that is, the PM is firing only when the patient's intrinsic rhythm decreases less than the preset rate.

Ventricular pacing is present when a QRS complex follows a pacer spike on the ECG (**Fig. 14**). Because the ventricular electrode is most commonly positioned in the right

Table 2		
Pacemaker nomenclature		
Position	**Specification**	**Specification Options**
I	Chamber paced	A = Atrium
		V = Ventricle
		D = Dual (A&V)
		O = None
II	Chamber sensed	A = Atrium
		V = Ventricle
		D = Dual (A&V)
		O = None
III	Response to sensed event	I = Inhibited
		T = Triggered
		D = Dual (I & T)
		O = None
IV	Rate modulation, programmability	R = Rate modulation
		P = Simple programmable
		M = Multiprogrammable
		C = Communicating
		O = None
V	Antitachydysrthythmia functions	P = Overdrive pacing
		S = Shock
		D = Dual (pacing and shock)
		O = None

Rate modulation gives the pacemaker the ability to increase the paced rate in response to cardiac demand, such as during exercise. Communicating refers to the device's ability to communicate with external equipment.

Data from Bernstein AD, Daubert JC, Fletcher RD, et al. The revised NASPE/BPEG generic code for antibradycardia, adaptive-rate, and multisite pacing. North American Society of Pacing and Electrophysiology/British Pacing and Electrophysiology Group. Pacing Clin Electrophysiol 2002;25:260.

Box 18
Symptoms of PM/ICD dysfunction

Dizziness

Syncope

Chest pain

Symptoms of congestive heart failure: orthopnea, paroxysmal nocturnal dyspnea, dyspnea on exertion, peripheral edema

Palpitations

Fatigue

Shortness of breath

Shocks

Hiccups

---

ventricle, the wave of conduction propagates from the right ventricle to the left ventricle, creating a QRS morphology resembling that of a left bundle branch block (LBBB).[64] In addition, as the wave of depolarization begins in the ventricles, there may be retrograde conduction through the atrioventricular (AV) node, which is seen

---

Box 19
Approach to the patient with potential PM/ICD complications

- Assess for hemodynamic instability
  - Altered mental status
  - Hypotension
  - Chest pain, myocardial ischemia
  - Respiratory distress
- Place patient on cardiac monitor and established peripheral venous access
- Obtain cardiac and general medical history
  - Medications
  - Elicit signs and symptoms of cardiac ischemia, heart failure, and infection
- Obtain device information
  - Type, model
  - Manufacturer
  - Date of implantation
  - Reason placed
- Conduct a thorough examination of the patient's cardiac and pulmonary systems
- Examination the pocket site
- Obtain posteroanterior and lateral chest radiograph
- Perform 12-lead electrocardiogram, and rhythm strip if necessary
- Measure serum electrolytes and cardiac enzymes
- Have device interrogated

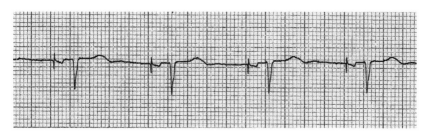

Fig. 13. Atrial pacing. There is 100% pacing with 100% capture—every P wave is preceded by a pacer spike and every pacer spike is followed by a P wave.

as P waves within the T wave, termed retrograde P waves.[68] If the patient has intrinsic atrial activity, there may be dissociated P waves as well. As with atrial pacing, there may be 100% pacing or demand pacing, depending on the patient's intrinsic rate and the PM settings.

Several ECG patterns may be identified in dual chamber PMs. In sequential dual chamber AV pacing, a pacer spike can be identified before each P wave and each QRS complex (**Fig. 15**). During biventricular pacing, the left ventricle is stimulated before the right ventricle, so the wave of depolarization is propagated from the left to right ventricle. The most reliable ECG finding to indicate biventricular pacing is a Q wave in lead I, as the wave of depolarization moves away from this lead. The ECG may also have a Q wave in leads V5 and V6, with a tall R wave in V1, although these findings are less reliable.[69]

Determining cardiac ischemia in paced rhythms is difficult. As discussed earlier, the ventricular pacer is often positioned in the right ventricle, giving rise to an LBBB pattern on ECG. Similar to evaluating patients for ischemic changes in the presence of a preexisting LBBB, Sgarbossa criteria may be used (**Box 20**).[70]

Magnet Application

Placement of a magnet over a PM eliminates sensing and returns the device to asynchronous pacing. Removal of the magnet returns the PM to its preprogrammed mode. If a patient presents with a native heart rate more than the threshold for pacing, no PM spikes are present on the ECG. To aid in assessing the function of the PM, place a magnet over the device (**Fig. 16**). If no pacing occurs, the battery is depleted. Removal of the magnet can induce PM-mediated tachycardia. Reapplying the magnet can treat this. In the case of an ICD, application of the magnet closes a switch in the generator, disabling tachyarrhythmia recognition and treatment. Most ICDs return to

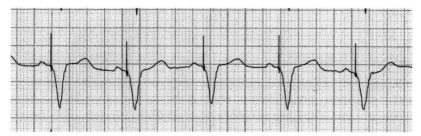

Fig. 14. Ventricular pacing. There is 100% pacing with 100% capture—every QRS complex is preceded by a pacer spike and every pacer spike is followed by a QRS complex.

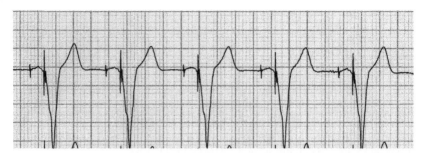

Fig. 15. AV sequential pacing. There is 100% pacing with 100% capture—there is a pacer spike followed by a P wave, then another pacer spike followed by a QRS complex.

normal function after the magnet is removed, but some are programmed to remain disabled. Therefore, it is necessary to have an ICD interrogated after a magnet is used to ensure it is functioning properly.

Chest Radiograph Findings

A chest radiograph is helpful in troubleshooting potential complications. Both poster-oanterior and lateral views should be obtained. It can reveal the presence of a hemo-thorax, pneumothorax, lead displacement, and lead fracture. An overpenetrated film can also identify the manufacturer and model of the device.[71] **Fig. 17** shows proper lead positioning. Similar to PMs, ICDs may have single, dual, or biventricular leads. In addition, there are one or more larger coils that help dissipate heat during high-voltage impulses.

PM AND ICD COMPLICATIONS

A list of pocket complications and their treatment are found in **Table 3** and includes hematomas, infections, wound dehiscence, and migration or erosion of the device through fascial planes.[72,73] Lead Complications may occur soon after implantation or may be delayed.[74,75] **Table 4** gives a list of these complications along with treatment recommendations.

Failure to Pace

Failure to pace can result from either a failure to capture or oversensing. Failure to capture is identified on ECG when a pacer spike is present but is not immediately followed by depolarization of the myocardium (**Fig. 18**). When this occurs immediately postimplantation, it is commonly due to lead dislodgement or malposition. Oversensing occurs when the PM interprets inappropriate signals, such as skeletal muscle

---

Box 20
Sgarbossa criteria: detecting acute myocardial ischemia in ventricular-paced rhythms

- ST-segment elevation of 1 mm or more concordant with (in the same direction as) the QRS complex
- ST-segment elevation of 5 mm or more discordant with (in the opposite direction from) the QRS complex
- ST-segment depression of 1 mm or more in lead V1, V2, or V3

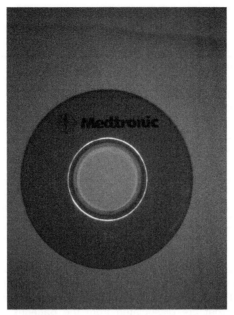

Fig. 16. Pacemaker/ICD magnet.

discharges, as intrinsic impulses, leading to inappropriate inhibition of pacing. This condition should be suspected if the patient's heart rate is lower than the set threshold without pacer spikes identified on ECG interpretation (**Fig. 19**). It can be confirmed by the application of a magnet over the PM pulse generator, which induces uninhibited pacing independent of the sensor function.[76]

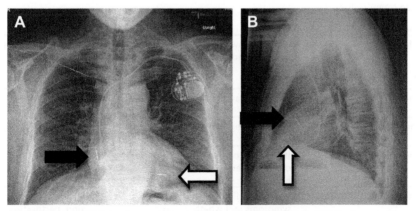

Fig. 17. Proper positioning of pacemaker leads on chest radiograph. (*A*) PA chest radiograph showing pacemaker device over the left upper chest and atrial lead (*solid arrow*) and ventricular lead (*hollow arrow*). (*B*) Lateral film. Atrial (*solid arrow*) and ventricular (*hollow arrow*) leads point toward the anterior chest wall.

Table 3
Pocket complications

Condition	Treatment	Notes
Hematoma	Surgical exploration	Common after implantation Do not attempt aspiration in the ED
Infection	Surgical removal of the device Empiric antibiotic therapy	Early infection—*Staphylococcus aureus* Late infection—*Staphylococcus epidermidis*
Wound dehiscence	Surgical debridement and reapproximation of the wound edges	Rare, occurs early after implantation
Migration	No treatment necessary if device is functioning properly	Happens slowly over time
Erosion	Relocation of the device	May cause PM failure

Inappropriate Pacing

With failure to sense or undersensing, the intrinsic atrial or ventricular beats are not recognized and the PM paces at its predetermined rate. In this situation, an ECG shows pacer spikes that are dissociated from the patient's intrinsic rhythm. As such, the interval between the intrinsic and paced complexes are variable (**Fig. 20**). There are a variety of causes for failure to pace and inappropriate pacing (**Box 21**).

COMPLICATIONS SPECIFIC TO PACEMAKERS

PM-mediated tachycardia (PMT) is seen with older dual chamber PMs and may occur spontaneously or after magnet application.[76] It is caused by a premature ventricular contraction that conducts retrograde through the AV node, which is interpreted by the PM as an intrinsic stimulus, and the PM stimulates the ventricles to depolarize.

Table 4
Lead complications

Condition	Treatment	Notes
Infection	Surgical removal of the leads Empiric antibiotics	Early infection—*Staphylococcus aureus* Late infection—*Staphylococcus epidermidis*
Hemothorax	Chest tube placement	Usually present within 48 h of implantation
Pneumothorax	Chest tube placement if >10%	Usually present within 48 h of implantation
Venous thrombosis	Anticoagulation with IV heparin or low-molecular-weight heparin	Surgery may be necessary in cases of superior vena cava syndrome
Dislodgement, migration	Varies depending on patient's symptoms and whether or not they are PM dependent; consult cardiologist	Can cause pulmonary embolism, PM dysfunction, perforation of the myocardium, cardiac tamponade
Erosion	Relocation of the device	May cause PM failure

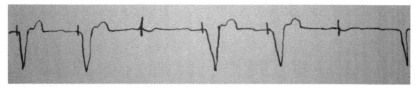

Fig. 18. Failure to capture. There are pacemaker spikes present without subsequent depolarization of the ventricles, as seen by no QRS complex following the pacer spike.

This stimulation establishes an inappropriate circuit or loop of depolarization. It can also occur on removal of a magnet over the device. When identified, a magnet should be applied to break the reentry dysrhythmia. If this fails, adenosine, carotid sinus massage, and TC pacing can also be used.[77,78] Newer PM models have algorithms that prevent or terminate PMT.

Runaway PM is caused by PM generator malfunction causing extreme tachycardia, including ventricular tachycardia (VT) or fibrillation.[76] This phenomenon is uncommon with modern PM technology. It should be managed with the placement of a magnet to induce a slower pacing rate and emergent reprogramming. It may necessitate disconnecting the generator from the leads if the patient is unstable.

PM syndrome is secondary to loss of AV synchrony.[76] Uncoordinated diastolic filling and emptying leads to decreased cardiac output and increased atrial pressures, which may lead to decreased coronary and systemic perfusion as well as congestive heart failure. Treatment involves upgrading the PM to a dual chamber model and treating the associated heart failure.

Twiddler syndrome is a twisting of the leads about the generator from patient manipulation of the pocket and generator,[76] which may cause lead fracture, dislodgement, or migration. Surgical correction is required.

MANAGEMENT OF IMPLANTABLE CARDIOVERTER-DEFIBRILLATION DISCHARGE

Patients who present to the ED after ICD discharge should be evaluated to determine if the discharge was appropriate or inappropriate. **Box 22** gives the management pathways for ICD discharge. It may be difficult to identify cardiac ischemia, as cardiac biomarker elevations may be present secondary to defibrillation.[79,80] ECG changes secondary to defibrillation should return to the patient's baseline in the absence of cardiac ischemia. Electrical storm is a term used to describe the occurrence of 3 or more dysrhythmic events resulting in ICD discharge in a 24-hour period. This event may be secondary to recurrent VT, supraventricular tachycardias (SVTs), or device malfunction.[81]

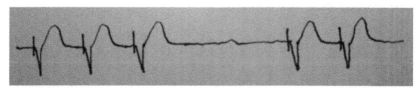

Fig. 19. Oversensing that results in a failure to pace, as seen by an inappropriate pause in pacemaker activity.

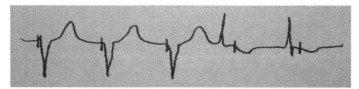

Fig. 20. Failure to sense. There are pacemaker spikes after the last 2 QRS complexes. The first 3 beats are pacemaker generated. Then a native beat follows, which is not sensed by the pacemaker, resulting in a pacer spike being generated after depolarization of the ventricles, at its preprogrammed rate.

Inappropriate ICD discharge is frequently secondary to SVTs.[81] Patients should be treated with standard therapies directed at the underlying rhythm abnormality. It may be necessary for sensing thresholds to be adjusted. **Box 23** lists the causes of ICD discharge.[82]

SUDDEN CARDIAC ARREST IN THE PRESENCE OF A PM OR ICD

Sudden cardiac arrest (SCA) in patients with PMs or ICDs should be managed following standard ACLS recommendations, with resuscitative efforts directed at the presenting dysrhythmia. Placement of external pads should be at least 8 cm away from the device, without compromising the efficacy of the defibrillation effort.[83] Antiarrhythmic drugs can affect the function of PMs, but ACLS protocols should still be followed. It may be necessary to deactivate the ICD during cardiac arrest, as this provides better control over defibrillation efforts. In addition, SVTs are common during cardiopulmonary resuscitation and can trigger ICD discharges that may induce VT or fibrillation.[84] The ICD should also be deactivated if resuscitative efforts are unsuccessful. To deactivate the ICD, a magnet is applied directly over the generator (see **Fig. 16**). It may be appropriate to secure the magnet to the chest with tape for continued effect, as most devices return to normal function when the magnet is removed. Devices should be assessed for damage after external defibrillation.[85]

Box 21
Common reasons for failure to pace or inappropriate pacing

- Battery depletion
- Lead fracture
- Lead migration, dislodgement
- Device thresholds set too high or too low
- Interference from skeletal myopotentials or electromagnetic fields
- Elevated pacing thresholds
  - Antiarrhythmia drugs, other medications
  - Acute myocardial ischemia
  - Electrolyte abnormalities
  - Defibrillation
  - Inflammation or fibrosis
  - Metabolic acidosis or alkalosis

Box 22
Management of ICD discharge in the ED

Asymptomatic, single discharge

• Outpatient follow-up with cardiologist

Symptomatic or multiple discharges

• Cardiac monitoring

• Measure electrolytes and cardiac enzymes

• Obtain 12-lead ECG

• Interrogate device

• Obtain PAL chest radiograph

• Consult with cardiology

• Admission or discharge depending on the results of the evaluation

---

MANAGEMENT OF TACHYARRHYTHMIAS IN THE ED

Tachyarrhythmias are not uncommon in the ED. Prompt recognition and treatment of the specific arrhythmia can be lifesaving. By having a standardized approach to these patients, the emergency physician can quickly and confidently make decisions to optimize the care of the patient while minimizing serious complications.

It is helpful to divide tachyarrhythmias into either narrow or wide QRS complex rhythms. Narrow complex tachycardias (NCTs) have a QRS duration less than 120 ms and are generally due to increased normal or abnormal automaticity and the presence of an accessory pathway ("reentry") that creates a circuit of electrical activity and depolarization or are triggered by medications or ischemia. **Table 5** shows a list NCTs and their specific features.

Wide complex tachycardias (WCTs) have a QRS complex greater than 120 ms and 4 main causes: VT, SVT in the presence of aberrant conduction that is either preexisting or rate related, or antidromic AV reentrant tachycardia from Wolfe Parkinson White (WPW) syndrome.[86] In WPW, electrical depolarization occurs along an accessory pathway in the antegrade direction and then along the Bundle of His/AV node or another accessory pathway in the retrograde direction, creating an endless loop of electrical

---

Box 23
Causes of ICD discharge

Appropriate

• In response to VT or fibrillation

Inappropriate

• In response to SVT

• Lead fracture

• Sensing of environmental electrical noise

Phantom

• Patients who have experienced a painful shock in the past may think they received a shock when they did not

Table 5
Narrow complex tachycarrhythmias

Rhythm	Mechanism	Features
ST	Accelerated sinus rate, usually in response to a stressor	P wave preceding every QRS, regular, rate 100–160 bpm
AT	Enhanced or abnormal automaticity	P wave preceding every QRS, regular, rate 120–250 bpm
JT	Abnormal enhanced automaticity	P waves may be retrograde, dissociated from the QRS or absent
MAT	Multiple atrial foci	Irregular, 3 different P waves present
AF	Irregular, chaotic depolarization of the atria	No P waves, irregularly irregular, rate 300–600 bpm
Afl	Reentry circuit involving a large area of the atrial myocardium	"Saw-toothed" P waves, rate 250–350 bpm, AV conduction often 2:1 with ventricular rate of 150
AVNRT	Reentry—2 distinct pathways with different electrical properties in the AV node	May have retrograde P waves but no P waves regularly associated with the QRS complex, 120–250 bpm, usually regular, most common form of PSVT
AVRT	Preexcitation due to an accessory pathway between the atria and ventricles	May have retrograde P waves, regular, 150–200 bpm, narrow QRS in orthodromic conduction, wide QRS in antidromic conduction

When P waves merge into the preceding T wave, they are called retrograde P waves. They occur because of retrograde conduction of the impulse from the ventricle to the atrium.

Abbreviations: AF, atrial fibrillation; Afl, atrial flutter; AT, atrial tachycardia; AVNRT, atrioventricular nodal reentry tachycardia; AVRT, atrioventricular reentry tachycardia; JT, junctional tachycardia; MAT, multifocal atrial tachycardia; PSVT, paroxysmal supraventricular tachycardia; ST, sinus tachycardia.

activity.[87] The treatments for these conditions are different, and the cause of a WCT should be determined. Inappropriate treatment of VT can result in sudden deterioration. If this determination is not possible, one should always assume the rhythm is VT and treat accordingly. **Table 6** gives the specific characteristics of WCT rhythms.

Hemodynamic stability must be quickly assessed in the presence of a tachyarrhythmia. Signs of instability are hypotension, altered mental status, pulmonary edema or respiratory distress, myocardial ischemia, or chest pain. If the patient is unstable, plans should be made for immediate cardioversion or defibrillation (**Fig. 21**). If the patient is stable, the next important step is close analysis of the ECG to determine the rhythm. It is also important to assess the patient's risk for, or known presence of, cardiac disease and obtain a complete list of medications including prescription, over-the-counter, and recreational drug use. **Box 24** provides a general outline of the approach to tachyarrhythmias.

Narrow Complex Tachycardias

If P waves are present for every QRS, then the rhythm is atrial tachycardia (AT), multifocal atrial tachycardia (MAT), or ST, and treatment is aimed at correcting the underlying cause. If the patient does not tolerate the tachycardia and it cannot be quickly corrected, IV beta-blockers (BBs) or calcium channel blockers (CCBs) are used cautiously to decrease the rate.[88]

For all other NCTs of undetermined rhythm, vagal maneuvers and adenosine can be tried, which may allow identification of the underlying rhythm by temporarily slowing the conduction through the AV node[89,90] In addition, reentry tachycardias often

Table 6
Ventricular tachycardias

Rhythm	Characteristics	Example
Monomorphic VT	Uniform QRS complexes	
Polymorphic VT	Changing QRS complexes	
Torsades de pointes	Twisting of the QRS peaks around the isoelectric baseline	
Ventricular flutter	Regular, monophasic, no isoelectric interval, rate 300 bpm	
Ventricular fibrillation	Rapid >300 bpm, grossly irregular, marked variability in QRS morphology and amplitude	

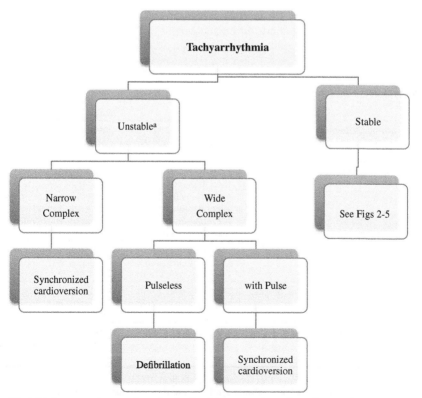

Fig. 21. Initial approach to tachyarrhythmias. [a] Hypotension, altered mental status, myocardial ischemia, chest pain, respiratory distress.

Box 24
Initial approach to tachyarrhythmias

Assess for hemodynamic instability

    Hypotension, altered mental status, myocardial ischemia, chest pain, respiratory distress

Obtain IV access, establish cardiopulmonary monitoring

If unstable, prepare for immediate defibrillation or synchronized cardioversion

If stable, complete evaluation

    Examine ECG to determine rhythm

    Assess for risk of, or presence of, heart disease

    Determine medications being taken by the patient including stimulant use

    Obtain chest radiograph and laboratory analysis of electrolytes, cardiac enzymes, renal function, complete blood count, and possibly thyroid function

Initiate treatment appropriate for the rhythm

Repeat ECG after rhythm converts or slows to identify underlying WPW or cardiac ischemia

Admit for further evaluation and treatment as indicated by the condition present[a]

[a] Patients with paroxysmal SVT are at extremely low risk for sudden death and can be discharged if the arrhythmia is terminated and they are asymptomatic.

---

terminate with resumption of normal sinus rhythm (NSR). It is often difficult to differentiate among the different SVTs, and electrophysiologic studies may be needed but typically do not affect the short-term management in the ED. If these methods do not terminate the rhythm, rate control should be attempted. **Table 7** lists the most

Table 7
Rate control medications

Drug	Mechanism	Dose	Notes
Metoprolol	Beta blocker	5 mg IV over 1–2 min q5-15 min maximum 15 mg	Onset immediately, peak effect at 20 min, duration 5–8 h
Esmolol	Beta blocker	0.5 mg/kg IV over 1 min then 0.05 mg/kg/min, increase by 0.05 mg/kg every 4 min up to 0.2 mg/kg/min can give up to 3 boluses	Use with caution in asthma, COPD and CHF; onset immediate, peak effect by 5 min, duration 10–30 min
Diltiazem	Calcium channel blocker	20 mg IV over 2 min then 5–15 mg/h infusion can repeat bolus q3 min	Onset in 2–3 min, peak effect at 2–7 min, half-life of 1–3 h
Verapamil	Calcium channel blocker	2.5–5 mg IV over 2 min can repeat q15–30 min	Onset 1–5 min, peak effect 10 min, duration 0.5–6 h
Digoxin	Cardiac glycoside	0.4–0.6 mg IV	Onset 5–30 min, peak effect 1.5–4 h, duration 3–4 d

Beta-blockers and calcium channel blockers are contraindicated in the presence of second- or third-degree heart block, Wolfe Parkinson White syndrome, and ventricular tachycardia.
Abbreviation: CHF, congestive heart failure.

common medications available for rate control. A summary of the approach to stable NCTs is found in **Fig. 22**.

An irregular rhythm without P waves suggests atrial fibrillation (AF) or atrial flutter (Afl).[89] If either rhythm is suspected, it is important to determine the duration of the tachycardia and the presence of LV dysfunction to guide further management. If the arrhythmia has been present for less than 48 hours, conversion to NSR is desirable and is accomplished with either electrical or pharmacologic methods.[86] If it has been for more than 48 hours, there is an increased risk of embolization from the presence of an atrial thrombus.[91,92] If rhythm control is still desired, the patient is administered warfarin for 3 weeks with subsequent electrical cardioversion or heparin in the ED with a transesophageal echocardiogram (TEE) to rule out atrial thrombus before electrical cardioversion.[93] Rate control is desired in the short term. If the patient has normal LV function, IV BBs and CCBs are first-line treatment, followed by amiodarone.[94] Digoxin may be used, but it has a much slower onset of action. If the patient's ejection fraction is less than 40%, digoxin is the first-line treatment.[94] BBs, CCBs, and amiodarone should be used with caution in this situation. **Fig. 23** summarizes the approach to rapid AF and Afl.

Disposition of patients presenting with NCTs depends on the underlying cause, persistence of symptoms or arrhythmia, and presence of underlying heart disease. The risk of sudden cardiac death (SCD) from a paroxysmal SVT is extremely small, and these patients can be discharged if the tachycardia has been terminated.[95] Patients with evidence of WPW require risk stratification to determine if they are at high risk of sudden death; this is typically done with cardiac electrophysiologic studies. The patient with new-onset AF/Afl is generally admitted to a monitored bed, although if the rhythm has converted and the patient is otherwise healthy, discharge is reasonable after consultation with the cardiologist. Certain patients with known paroxysmal AF who have converted to NSR may also be discharged after consultation with the cardiologist.

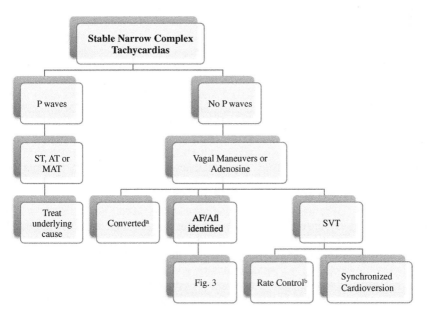

Fig. 22. Treatment of stable narrow complex tachycardias. [a] Likely a supraventricular tachycardia, [b] with calcium channel blocker or beta blocker.

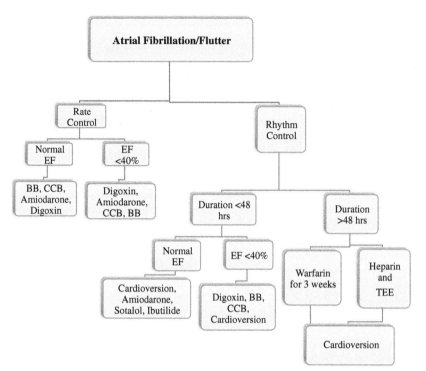

Fig. 23. Treatment of atrial fibrillation and atrial flutter. EF, ejection fraction; TEE, transeso-phageal echocardiogram. BB, beta blocker; CCB, calcium channel blocker.

Wide Complex Tachycardias

WCTs are either ventricular or supraventricular in origin. In unselected populations, a WCT is VT about 80% of the time and almost always (95%) if the patient has had a previous myocardial infarction.[96–98] **Table 8** lists elements of the history and ECG that strongly suggest the rhythm is VT.[99,100] There are also algorithms available to help diagnose VT from other WCTs, but they are complex, time consuming to sort through, difficult to remember, and not completely sensitive or specific.[100–103] VT and antidromic atrioventricular reentry tachycardia (AVRT) (WPW) are particularly difficult to differentiate. AVRT is uncommon, occurring about 6% of the time.[104] If the diagnosis is still unclear after evaluation of the ECG, the safest approach is to treat it as VT, as therapies for SVTs can precipitate cardiac arrest in patients with VT.[96,97,105] If the emergency physician is certain that the rhythm is SVT with aberrancy, it can be treated in the standard approach for SVTs.

Monomorphic VT is treated with immediate synchronized cardioversion, or if the patient is stable, antiarrhythmic medications are initiated (**Fig. 24**). Polymorphic VT (pVT), also known as torsades de pointes, has a continuously varying QRS complex. It should be treated with synchronized cardioversion. Higher energies may be needed with WCTs than with NCTs. Sedation and/or analgesia should be provided before therapy. Treatment of recurrent or refractory pVT depends on the baseline QT interval; if it is prolonged, overdrive pacing, magnesium, isoproterenol, lidocaine, or BBs can be used. Withdrawing the offending agent and correcting electrolyte abnormalities should be a priority. **Box 25** gives a list of drugs that can prolong the QT interval. If

Table 8
Differentiating ventricular tachycardia from other wide complex tachycardias

Characteristic	VT	SVT
More common	X	
History of heart disease or physical findings suggestive of heart disease—sternotomy scar, PM/ICD, signs of PAD, CHF	X	
Presence of ICD	X	
History of SVT		X
Age < 35 y		X
QRS morphology similar to morphology during NSR		X
Slight rhythm irregularity	X	
QRS duration > 160 ms	X	
Variation in the QRS and ST-T shape	X	
Concordance		
QRS complexes in V1-V6 are monophasic with the same polarity	X	
AV dissociation—Atrial activity that is independent of ventricular activity		
Dissociated P waves—P waves not consistently coupled to QRS	X	
Fusion beats—QRS complex intermediate to sinus beat & ventricular complex	X	
Capture beats—QRS complexes during WCT that are identical to sinus complex	X	

These features are more characteristic of the rhythm indicated, but their absence does not exclude that rhythm.
Abbreviations: CHF, congestive heart failure; PAD, peripheral artery disease.

the QT interval is normal, antiarrhythmic medications should be used. Class I and III antiarrhythmic drugs are usually reserved for refractory or recurrent arrhythmias as a result of their side-effect profile (**Table 9**). Frequent episodes of VT requiring cardioversion is called "VT storm." The single most effective treatment of this condition is IV BB agents.[106] **Fig. 25** gives an algorithm for the treatment of pVT. A patient presenting with VT will require cardiology consultation and admission to a monitored bed or intensive care unit (ICU) if arrhythmia is recurrent or refractory.

TACHYARRHYTHMIAS IN CHILDREN

The initial approach is similar to that in adults. First, determine hemodynamic stability. In infants, this may present as irritability, tachypnea, or poor feeding; if unstable, initiate cardioversion with 0.5 to 2.0 J/kg.[107] If stable, continue evaluation by scrutinizing the ECG and using vagal maneuvers and adenosine for NCTs to help identify or convert the rhythm. The most common causes of SVT in children are reentry tachycardia due to AVRT (WPW) and atrioventricular nodal reentry tachycardia (AVNRT).

SPECIFIC THERAPIES

If the patient is stable, an attempt should be made to identify or convert the narrow complex tachyarrhythmia. Vagal maneuvers generally work by temporarily slowing the conduction through the sinoatrial or the AV node. **Table 10** gives a list of vagal maneuvers along with their indications and contraindications. Adenosine slows conduction through the AV node and is effective at terminating AVNRT and AVRT and at unmasking atrial activity that is difficult to appreciate at rapid rates. It does not have any effect on ST or AT and usually does not terminate AF or Afl. Adenosine

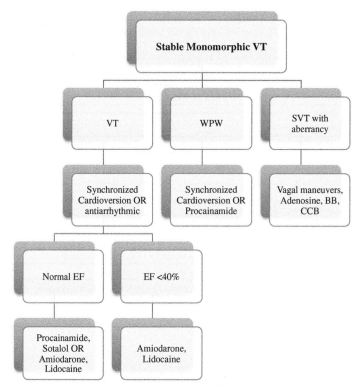

Fig. 24. Treatment of monomorphic VT. EF, ejection fraction.

has been contraindicated in VT, but a recent retrospective analysis showed that in 197 patients receiving it for undifferentiated WCT, there were no dysrhythmia complications. Only 2% of those who were determined to have had VT converted after administration adenosine, while 90% of those with SVT converted. The investigators suggest that adenosine is safe and useful as a diagnostic aid in undifferentiated WCTs.[108] There is only one case report in the literature of adenosine-induced VF in a patient with stable VT.[109] **Box 26** gives details regarding adenosine. These therapies can have complications and should be performed under continuous cardiac monitoring with IV access established and resuscitative equipment at hand.

SPECIAL CONSIDERATIONS

Arrhythmias secondary to digitalis toxicity have a unique treatment algorithm. Minor cases are managed by discontinuation of the drug and monitoring. If there are sustained ventricular arrhythmias, the patient should receive digoxin-specific Fab antibody. Temporary pacing, or emergent dialysis if there is concomitant hyperkalemia, may be necessary. Atrial fibrillation in patients with underlying WPW can degenerate into VF with adenosine, so it should be used with caution if WPW is a possible mechanism. Adenosine has been reported to cause a variety of arrhythmias, such as bradycardia, complete heart block, nonsustained VT, transient asystole, and AF.[110–113] Caution should be used when using more than one rate control or antiarrhythmic medication on a patient, as it can precipitate arrhythmias. **Box 27** shows a list of important points to remember in diagnosing and treating tachyarrhythmias.

Box 25
Drugs known to prolong the QT interval

- Antiarrhythmics
  - Amiodarone, disopyramide, dofetilide, flecainide, ibutilide
  - Procainamide, quinidine, sotalol
- Antiinfectives
  - Chloroquine, clarithromycin, erythromycin, moxifloxacin
  - Pentamidine, sparfloxacin
- Antipsychotics
  - Chlorpromazine, haloperidol, mesoridazine, pimozide, thioridazine
- Citalopram
- Levomethadyl
- Methadone
- Probucol
- Tefenadine
- Vendetanib

Drugs that may prolong the QT interval

- Antiinfectives
  - Amantadine, azithromycin, foscarnet, gatifloxacin, levofloxacin
  - Ofloxacin, telithromycin
- Antipsychotics
  - Clozapine, quetiapine, risperidone, ziprasidone
- Octreotide
- Atazanavir
- Chloral hydrate
- Dolasetron
- Escitalopram
- Famotidine
- Fosphenytoin
- Lithium
- Nicardipine
- Ondansetron
- Oxytocin
- Ranolazine
- Tacrolimus
- Tamoxifen
- Tizanidine
- Vardenafil
- Venlafaxine

---

[a] Diuretics can cause prolongation of the QT indirectly by causing hypomagnesemia and hypokalemia. Ives, HE. "Loop Diuretics." In: Basic and Clinical Pharmacology. Ed Katzung BG, 12th edition. USA: McGraw Hill 2012. p. 258–60.
[b] Digoxin toxicity can induce torsades de pointes.
  Data from Arizona Center for Education and Research on Therapeutics. Available at: www.azcert.org, "QT Drug Lists". Accessed November 12, 2011.

Table 9
Antiarrhythmic medications

Drug	Dose	Side Effects
Amiodarone	150 mg IV over 10 min, then 1 mg/min for 6 h, then 0.5 mg/mg for 18 h, Peds: 5 mg/kg IV over 30 min, then 5–15 mcg/kg/min infusion	Can repeat the bolus; maximum 2.2 g in 24 h. Pediatric dosing is off-label. Can cause hypotension (infusion rate dependent), long half-life. Contraindicated in second- and third-degree heart block
Procainamide	20–50 mg/min IV to total of 17 mg/kg Peds: 15 mg/kg IV over 30 min, then 0.02–0.08 mg/kg/min IV	Hypotension, QT prolongation. Reduce dose for renal or cardiac impairment, contraindicated in second- and third-degree heart block
Lidocaine	1–1.5 mg/kg over 2–3 min, then 1–4 mg/min infusion, Peds: 0.5–1 mg/kg slow IV, then 20–50 µg/kg/min infusion	Can repeat the bolus, maximum dose 3 mg/kg. Can cause hypotension, gastrointestinal upset. Contraindicated in second- and third-degree heart block
Sotalol	75 mg IV	May prolong QT interval, cause dizziness, dyspnea, chest pain. Avoid in second- and third-degree heart block, asthma, and hypokalemia

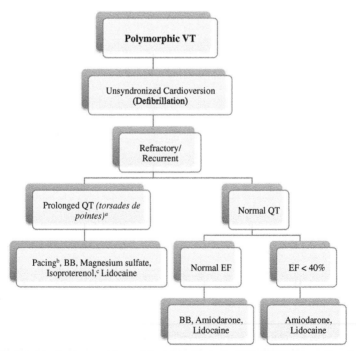

Fig. 25. Treatment of polymorphic ventricular tachycardia (VT). [a] Withdraw offending agent and correct electrolytes. [b] For drug-induced prolongation. [c] For noncongenital prolongation. EF, ejection fraction.

Table 10
Vagal maneuvers

Maneuver	Indications	Contraindications	Complications
Diving Reflex Place bag of ice and water on face for 15–30 s, or submerge face in water or drip cold water down the nares	Children	—	—
Rectal stimulation Insert rectal thermometer	Infants	—	—
Carotid massage With patient supine, head turned away, apply vigorous circular pressure over carotid artery at level of cricoid cartilage	Adults	History of TIA or CVA Children, Infants Carotid bruit MI in past 6 mo History of VT or VF Digoxin toxicity	Profound hypotension and bradycardia Loss of consciousness TIA CVA Arrhythmia
Valsalva Exhale against a closed glottis, cough	Children Adults	—	—
Lowering the head of the bed occasionally converts an SVT, presumably by stretching the carotid bulb	Infant Children Adults	—	—

Abbreviations: CVA, cerebrovascular accident; MI, myocardial infarction; TIA, transient ischemic attack.

CARDIOVERSION, DEFIBRILLATION, AND CARDIAC ARREST IN THE ED
Cardioversion and Defibrillation

Cardioversion involves the application of electrical energy across the chest wall and myocardium that is synchronized with the QRS complex.[58] The brief burst of electrical current momentarily causes depolarization of most of the cardiac cells and allows the

Box 26
Adenosine

Adenosine blocks AV nodal conduction. It is useful in converting SVTs by interrupting the accessory pathway. It may also slow down the ventricular response sufficiently to identify the underlying rhythm. It has an onset of 20 to 30 seconds and a duration of 10 seconds and is cleared in 30 seconds. Patients often experience flushing, chest pain, or dizziness. It can cause hypotension, second- or third-degree heart block, AF or Afl, VT, or VF. It often results in 2 to 3 seconds of asystole, but occasionally is more prolonged than that.

The dose is 6 mg IVP over 1 to 3 seconds immediately followed by 20 mL normal saline flush. It should be administered as proximally as possible to the central circulation because of its short half-life of less than 10 seconds. The dose is doubled to 12 mg and repeated after 2 minutes if there is no response from the initial dose. If the patient weighs less than 50 kg, start with 0.1 mg/kg. If uneffective, double the dose and repeat. The maximum dose is 0.3 mg/kg/dose.

It is contraindicated in patients taking digoxin and dipyridamole. It should also not be used in patients with WCTs who are irregular or have a history of WPW. Avoid if patient has second- or third-degree heart block. It is a pregnancy class C drug.

Box 27
Important points to remember in diagnosing and treating tachyarrhythmias

- If there is any doubt about whether the WCT is VT, treat it as VT.

- Adenosine, BBs and CCBs are contraindicated in VT and antidromic (wide complex) WPW syndrome.

- Obtain an ECG after the rhythm converts or slows to look for cardiac ischemia or evidence of underlying WPW syndrome.

- Procainamide exacerbates heart failure and prolongs the QT; therefore, it is contraindicated with LV dysfunction and torsades de pointes.

- Rapid AF caused by a preexcitation syndrome such as WPW syndrome can degenerate into VF after administration of AV nodal blocking agents by increasing the conduction via the accessory pathway.

- Arrhythmias secondary to digoxin toxicity should be treated with digoxin-specific Fab antibody and temporary TC or TV pacing.

- Using multiple AV nodal blocking agents and/or antiarrhythmia drugs in the same patient should be performed only when absolutely necessary and with caution, as it can precipitate other dysrhythmias.

---

sinus node to resume normal PM function, or in the case of reentry tachyarrhythmias, by interrupting the self-perpetuating circuit. In contrast to defibrillation, this delivery of electrical energy is synchronized with the peak of the R wave, when the ventricles are in an absolute refractory period. Synchronization is imperative, as attempted depolarization during the vulnerable refractory phase of the ventricles can generate disorganized ventricular myocyte excitation, leading to VT or fibrillation.[58]

Defibrillation is the nonsynchronized delivery of electrical energy across the chest wall and myocardium used to terminate chaotic or rapid ventricular activity by depolarizing the myocardium.[58] The unorganized electrical activity that occurs during VF produces inadequate pump function and cardiac output. This rhythm is rapidly fatal, leading to SCA if not abolished immediately. VT is a more organized rapid ventricular rhythm that carries a high potential to degenerate into VF, although this rhythm may be tolerated for some time without clinical decompensation. Pulseless VT indicates cardiac pump failure and should be treated in the same manner as VF.

SCA Overview

Each year in the United States, there are 400,000 to 460,000 unexpected SCDs.[114] The median survival for out-of-hospital cardiac arrest is less than 10%.[115] SCD is the cessation of cardiac activity in the setting of hemodynamic collapse most often due to sustained VF or tachycardia.[116] Hypoperfusion of the heart and brain occurs, which clinically manifests as loss of consciousness, apnea, or agonal respirations and loss of pulses. If not reversed rapidly, SCD ensues. The most common cause is structural heart disease, usually coronary heart disease.[114,117] Management of SCD in the ED involves identification of cardiac dysrhythmias, appropriate use of cardiac defibrillation, identification and treatment of reversible causes of SCA, and immediate postresuscitative care in the event of return of spontaneous circulation (ROSC).

Indications for cardioversion are listed in **Box 28**. An unstable tachycardia is defined as one in which the patient is experiencing hypotension, chest pain or myocardial ischemia, respiratory distress, signs of heart failure, or altered mental status.

Box 28
Indications for synchronized electrical cardioversion

Unstable VT with a pulse

Unstable SVTs

    AV nodal reentrant tachycardia

    AV reentrant tachycardia (preexcitation syndromes: WPW, LGL)

    AF with rapid ventricular response

    Afl with rapid ventricular response

Failed pharmacologic cardioversion/rate control of tachyarrhythmias

Anticipated complications from prolonged tachycardia—ischemia, clot formation

Abbreviation: LGL, Lown-Ganong-Levine syndrome.

Indications for immediate defibrillation are listed in **Box 29**. pVT is identified by beat-to-beat variations in QRS morphology, as compared with the uniform appearance of QRS complexes in monomorphic VT (**Fig. 26**). In cases of SCA for greater than 4 to 5 minutes or if down time is unknown, current guidelines recommend cardiopulmonary resuscitation (CPR) be performed for 2 minutes before attempted defibrillation.[51,118] In theory, this increases coronary perfusion and chances of successful ROSC.

Contraindications to cardioversion include tachycardias secondary to enhanced automaticity such as sinus tachycardia or digitalis toxicity. If AF and Afl with rapid ventricular response have been present for greater than 48 hours, cardioversion is not recommended until the absence of an atrial thrombus is established by transesophageal echocardiography or the patient is sufficiently anticoagulated.[91,94]

Contraindications to defibrillation include PEA, asystole, presence of a pulse, and institution of a do not resuscitate (DNR) order (**Box 30**).

The list of equipment necessary for cardioversion and defibrillation is found in **Box 31**. There are a variety of different defibrillators in use today. Most commonly used defibrillators include a cardiac monitor and have both defibrillation and cardioversion capabilities. When using a defibrillator with an intrinsic cardiac monitor, it is necessary to ensure that the patient is connected to the electrodes specific to that monitor for the defibrillator to detect the patient's rhythm. The capacitor is charged to a prespecified energy level, which is delivered via electrodes applied to the patient. **Fig. 27** shows proper placement of the adhesive pad or paddles. Current waveforms may be monophasic or biphasic, although biphasic defibrillators have largely replaced monophasic defibrillators, as they have been shown to be slightly more effective and require lower energy.[119–121] **Table 11** depicts the recommended energy levels. It is important to become familiar with the specific equipment available in one's work place before the need to use it.

Box 29
Indications for defibrillation

VF

Pulseless VT

Unstable pVT (torsades de pointes)

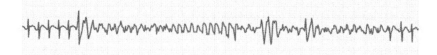

Fig. 26. Beat-to-beat variations in QRS morphology, as compared with the uniform appearance of QRS complexes in monomorphic VT. (*From* White RD, Wood DL. Out-of-hospital pleomorphic ventricular tachycardia and resuscitation: association with acute myocardial ischemia and infarction. Ann Emerg Med 1992;21:1282; with permission.)

The basic steps for cardioversion/defibrillation are found in **Box 32**. Before cardioversion, if the clinical situation allows, IV analgesia or sedation should be used, as shock delivery is painful. A list of commonly used medications is found in **Table 12**. Most of these medications can cause hypotension and respiratory depression, which may be problematic in a patient who is already hemodynamically unstable. Caution should be used in choosing an agent in this situation. It is good practice to have the defibrillator on and pads in place before medication administration in the event of further clinical decline. Airway equipment should also be readily available. **Box 33** provides tips and suggestions for effective cardioversion and defibrillation.

After shock delivery, the rhythm may degenerate to unstable VT or VF, bradycardia, AV blocks, or asystole.[127] Chest wall burns, usually superficial partial thickness, can occur. Sedation and analgesia administration can result in hypotension, respiratory depression, apnea, bradycardia, and laryngospasm. Mild shocks to health care workers may also occur but are harmless.

Rapid loss of consciousness, pulse, and normal respiration should indicate a patient is suffering SCA. CPR should be instituted immediately while a second member of the health care team is sent for the defibrillator and code cart. The patient should be connected to the cardiac monitor and defibrillator without interrupting chest compressions. IV access should be established and respirations assisted with a bag-mask ventilation device. The cardiac rhythm should be assessed.

If the arrhythmia is identified as PEA or asystole, standard CPR should be continued (**Box 34**). Identification of reversible causes should be sought. A helpful mnemonic can be found in **Box 35**. If VF or pulseless VT is identified, immediate defibrillation should

Box 30
Contraindications for cardioversion and defibrillation
Cardioversion
Tachycardia due to enhanced automaticity (ST, AT, drug toxicity)
AF with RVR present for more than 48 hours
Pulseless VT
Defibrillation
PEA
Asystole
Presence of a pulse
DNR order
Abbreviations: RVR, rapid ventricular response; ST, sinus tachycardia.

| **Box 31** |
| **Cardioversion/defibrillation equipment** |
| Defibrillator |
| Cardiac monitor |
| Pads or paddles |
| Conducting gel, if using paddles |
| Patient interface cables that connect to the defibrillator/cardiac monitor |
| Analgesic/sedating medications |

A

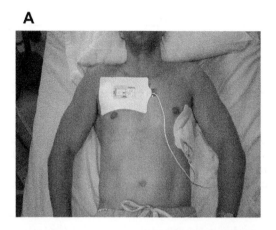

B

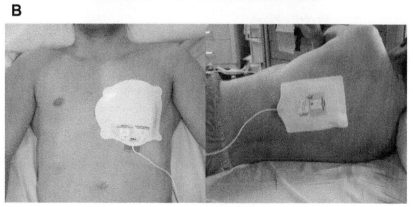

C

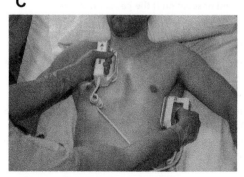

Fig. 27. (*A*) Pad placement for cardioversion/defibrillation. (*B*) Alternate anteroposterior placement. (*C*) Paddle placement.

Table 11
American Heart Association's recommendations for initial energy level for defibrillation/cardioversion

Rhythm	Biphasic (J)	Monophasic (J)
VF or unstable VT	120–200 (Unsynchronized)	360 (Unsynchronized)
Stable monomorphic VT	200	100
AVNRT or AVRT		
Narrow regular	50–100	50–100
Narrow irregular	120–200	200
Wide regular	100	100
Wide irregular	120–200 (Unsynchronized)	360 (Unsynchronized)
Atrial fibrillation	120–200	200
Atrial flutter	50–100	100

Energies are for synchronized mode unless otherwise specified.

occur. If ROSC does not occur, resuscitative efforts should be continued. **Box 36** shows the steps in the treatment of pulseless VT/VF. If there is ROSC, as evidenced by a perfusing cardiac rhythm, immediate postresuscitative care should be begun. **Box 37** contains some tips for optimizing resuscitation. Refer to the American Heart

Box 32
Steps for cardioversion/defibrillation

1. Turn on the defibrillator.
2. Place pads on the patient or prepare paddles.
   a. If using adhesive pads, place them on the patient in the anterolateral or anteroposterior position (see **Fig. 26**). Alternative placement is shown in **Fig. 26**.
   b. If using paddles, remove them from the device and apply a liberal amount of conductive gel to the paddle surfaces. Do not use ultrasonography gel. Rub paddles together to evenly distribute the gel. Hold paddles firmly to the patient's chest wall in the anterolateral position (see **Fig. 26**).
3. Connect the patient interface cables from the defibrillator to the adhesive pads or paddles.
4. Connect the patient to the cardiac monitor using the electrodes attached to the device.
5. Interpret the rhythm.
6. Provide analgesia and/or sedation if the patient is awake.
7. Select the DEFIBRILLATION operating mode.
8. Select the desired energy level (see **Table 11**).
9. Choose synchronized (cardioversion) or unsynchronized (defibrillation) shock delivery based on the rhythm as discussed earlier.
10. Charge the capacitor by pressing the CHARGE button.
11. When the defibrillator is charged, ensure no one is in contact with the patient or stretcher; this is best accomplished by stating, "All clear."
12. Press the shock button on the defibrillator or on the paddles and hold for several seconds, as there may be a delay in shock delivery.
13. Reassess rhythm.

Table 12
Commonly used medications for analgesia/sedation

Agent	Dose	Disadvantage	Advantage
Etomidate	0.15 mg/kg	Painful injection, myoclonus	Rapid onset, short duration, minimal cardiovascular effects
Midazolam	0.15 mg/kg	Hypotension, delayed onset	Can be reversed
Propofol	1 mg/kg	Respiratory depression/apnea, hypotension, painful injection	Rapid onset and short duration
Fentanyl	50–100 μg[a]	Bradycardia, chest wall rigidity	Can be reversed
Methohexital	1 mg/kg	Hypotension, laryngospasm	Short duration

[a] Use 2 μg/kg if age <12 y. Dose routes are IV.

Association's guidelines for Advanced Cardiac Life Support (ACLS) to review the complete algorithms available to manage cardiac arrest.[128]

No ACLS drug has been shown to improve the long-term outcome in cardiac arrest.[129–131] There is new emphasis on quality chest compressions during resuscitation.

Box 33
Tips and suggestions for successful cardioversion/defibrillation

- The efficacy of shock delivery is decreased by increased transthoracic impedance such as the inspiratory phase of ventilation, tissue scarring or edema of the thoracic cage, pleural effusion, and hyperinflation.

- Less-organized rhythms that have persisted for longer periods are more difficult to abolish and may require higher energy levels.

- If you are attempting synchronized cardioversion and the machine does not fire, it may not be able to detect the R wave. Change the amplitude or leads. If still unsuccessful, reassess the rhythm to determine whether cardioversion or defibrillation is appropriate.

- Defibrillator machines convert to the unsynchronized mode after shock delivery. Always reset to synchronized mode before additional attempts at cardioversion.

- Pads are applied either in the anterolateral or anteroposterior position, without clear advantage of one position over the other for shock efficacy.[122,123] Paddles have been shown in some studies to be more effective than pads. Larger pads, up to a certain point, have been shown to be more effective at terminating VF.[124]

- If using the paddles, be sure that ample conducting gel is applied and distributed over the entire surface of the paddles. Disposable gel pads can also be used. It requires about 25 pounds of force for good shock delivery.

- If an internal PM is present, the pads should be placed at least 8 cm from the device. The device needs to be interrogated later to ensure proper function.

- Most defibrillator devices include pediatric size paddles or adhesive pads. Use adult-sized paddles/pads if the child is greater than 10 kg.[125] Defibrillation is still recommended if size-appropriate equipment is not available.

- Shocks should not result in elevated troponin levels, although they may elevate creatinine kinase levels.[126]

- If the rhythm degenerates to VF after synchronized cardioversion, give a second unsynchronized shock immediately.

- Be familiar with your equipment *before* having to use it.

Box 34
Treatment of asystole and PEA arrest

1. CPR × 2 minutes[a]
2. Give epinephrine or vasopressin during CPR
   a. Epinephrine 1 mg IV/IO every 3 to 5 minutes
   b. Vasopressin 40 U IV/IO × 1 dose, to replace first or second epinephrine
3. Consider atropine
   a. Atropine 1 mg IV/IO every 3 to 5 minutes; up to 3 doses
4. Reassess rhythm. If PEA or asystole persists
5. Resume CPR × 2 minutes
6. Reassess rhythm. If PEA or asystole persists, return to step 2
7. If there is ROSC, initiate postresuscitative care

Abbreviation: IO, intraosseous.
[a] 100 compressions/min.

Mounting evidence indicates that patients do better with continuous chest compressions rather than compressions interrupted by ventilations,[132–134] which is thought to be due to maintaining a higher coronary perfusion pressure. In a swine model, Kern and colleagues[135] found a 13% survival rate with standard CPR and 80% survival with normal neurologic function in the arm receiving continuous chest compression.

Immediate postresuscitative care of patients with ROSC after cardiac arrest is paramount for survival with optimal neurologic function. Immediately after ROSC, there should be emphasis on maintaining the patient's intrinsic rhythm and providing hemodynamic support. **Box 38** provides a postresuscitation checklist.

Box 35
Mnemonic for causes of PEA/asystole

H's

Hypovolemia

Hypothermia

Hypoxia

Hydrogen ion (acidosis)

Hypokalemia/hyperkalemia

Hypoglycemia

T's

Thrombosis (coronary or pulmonary)

Tamponade

Tension pneumothorax

Trauma

Toxins

Box 36
Treatment of pulseless VT/VF

1. Give 1 shock—120 to 200 J biphasic, 360 J monophasic
2. Resume CPR × 2 minutes
3. Reassess rhythm. If ROSC, initiate postresuscitative care. If VT/VF persists
4. Give 1 shock—same or higher joules as first shock
5. Resume CPR × 2 minutes
6. Give epinephrine or vasopressin during CPR
   a. Epinephrine 1 mg IV/IO every 3 to 5 minutes
   b. Vasopressin 40 U IV/IO × 1 dose; replaces first or second dose of epinephrine
7. Reassess rhythm. If VT/VF persists
8. Give 1 shock at highest energy dose
9. Resume CPR × 2 minutes
10. Reassess rhythm. If VT/VF persists
11. Continue resuscitative efforts
12. Consider antiarrhythmic—amiodarone, lidocaine, magnesium if torsades de pointes
    a. Amiodarone 300 mg IV/IO once, may repeat 150 mg IV/IO once
    b. Lidocaine 1 to 1.5 mg/kg IV/IO, then 0.5 to 0.75 mg/kg IV/IO; maximum 3 doses or 3 mg/kg
    c. Magnesium 1 to 2 g IV/IO

Abbreviation: IO, intraosseous.

If a definitive airway was not established during the resuscitative efforts, this should be established. The Fio_2 should be weaned as soon as possible to prevent damage from prolonged hyperoxia.[136] It is not uncommon for patients to require blood pressure support with one or several vasopressors. **Table 13** provides details regarding

---

Box 37
Optimizing resuscitation

- Effective chest compressions are hard and fast at a rate of 100 compressions per minute. The chest wall should be compressed to one-third the anteroposterior diameter of the chest, with complete chest recoil allowed between compressions.

- One breath every 6 to 10 seconds should be given by bag-valve-mask with continuous chest compressions. Effective chest compressions should be given priority over ventilation.

- Chest compressions should be interrupted as little as possible.

- In pediatric patients, if the child is pulseless, follow CPR recommendations as in adults. If the child regains a pulse, one breath every 3 to 5 seconds should be delivered. If the heart rate remains less than 60 bpm, chest compressions should be continued.[117]

- After defibrillation, CPR should be resumed immediately for 2 minutes before pulse check and rhythm analysis, as the myocardial cells may be stunned after defibrillation and cardiopulmonary support is still necessary.

- Search for a reversible cause of the SCA.

> **Box 38**
> **Postresuscitation checklist**
>
> - Provide blood pressure support; this may require vasopressors. See **Box 9** for a list of options.
> - Arterial blood pressure monitoring should be considered.
> - Maximize oxygenation and ventilation. If the patient remains unconscious, intubation should be performed. Periodic arterial blood gas sampling should occur.
> - Central venous access may be necessary as there are often multiple infusions necessary at the same time. Place a central line.
> - Periodic electrolyte and glucose measurements should be performed with replacement as needed.

common vasopressors. Central venous access may be necessary to accommodate multiple infusions.

The literature supports the use of therapeutic hypothermia in patients with ROSC to improve neurologic function after cardiac arrest.[137–139] Moderate therapeutic hypothermia of 32 to 33.9°C (90–93°F) for 12 to 24 hours should be instituted within 6 hours of ROSC. It is indicated in patients with nonperfusing VT/VF and patients with asystole/PEA thought to be cardiac in origin with ROSC and who remain unconscious. It can also be considered in patients who regain consciousness but are unable to follow commands. A mean arterial pressure greater than 65 mm Hg must be obtained, although the use of vasopressor support is allowed. **Box 39** shows exclusion criteria for induced hypothermia. Internal or external cooling systems may be used with continuous temperature monitoring depending on one's institutional resources. There is limited evidence that suggests that percutaneous coronary intervention during hypothermia is feasible and safe.[129] Patients should be admitted to the ICU for close monitoring.

Table 13
Common vasopressors used in postresuscitative care

Agent	Dose	Mechanism	Notes
Dopamine	5 µg/kg/min IV; increase 5–10 µg/kg/min, max 20 µg/kg/min	α and β₁ stimulation, inotropy and peripheral vasoconstriction	Increases heart rate, contraindicated when tachyarrhythmia or pheochromocytoma
Norepinephrine	2–12 µg/min IV; titrate to effect, maximum 30 µg/min	α and β₁ stimulation, inotropy, chronotropy, peripheral vasoconstriction	Ventricular irritability, hypotension with MAOIs and TCAs
Phenylephrine	100–200 µg/min IV; titrate to effect	α Receptor stimulation, vasoconstriction alone	Reflex bradycardia
Epinephrine	2–10 µg/min IV of 1:10,000 solution; titrate to effect	α, β₁, and β₂ stimulation, inotropy, chronotropy, vasoconstriction	Can cause tachycardia, arrhythmias, and cardiac ischemia

Abbreviations: MAOI, monoamine oxidase inhibitor; TCA, tricyclic antidepressant.

Box 39
Exclusion criteria for induced hypothermia

- DNR advance directive, MOLST, poor baseline health status, or terminal disease

- Traumatic cause for the arrest

- Active bleeding or known intracranial bleeding (relative)

- Cryoglobulinemia (relative)

- Pregnancy (relative)

- Recent major surgical procedure (relative)

- Severe sepsis or septic shock as cause of arrest (relative)

Abbreviation: MOLST, medical orders for life-sustaining treatment.

SUMMARY

Emergency physicians must be able to quickly evaluate and manage cardiac emergencies. This ability requires having skills in various cardiac procedures. Knowledge of the indications, contraindications, techniques, and complications of these procedures can minimize morbidity and mortality, thus optimizing patient outcomes.

REFERENCES

1. Kilpatrick Z, Chapman C. On pericardiocentesis. Am J Cardiol 1965;16:622.
2. Tsang TS, Oh JK, Seward JB. Diagnosis and management of cardiac tamponade in the era of echocardiography. Clin Cardiol 1999;22:446–52.
3. Tayal VS, Moore CL, Rose GA. Cardiac. In: Ma OJ, Mateer JR, editors. Emergency ultrasound. USA: McGraw-Hill; 2003. p. 89–127.
4. Beck CS. Two cardiac compression triads. JAMA 1935;104(9):714–6.
5. Guberman BA, Fowler NO, Engel PJ, et al. Cardiac tamponade in medical patients. Circulation 1981;64(3):633–40.
6. Mandavia DP, Hoffner RJ, Mahaney K, et al. Bedside echocardiography by emergency physicians. Ann Emerg Med 2001;38(4):377–82.
7. Labovitz AJ, Noble VE, Bierig M, et al. Focused cardiac ultrasound in the emergent setting: a consensus statement of the American Society of Echocardiography and American College of Emergency Physicians. J Am Soc Echocardiogr 2010;23(12):1225–30.
8. Tayal TS, Kline JA. Emergency echocardiography to detect pericardial effusions in patients in PEA and near-PEA states. Resuscitation 2003;59:315–8.
9. Reichman E, Simon R. Pericardiocentesis. In: Roberts JR, Hedges JR, editors. Emergency medicine procedures. 4th edition. Philadelphia USA: McGraw Hill; 2004. p. 204–16.
10. Tsang TS, Enriquez-Sarano M, Freeman WK, et al. Consecutive 1127 therapeutic echocardiographically guided pericardioceteses: clinical profile, practice patterns, and outcomes spanning 21 years. Mayo Clin Proc 2002;77(5):429–36.
11. Yarlagadda C. "Cardiac tamponade". In: Fredi JL, editor. Medscape Reference. Updated August 2, 2012. Available at: http://emedicine.medscape.com/article/152083. Accessed November 2, 2012.

12. Isselbacher EM, Cigarroa JE, Eagle KA. Cardiac tamponade complicating prox-imal aortic dissection: is pericardiocentesis harmful? Circulation 1994;90: 2375–8.
13. Erbel R, Alfonso F, Boileau C, et al. Diagnosis and management of aortic dissec-tion. Eur Heart J 2001;22(18):1642–81.
14. Mellwig KP, Vogt J, Schmidt HK, et al. Acute aortic dissection (Stanford A) with pericardial tamponade–extension of the dissection after emergency pericardial puncture. Z Kardiol 1998;87(6):482–6.
15. Coats TJ, Keogh S, Clark H, et al. Prehospital resuscitative thoracotomy for cardiac arrest after penetrating trauma: rationale and case series. J Trauma 2001;50:670–3.
16. Powell DW, Moore EE, Cothren CC, et al. Is emergency department resuscitative thoracotomy futile care for the critically injured patient requiring prehospital cardiopulmonary resuscitation? J Am Coll Surg 2004;199:211–5.
17. Lewis G, Knottenbelt JD. Should emergency room thoracotomy be reserved for cases of cardiac tamponade? Injury 1991;22:5–6.
18. Harris DG, Papagiannopoulos KA, Pretorius J, et al. Current evaluation of cardiac stab wounds. Ann Thorac Surg 1999;68(6):2119–22.
19. Breaux EP, Dupont JB, et al. Cardiac tamponade following penetrating medias-tinal injuries: improved survival with early pericardiocentesis. J Trauma 1979; 19(6):461–6.
20. Sagrista-Sauleda J, Angel J, Juame M, et al. Hemodynamic effects of volume expansion in patients with cardiac tamponade. Circulation 2008; 117:1545–9.
21. Kerber RE, Gascho JA, Litchfield R, et al. Hemodynamic effects of volume expansion and nitroprusside compared with pericardiocentesis in patients with acute cardiac tamponade. N Engl J Med 1982;307:929–31.
22. Zhang H, Spapen H, Vincent JL, et al. Effects of dobutamine and norepineph-rine on oxygen availability in tamponade-induced stagnant hypoxia: a prospec-tive, randomized, controlled study. Crit Care Med 1994;22(2):299–305.
23. Martin JB, Manual WJ, et al. Comparative effects of catecholamines in cardiac tamponade; experimental and clinical studies. Am J Cardiol 1980;46:59–63.
24. Seldinger SI. Catheter replacement of the needle in percutaneous angiography: a new technique. Acta Radiol 1953;39:368.
25. Ball JB, Morrison WL. Cardiac tamponade. Postgrad Med J 1997;73:141–5.
26. Krikorian JG, Hancock EW. Pericardiocentesis. Am J Med 1978;65:808–11.
27. Wong B, Murphy J, Chang CJ, et al. The risk of pericardiocentesis. Am J Cardiol 1979;44(6):1110–4.
28. Maisch B, Seferovic PM, Ristic AD, et al. Guidelines on the diagnosis and management of pericardial disease executive summary: the Task Force on the diagnosis and management of pericardial diseases of the European Society of Cardiology. Eur Heart J 2004;25:587–610.
29. Tsang TS, Freeman WK, Sinak JL, et al. Echocardiographically guided pericar-diocentesis: evolution and state-of-the-art technique. Mayo Clin Proc 1998;73: 647–52.
30. Salem K, Mulji A, Lonn E, et al. Echocardiographically guided pericardiocente-sis: the gold standard for the management of pericardial effusion and cardiac tamponade. Can J Cardiol 1999;15:1251–5.
31. Susini G, Pepi M, Sisillo E, et al. Percutaneous pericardiocentesis versus subxi-phoid pericardiotomy in cardiac tamponade due to postoperative pericardial effusion. J Cardiothorac Vasc Anesth 1993;7:178–83.

32. Quinones MA, Douglas PS, Foster E, et al. ACC/AHA clinical competence statement on echocardiography. A report of the American College of Cardiology/American Heart Association/American College of Physicians–American Society of Internal Medicine Task Force on Clinical Competence. J Am Coll Cardiol 2003;41:S735–1097.
33. Treasure T, Cottler L. Practical procedures: how to aspirate the pericardium. Br J Hosp Med 1980;24:488.
34. Synovitz CK, Brown EJ. Pericardiocentesis. In: Tintinalli JE, editor. Tintinalli's emergency medicine. 7th edition. USA: McGraw; 2010. p. 250–7.
35. Blaivas M. Incidence of pericardial effusion in patients presenting to the emergency department with unexplained dyspnea. Acad Emerg Med 2001;8(12): 1143–6.
36. Shabetai R. Pericardial effusion: haemodynamic spectrum. Heart 2004;90: 255–6.
37. Vandyke WH Jr, Cure J, Chakko CS, et al. Pulmonary edema after pericadiocentesis for cardiac tamponade. N Engl J Med 1983;309:595–6.
38. Armstrong WF, Feigenbaum H, Dillon JC, et al. Acute right ventricular dilation and echocardiographic volume overload following pericardiocentesis for relief of cardiac tamponade. Am Heart J 1984;107(6):1266–70.
39. Chandraratna PA. Echocardiography and Doppler ultrasound in the evaluation of pericardial disease. Circulation 1991;84(Suppl I):1303–10.
40. Demetriades D. Cardiac wounds. Experience with 70 patients. Ann Surg 1986; 203:315–7.
41. Arom KV, Richardson JD, Webb G, et al. Subxiphoid pericardial window in patients with suspected traumatic pericardial tamponade. Ann Thorac Surg 1977;23:545–9.
42. Zoll PM, Linenthal AJ, Norman LR, et al. Treatment of unexpected cardiac arrest by external electric stimulation of the heart. N Engl J Med 1956;254:511.
43. Zoll PM, Linenthal AJ, Norman LR. Treatment of Stokes-Adams disease by external stimulation of the heart. Circulation 1954;9:482.
44. Zoll PM, Linenthal AJ, Norman LR, et al. External electric stimulation of the heart in cardiac arrest. Arch Intern Med 1955;96:639.
45. Chardack WM, Gage AA, Greatbatch W. A transistorized, self-contained, implantable pacemaker for the long-term correction of complete heart block. Surgery 1960;48:643.
46. Dalsey WC, Syverud SA, Trott A. Transcutaneous cardiac pacing. J Emerg Med 1984;1:201.
47. Clinton JE, Zoll PM, Zoll R, et al. External noninvasive cardiac pacing. J Emerg Med 1985;2:155.
48. Bessman ES. Emergency cardiac pacing. In: Roberts JR, Hedges JR, editors. Clinical procedures in emergency medicine. 5th edition. USA: Saunders Elsevier; 2010. p. 269–86.
49. Hindman MC, Wagner GS, JaRo M, et al. The clinical significance of bundle branch block complicating acute myocardial infarction: clinical characteristics, hospital mortality, and one-year follow-up. Circulation 1978;58:679.
50. Beland MJ, Hesslein PS, Finlay CD, et al. Noninvasive transcutaneous cardiac pacing in children. Pacing Clin Electrophysiol 1987;10:1262.
51. Hazinski MF, Nolan JP, Billi JE, et al. Part 1: executive summary: 2010 International consensus on cardiopulmonary resuscitation and emergency cardiovascular care science with treatment recommendations. Circulation 2010;122(2): S250–75.

52. Hofer CA, Smith JK, Tenholder MF. Verapamil intoxication: a literature review of overdoses and discussion of therapeutic options. Am J Med 1993;95:431.
53. Taboulet P, Cariou A, Berdeaux A, et al. Pathophysiology and management of self poisoning with beta-blockers. J Toxicol Clin Toxicol 1993;31:531.
54. Taboulet P, Baud FJ, Bismuth C, et al. Acute digitalis intoxication: is pacing still appropriate? J Toxicol Clin Toxicol 1993;31:261.
55. Ramoska EA, Spiller HA, Myers A. Calcium channel blocker toxicity. Ann Emerg Med 1990;19:649.
56. ECC Committee, Subcommittees and Task Forces of the American Heart Association. 2005 American Heart Association guidelines for cardiopulmonary resuscitation and emergency cardiovascular care, Part 10.2: toxicology in ECC. Circulation 2005;112:IV126–32.
57. Hazard PB. Transvenous cardiac pacing in cardiopulmonary resuscitation. Crit Care Med 1981;9:666.
58. ECC Committee, Subcommittees and Task Forces of the American Heart Association. 2005 American Heart Association guidelines for cardiopulmonary resuscitation and emergency cardiovascular care, Part 5: electrical therapies: automated external defibrillators, defibrillation, cardioversion, and pacing. Circulation 2005;112:IV35–46.
59. Dronen S, Thompson B, Nowak R, et al. Subclavian vein catheterization during cardiopulmonary resuscitation. JAMA 1982;247(23):3227–30.
60. Laczika K, Thalhammer F, Locker G, et al. Safe and efficient emergency transvenous ventricular packing via the right supraclavicular route. Anesth Analg 2000;90(4):784–9.
61. Syverud SA, Dalsey WC, Hedges JR, et al. Radiographic assessment of transvenous pacemaker placement during CPR. Ann Emerg Med 1986; 15(2):131–7.
62. Mey U, Glasmacher A, Hahn C, et al. Evaluation of an ultrasound-guided technique for central venous access via the internal jugular vein in 493 patients. Support Care Cancer 2003;11:148.
63. Alderson PJ, Burrows FA, Stemp LI, et al. Use of ultrasound to evaluate internal jugular vein anatomy and to facilitate central venous cannulation in paediatric patients. Br J Anaesth 1993;70:145.
64. Cajozzo M, Quintini G, Cocchiera G, et al. Comparison of central venous catheterization with and without ultrasound guide. Transfus Apher Sci 2004; 31:199.
65. Whalen RE, Starmer CF, et al. Electrical hazards associated with cardiac pacemaking. Ann N Y Acad Sci 1964;111:922–31.
66. Epstein AW, DiMarco JP, Ellenbogen KA, et al. AHA Practice Guidelines. ACC/AHA/HRS 2008 Guidelines for device-based therapy of cardiac rhythm abnormalities. Circulation 2008;117(21):e350–408.
67. Bernstein AD, Daubert JC, Fletcher RD, et al. The revised NASPE/BPEG generic code for antibradycardia, adaptive-rate, and multisite pacing. North American Society of Pacing and Electrophysiology/British Pacing and Electrophysiology Group. Pacing Clin Electrophysiol 2002;25:260.
68. Furman S, Fisher JD. Endless loop tachycardia in an AV universal (DDD) pacemaker. Pacing Clin Electrophysiol 1982;5(4):486–9.
69. Scher D. Troubleshooting pacemakers and implantable cardioverter defibrillators. Curr Opin Cardiol 2004;19(1):36–46.
70. Sgarbossa EB, Pinski SL, Barbagelata A, et al. Electrocardiographic diagnosis of evolving acute myocardial infarction in the presence of left bundle-branch block.

GUSTO-1 (global utilization of streptokinase and tissue plasminogen activator for occluded coronary arteries) Investigators. N Engl J Med 1996;334(8):481.

71. Cardall TY, Chan TC, Brady WJ, et al. Permanent pacemakers: issues relevant to the emergency physician, part I. J Emerg Med 1999;17(3):479–89.
72. Pavia S, Wilkoff B. The management of surgical complications of pacemaker and implantable cardioverter-defibrillators. Curr Opin Cardiol 2001;16(1):66–71.
73. Sohail MR, Uslan DZ, Khan AH. Risk factor analysis of permanent pacemaker infection. Clin Infect Dis 2007;45(2):166–73.
74. Hauser RG, Hayes DL, Kallinen LM, et al. Clinical experience with pacemaker pulse generators and transvenous leads: an 8-year prospective multicenter study. Heart Rhythm 2007;4(2):154–60.
75. Parsonnet V, Bilitch M, Furman S, et al. Early malfunction of transvenous pacemaker electrodes. A 3 center study. Circulation 1979;60(3):590–6.
76. Cardall TY, Brady WJ, Chan TC, et al. Permanent cardiac pacemakers: issues relevant to the emergency physician, part II. J Emerg Med 1999;17(4):697–709.
77. Conti JB, Curtis AB, Hill JA, et al. Termination of pacemaker-mediated tachycardia by adenosine. Clin Cardiol 1994;17:47–8.
78. Barold SS, Falkoff MD, Ong LS, et al. Pacemaker endless loop tachycardia: termination by simple techniques other than magnet application. Am J Med 1988;85:817–22.
79. Rao SP, Miller S, Rosenbaum R, et al. Cardiac troponin I and cardiac enzymes after electrophysiologic studies, ablations and defibrillator implantations. Am J Cardiol 1999;84(4):470 A9.
80. Hurst TM, Hinrichs M, Breidenbach C, et al. Detection of myocardial injury during transvenous implantation of cardioverter-defibrillators. J Am Coll Cardiol 1999;34(2):402–8.
81. Proietti R, Sagone A. Electrical storm: incidence, prognosis and therapy. Indian Pacing Electrophysiol J 2011;11(2):34–42.
82. Stevenson WG, Chaitman BR, Ellebnogen KA, et al. Clinical assessment and management of patients with implanted cardioverter-defibrillators presenting to nonelectrophysiologists. Circulation 2004;110(25):3866–9.
83. Jacobs I, Sunde K, Deakin CD, et al. 2010 International consensus on cardiopulmonary resuscitation and emergency cardiovascular care science with treatment recommendations. Part 6: defibrillation. Circulation 2010;122:S325–37.
84. Levine PA, Barold SS, Fletcher RD, et al. Adverse acute and chronic effects of electrical defibrillation and cardioversion on implanted unipolar cardiac pacing systems. J Am Coll Cardiol 1983;1:1413–22.
85. Pinski SL. Emergencies related to implantable cardioverter-defibrillators. Crit Care Med 2000;10(Suppl):N174–80.
86. Podrid PJ. Overview of the acute management of tachyarrhythmias. In: Ganz L, Hoekstra J, editors. UpToDate. Updated October 2, 2008. Available at: www.uptodate.com/contents/overview-of-the-management-of-tachyarrhythmias. Accessed November 18, 2011.
87. Atie J, Brugada P, Brugada J, et al. Clinical and electrophysiologic characteristics of patients with antidromic circus movement tachycardia in the Wolff-Parkinson White syndrome. Am J Cardiol 1990;66:1082–91.
88. Minezak BM. Techniques for supraventricular tachycardia. In: Roberts JR, Hedges JR, editors. Clinical procedures in emergency medicine. 5th edition. Saunders Elsevier; 2010. p. 197–211.
89. Ganz LI. Approach to the diagnosis of narrow QRS complex tachycardias. In: Knight BP, Goldberger AL, Hoestra J, Editors. Online Medical Reference.

90. Deakin CD, Morrison LJ. 2010 International consensus on cardiopulmonary resuscitation and emergency cardiovascular care science with treatment recommendations. Part 8: advanced life support. Resuscitation 2010;81(Suppl 1):e93–174.

91. Gentile F, Elhendy A, Khandheria BK, et al. Safety of electrical cardioversion in patients with atrial fibrillation. Mayo Clin Proc 2002;77(9):897–904.

92. Albers GW, Dalen JE, Laupacis A, et al. Antithrombotic therapy in atrial fibrillation. Chest 2001;119(Suppl 1):194S–206S.

93. Singer DE, Albers GW, Dalen JE, et al. Antithrombotic therapy in atrial fibrillation: the 7th ACCP conference on antithrombotic and thrombolytic therapy. Chest 2004;126(Suppl 3):429S–56S.

94. Fuster V, Ryden LE, Cannom DS, et al. ACC/AHA/ESC 2006 Guidelines for the management of patient with atrial fibrillation. A report of the American College of Cardiology/American Heart Association Task Force on practice guidelines and the European Society of Cardiology Committee for Practice Guidelines (Writing Committee to Revise the 2001 Guidelines for the Management of Patients with Atrial Fibrillation). Circulation 2006;114:700–52.

95. Luber S, Brady WJ, Joyce T, et al. Paroxysmal supraventricular tachycardia: outcome after ED care. Am J Emerg Med 2001;19(1):40–2.

96. Steward RB, Bardy GH, Greene HL. Wide complex tachycardia: misdiagnosis and outcome after emergent therapy. Ann Intern Med 1986;104:766.

97. Akhtar M, Shenasa M, Jazayeri M, et al. Wide QRS complex tachycardia. Reappraisal of a common clinical problem. Ann Intern Med 1988;109:905.

98. Gupta AK, Thakur RK. Wide QRS complex tachycardias. Med Clin North Am 2001;85:245.

99. Tchou P, Young P, Mahmud R, et al. Useful clinical criteria for the diagnosis of ventricular tachycardia. Am J Med 1988;84:53.

100. Wellens HJ. Electrophysiology: ventricular tachycardia: diagnosis of broad QRS complex tachycardia. Heart 2001;86:579.

101. Lau EW, Pathamanathan RK, Ng GA, et al. The Bayesian approach improves the electrocardiographic diagnosis of broad complex tachycardia. Pacing Clin Electrophysiol 2000;23:1519.

102. Brugada P, Brugada J, Mont L, et al. A new approach to the differential diagnosis of a regular tachycardia with a wide QRS complex. Circulation 1991;83:1649.

103. Vereckei A, Duray G, Szenasi G, et al. Application of a new algorithm in the differential diagnosis of wide QRS complex tachycardia. Eur Heart J 2007;28:589.

104. Miller JM, Hsia HH, Rothman SA, et al. Ventricular tachycardia versus supraventricular tachycardia with aberrancy: electrocardiographic distinctions. In: Zipes DP, Jalife J, editors. Cardiac electrophysiology from cell to bedside. Philadelphia: WB Saunders; 2000. p. 696.

105. Buxton AE, Marchlinski FE, Doherty JU, et al. Hazards of intravenous verapamil for sustained ventricular tachycardia. Am J Cardiol 1987;59:1107.

106. Zipes DP, Camm AJ, Borggrefe M, et al. ACC/AHA/ESC 2006 Guidelines for management of patients with ventricular arrhythmias and the prevention of sudden cardiac death—executive summary. A report of the American College of Cardiology/American Heart Association Task Force and the European Society of Cardiology Committee for Practice Guidelines (Writing Committee to Develop Guidelines for Management of Patients With Ventricular Arrhythmias and the Prevention of Sudden Cardiac Death). Circulation 2006;114:1088–132.

107. ECC Committee, Subcommittees and Task Forces of the American Heart Association. 2005 American Heart Association guidelines for cardiopulmonary resuscitation and emergency cardiovascular care. Part 12: pediatric advanced life support. Circulation 2005;112(Suppl 24):IV167–87.

108. Marill KA, Wolfram S, deSouza IS, et al. Adenosine for wide-complex tachycardia: efficacy and safety. Crit Care Med 2009;37(9):2512–8.

109. Parham WA, Mehdirad AA, Biermann KM, et al. Case report: adenosine induced ventricular fibrillation in a patient with stable ventricular tachycardia. J Interv Card Electrophysiol 2001;5:71–4.

110. Strickberger SA, Man KC, Daoud EG, et al. Adenosine-induced atrial arrhythmia: a prospective analysis. Ann Intern Med 1997;127:417.

111. Rankin AC, Brooks R, Ruskin JN, et al. Adenosine and the treatment of supraventricular tachycardia. Am J Med 1992;92:655–64.

112. DiMarco J, Sellers TD, Berne R, et al. Adenosine: electrophysiologic effects and therapeutic use for terminating paroxysmal supra-ventricular tachycardia. Circulation 1983;68:1254–63.

113. Garratt CJ, O'Nunain S, Griffith M, et al. Effects of intravenous adenosine in patients with preexcited junctional tachycardias: therapeutic efficacy and incidence of proarrhythmic events. Am J Cardiol 1994;74:401–4.

114. Centers for Disease Control and Prevention (CDC). State-specific mortality from sudden cardiac death – United States, 1999. MMWR Morb Mortal Wkly Rep 2002;51:123 Academic One File. Web. 14 Dec. 2011.

115. Nichol G, Thomas E, Callaway CW, et al. Resuscitation outcomes consortium investigators. JAMA 2008;300(12):1423–31.

116. Bayes de Luna A, Coumel P, Leclercq JF, et al. Ambulatory sudden cardiac death: mechanisms of production of fatal arrhythmia on the basis of data from 157 cases. Am Heart J 1989;117:151–9.

117. Rea TD, Pearce RM, Raghunathan TE, et al. Incidence of out-of-hospital cardiac arrest. Am J Cardiol 2004;93:1455.

118. Efestol T, Wik L, Sunde K, et al. Effects of cardiopulmonary resuscitation on predictors of ventricular fibrillation success during out-of-hospital cardiac arrest. Circulation 2004;110:10.

119. Leng CT, Paradis NA, Calkins H, et al. Resuscitation after prolonged ventricular defibrillation with the use of monophasic and biphasic waveform pulses for external defibrillation. Circulation 2000;101(25):2968–74.

120. Van Alem AP, Chapman FW, Lank P, et al. A prospective, randomized and blinded comparison of first shock success of monophasic and biphasic waveforms in out of hospital cardiac arrest. Resuscitation 2003;58:17.

121. Schneider T, Martens PR, Paschen H, et al. Multicenter, randomized, controlled trial of 150-J biphasic shocks compared with 200- to 360-J monophasic shocks in the resuscitation of out-of-hospital cardiac arrest victims. Optimized Response to Cardiac Arrest (ORCA) Investigators. Circulation 2000;102:1780.

122. Mathew TP, Moore A, McIntyre M, et al. Randomized comparison of electrode positions for cardioversion of atrial fibrillation. Heart 1999;81:576.

123. Kerber RE, Jensen SR, Grayzel J, et al. Elective cardioversion: influence of paddle-electrode location and size on success rates and energy requirements. N Engl J Med 1981;305:658.

124. Dalzell GW, Cunningham SR, Anderson J, et al. Electrode pad size, transthoracic impedance and success of external ventricular defibrillation. Am J Cardiol 1989;64:741.

125. Atkins DL, Kerber RE. Pediatric defibrillation: current flow is improved by using "adult" electrode paddles. Pediatrics 1994;94:90.
126. Reiffel J, McCarthy DM, Leahey EB. Does DC cardioversion affect isoenzyme recognition of myocardial infarction? Am Heart J 1979;97:6.
127. Waldecker B, Brugada P, Zehender M, et al. Dysrhythmias after direct-current cardioversion. Am J Cardiol 1986;57:120.
128. AHA 2010 Guidelines for CPR and ECC. American Heart Association, USA. January 28, 2010. Print. November 2010;122(18 Suppl 3).
129. Morrison LJ, Deakin CD, Morley PT, et al. Part 8: advanced life support: 2010 International consensus on cardiopulmonary resuscitation and emergency cardiovascular care science with treatment recommendations. Circulation 2010;122(16):S345–421.
130. Olasveengen TM, Sunde KS, et al. Intravenous drug administration during out-of-hospital cardiac arrest. JAMA 2009;302(20):2222–9.
131. Stiell IG, Wells GA, Field B, et al. Advanced cardiac life support in out-of-hospital cardiac arrest. N Engl J Med 2004;351(7):647–56.
132. Eftestol T, Sunde K, Steen PA, et al. Effects of interrupting precordial compressions on the calculated probability of defibrillation success during out-of-hospital cardiac arrest. Circulation 2002;105(19):2270–3.
133. Yu T, Weil MH, Tang W, et al. Adverse outcomes of interrupted precordial compression during automated defibrillation. Circulation 2002;106(3):368–72.
134. Sayre MR, Berg RA, Cave DM, et al. Hands-only (compression-only) cardiopulmonary resuscitation: a call to action for bystander response to adults who experience out-of-hospital sudden cardiac arrest. Circulation 2008;117(16):2162–7.
135. Kern KB, Hilwig RW, Berg RA, et al. Importance of continuous chest compressions during cardiopulmonary resuscitation. Improved outcome during a simulated single lay-rescuer scenerio. Circulation 2002;105(5):645–9.
136. Kilgannon JH, Jones AE, Shapiro NI, et al. Association between arterial hyperoxia following resuscitation from cardiac arrest and in-hospital mortality. JAMA 2010;303:2165.
137. Constantine M. Current evidence in therapeutic hypothermia for postcardiac arrest care. Emerg Med Pract 2011;13(4):1–21.
138. Van der Wal G, Brinkman S, Bisschops LL, et al. Influence of mild therapeutic hypothermia after cardiac arrest on hospital mortality. Crit Care Med 2011;39(1):84–8.
139. International Liaison Committee on Resuscitation. 2005 International consensus on cardiopulmonary resuscitation and emergency cardiovascular care science with treatment recommendations. Circulation 2005;112:IV51.

Critical Obstetric and Gynecologic Procedures in the Emergency Department

Joanna Mercado, MD, MSc[a],*, Isabel Brea, MD[b],
Brian Mendez, MD[c], Hilsa Quinones, MD[c], David Rodriguez, MD[c]

KEYWORDS

- Labor • Delivery • Episiotomy • Breech presentation • Bartholin abscess

KEY POINTS

- The emergency medicine physician should be prepared to manage imminent delivery at any time in the emergency department.
- Malpresentation, shoulder dystocia, or multiple gestation could complicate any delivery in the emergency department. The emergency medicine physician should be familiarized with the different maneuvers, from alleviation of shoulder dystocia to breech delivery maneuvers.
- The emergency department is a dynamic and challenging setting in which time matters; knowledge of and proficiency in the obstetric and gynecology procedures enable physicians to develop strategies to treat patients and the complications.

OBSTETRICS PROCEDURES

Labor

Active labor is defined by consecutive, rhythmic, involuntary uterine contractions that result in dilation and effacement of the cervix.[1,2] Active labor is divided into 3 stages. The first stage begins when uterine contractions have sufficient frequency, intensity, and duration to result in effacement and progressive dilation of the cervix, and ends when the cervix is fully dilated (10 cm) to allow passage of the fetal head (**Fig. 1**).[3] The second stage begins when full cervix dilation is achieved, and ends when the fetus is delivered. The third stage begins when the fetus is separated from the mother, and ends with placenta delivery.

Evaluation

On arrival of the patient to emergency department, the evaluation begins with an adequate history and physical examination. Pertinent information to obtain includes

[a] Research Section, Department of Emergency Medicine, University of Puerto Rico, San Juan, PR, USA; [b] Department of Emergency Medicine, Life Lion & Critical Care Transport, Penn State Hershey Medical Center, College of Medicine, Hershey, PA, USA; [c] Department of Emergency Medicine, University of Puerto Rico, San Juan, PR, USA
* Corresponding author.
E-mail address: jmercadoa@gmail.com

Emerg Med Clin N Am 31 (2013) 207–236
http://dx.doi.org/10.1016/j.emc.2012.09.005
0733-8627/13/$ – see front matter © 2013 Elsevier Inc. All rights reserved.

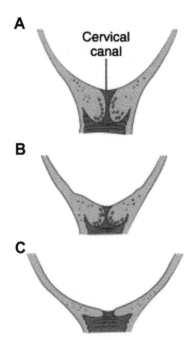

Fig. 1. Effacement of the cervix; (*A*) 0%, (*B*) 50%, and (*C*) 100%. (*From* Romney S, Gray MK, Little AB, et al [eds]: Gynecology and Obstetrics: The Health Care of Women. New York: McGraw-Hill, 1975; with permission.)

frequency of contractions, vaginal discharge or bleeding, and prenatal history. In addition, a focused physical examination is essential to determine the position and presentation of the fetus (**Fig. 2**).

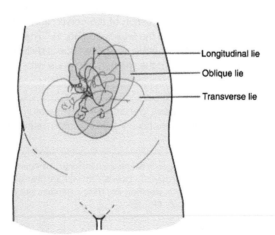

Fig. 2. Different presentations of the fetus. (*From* Lanni SM, Seeds JW. Malpresentations and shoulder dystocia. In: Gabbe SG, ed. Obstetrics: Normal and Problem Pregnancies. Philadelphia, Elsevier Churchill Livingstone, 2007; with permission.)

Presentation

Presentation (presenting part) refers to which part of the fetus is nearest to or foremost in the birth canal. To determine the presenting part, a sterile vaginal examination should be performed. Head, buttocks, or feet could be the presenting part. However, if the fetus is in transverse lie, the presenting part is the shoulder (**Table 1**).

Next, the position of fetus should be determined, which is identified by the relationship of the presenting part to the birth canal. This evaluation is performed by palpating the abdomen using Leopold maneuvers (**Fig. 3**).

Vaginal examination

The patient should be examined in a lithotomy position. Unless excessive blood is evident, a manual vaginal examination is indicated. The vulva and perineal area should be prepared for evaluation by cleaning the area with gauze soaked in providone-iodine.[4,5] The index and middle fingers of the nonsterile gloved hand should be used to expose the vaginal opening to avoid sterile-gloved fingers touching the labia. The sterile-gloved hand should then be used to examine the cervix.

Effacement, which ranges from 0% through 100%, should be assessed by palpating the cervix (see **Fig. 1**).[5] Cervical dilation is then determined by estimating the average diameter of the cervical os using the examiner fingers. Cervical dilation is expressed in centimeters, with 10 cm indicating full dilatation. Once the cervix is examined, the position of the fetus head with respect to the ischiatic spine should be determined.

Position

Zero station refers to when the infant's head is located between both ischiatic spines. The station should increase as the head reaches the birth canal, from −3 (head is above ischiatic spines) to +3 (just before crowning). A new station classification based on a scale of −5 through +5 also has been described in more recent literature, as shown in **Fig. 4**.[6]

Emergent Vaginal Delivery

Precipitous delivery in the emergency department is uncommon because most patients in active labor are immediately transported to the labor and delivery room for evaluation. However, emergency department physicians may sometimes need to manage an emergent delivery. Once the patient has arrived to the emergency department, the physician should perform the examination as discussed unless evidence of bleeding is present, in which a focused assessment of the vulvar area is strongly recommended. While the patient is being examined, obstetric and pediatric consults should be requested without delay.[7] The patient should then be placed in the lithotomy position. If the head is visible in the vaginal outlet or the vulvar area encircles the fetal head (*crowning*), the physician should prepare for imminent emergent delivery. The

Table 1 Types of presentation	
Cephalic	Relation of fetal head to the body as fetus flex the neck
Vertex	Occipital fontanelle is palpated
Face	Palpate frontal fontanelle
Breech	Presenting other part than head
Frank	
Complete	
Footling	
Incomplete	

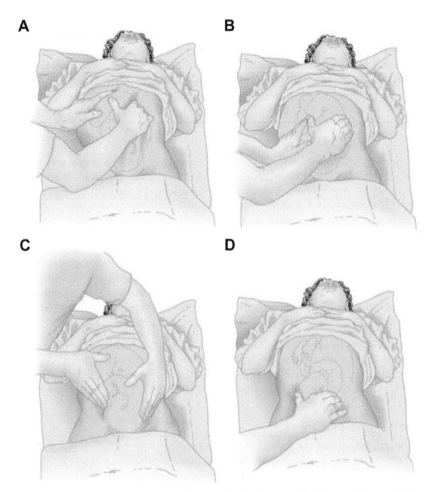

Fig. 3. Leopold maneuvers. (*A*) First palpate the fundus part, (*B*) then palpate the lateral abdomen to find the fetus back, (*C*) then palpate the other lateral parts, (*D*) then palpate the presenting part. (*From* Desai S, Henderson O, Mallon WK. Labor and delivery and their complications. In: Marx JA, Hockberger RS, Walls RM, et al, editors. Marx: Rosen's emergency medicine. 7th edition. Elsevier; 2010. p. 2327–47; with permission.)

physician should be aware that an episiotomy cannot be performed in this situation, because it will cause perineum tearing.[5,6]

Every emergency department should be prepared for emergent vaginal deliveries, including maintaining ready access to the adequate equipment (**Box 1**). The delivery should be performed using the Ritgen maneuver (**Fig. 5**). Once the fetus head is crowning and the diameter of introitus is opened more than 5 cm, the gloved hand might be draped with a towel to avoid the fetal face coming in contact with the mother's anus.[5,8] Then, forward pressure should be placed on the fetal chin with one hand, and pressure put over fetal occiput with the other. This maneuver will avoid "popping," and the physician will maintain control of the delivery. The neck extension is favored, allowing the head delivery to be slow; the occiput passes through the symphysis pubis, and the face and anterior fontanelle pass over the perineum (see **Fig. 5**).[5,7,8]

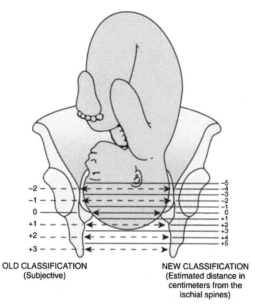

OLD CLASSIFICATION
(Subjective)

NEW CLASSIFICATION
(Estimated distance in
centimeters from the
ischial spines)

Fig. 4. Station of the fetus. (*From* Lanni SM, Seeds JW. Malpresentations and shoulder dystocia. In: Gabbe SG, ed. Obstetrics: Normal and Problem Pregnancies. Philadelphia, Elsevier Churchill Livingstone, 2007; with permission.)

After the head is completely outside the vagina, immediate clearing of nasopharynx should be performed before the rest of the body is delivered[5,7,8] to prevent aspiration. For clearing the nasopharynx, the physician may use an infant nasogastric tube (5 French) attached to a syringe, or a suction bulb. The infant should be checked for

Box 1
Equipment for emergent vaginal delivery
Sterile gloves
Sterile gown
Towels
Hemostats
Placenta basin
Cord clamps[2]
Surgical scissors
Suction bulb
Infant nasogastric tube
Syringes
Neonatal air bag
Needles
Gauzes
Neonatal warmer

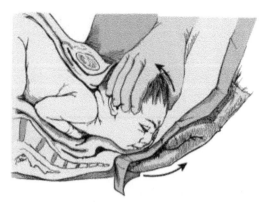

Fig. 5. Ritgen maneuver. (*From* Seils A, et al [eds]: Williams Obstetrics, 22nd ed. New York: McGraw-Hill Medical Publishing Division, 2005; with permission.)

meconium aspiration and the amount should be recorded. If meconium is obtained, suction should be established and pediatrics consulted.[5]

Once the head is delivered and nasopharynx cleared, the physician should use a finger to examine the exterior neck for the umbilical cord (**Fig. 6**). If the cord is present about the neck, the finger should be placed between the neck and umbilical cord for detangling. The umbilical cord may pass over the infant's head easily, but sometimes the nuchal cord is too tight. In this case, the umbilical cord should be clamped on 2 sides and cut in between to deliver the infant promptly.[5,8]

In most cases, the occiput turns to one side of the mother's thigh. Then, the shoulders begin to appear at the vulva, and in some cases deliver spontaneously. In other cases, a delay may occur and manipulation should be performed for deliver them. The infant's head should be grasped with both hands and gently pulled downward until anterior shoulder passes under the pubis. With an upward movement, the posterior shoulder is delivered, followed by the anterior shoulder.[5,9] The rest of the body usually follows the shoulder, but if not, moderate traction on the infant's head and pressure on the uterine fundus allow completion of the delivery. If any traction is needed, it should

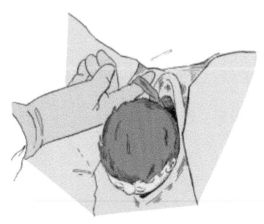

Fig. 6. Assessment of umbilical cord entanglement. (*From* Probst BD. Emergency childbirth. In: Roberts JR, Hedges JR, eds. Clinical Procedures in Emergency Medicine, 5th ed. Philadelphia: Elsevier 2009; with permission.)

be performed in the long axis of the infant's neck, and placing a finger below the axilla should be avoided because brachial nerve injury may occur.[5] At this time, the second stage of labor ends.

The third stage of labor begins when the umbilical cord is clamped and cut. The clamp may be placed approximately 4 to 5 cm from the infant abdomen.[6] A segment should be reserved for blood gas analysis. Once the umbilical cord is cut, the infant should be placed in a heated unit.

Placenta delivery

A gush of blood marks this part of the third stage of labor (**Box 2**). Bleeding will inevitably occur when the placenta separates from the uterus.[6] This may take up to 5 to 15 minutes after fetal delivery.[6] Once the blood comes out of the vagina, the uterus should be massaged to achieve uterus contraction. The cord may become slack. If the placenta does not descend at this time, manual removal is mandatory.

If the placenta does not descend in more than 5 minutes, the mother will be asked to bear down, cough, or push—maneuvers that increase the intra-abdominal pressure. Meanwhile, the physician should still massage the fundus.[5,6] Pressure or traction on the umbilical cord should be avoided; the placenta should never be forced to separate. One of the most frightening complications is uterus inversion, which could be caused by forceful placenta separation.[5]

Pressure to the abdomen should be stopped as the placenta is delivered. Careful examination of placenta is mandatory to assess for retained membranes. If any membrane is tearing, it should be grasped with ring forceps and removed with gentle traction.

Oxytocin should be started when the placenta is delivered, which is among the most used agents for myometrium contraction. Its principal indication is myometrium contraction to achieve hemostasis and a well-contracted uterus.[6] Other available agents include ergonovine, methylergonovine. The preferred agent depends on the institution and the timing of administration. Oxytocin infusion should be started after the placenta delivery. Some cases have been reported in which oxytocin was started before delivery because of entrapment of the placenta or because of the possibility that an undiagnosed twin delivery may entrap one of the infants inside the uterus.[5]

The dose for oxytocin is 20 units (2 mL) per liter at a rate of 10 mL/min until the uterus is well contracted and bleeding is well controlled. The infusion rate should be changed to 1 to 2 mL/min until the mother can be transferred to a recovery suite, at which time the infusion should be discontinued.[6] Careful observation should occur through 1 hour after placenta delivery. Bleeding may occur from uterus relaxation; the mother should be examined for vaginal or introitus laceration, which may cause excessive bleeding.

Episiotomy

Episiotomy (perineotomy) is an incision on the perineum and the posterior vaginal wall to enlarge the vaginal introitus to facilitate the passage the fetus head. In past

---

Box 2
Signs of placental separation

Uterus is globular and firmer

Gush of blood

Uterus rises in abdomen

Umbilical cord is slack, farther out of the vagina

decades, it was thought to prevent traumatic vaginal tears during delivery. Among others benefits of the episiotomy procedure, it can minimize compression and fetal head trauma, facilitate the second stage of labor, and remove the resistance of pudendal musculatures.[5]

Currently, the American College of Obstetrics and Gynecology (ACOG) does not recommend episiotomy as a routine procedure,[10] because no evidence shows it enables a better outcome of delivery. Moreover, it is less often performed because of many complications, including bleeding, hematoma formation, third- and fourth-degree lacerations, incontinence, infections, swelling, and dyspareunia.[11,12] Thus, the routine episiotomy is no longer recommended, but a selective approach is now encouraged.[13] Indications for selective episiotomy[14] include breech delivery, preterm labor, and imminent perineal tearing (**Box 3**).

Two different approaches exist for the incision: midline (median) or mediolateral. Controversy persists regarding which approach is preferable, but mediolateral is still most recommended by the ACOG.[10,15] Either way, mediolateral has many disadvantages, including increased blood loss, postpartum discomfort, and dyspareunia. Although median episiotomy has an increase risk of anal sphincter injury, it is reported to have a better healing rate and satisfactory repair in selective cases.[11]

The median episiotomy can be complicated by traumatic extensions, such as first-, second-, third-, and fourth-degree tears (**Fig. 7**).

Technique

In the vertex presentation, the episiotomy should be performed when the fetal head is distending the perineum 3 to 4 cm with every contraction and the caput is seen through the vagina.[5] When the fetus is in the breech presentation, episiotomy should be performed just before the delivery.[5,6]

As the head is descending through vagina canal, the physician's index and second fingers are placed in the posterior vaginal fourchette, inside the introitus, and in the perineal area. Using Mayo scissors or blades, a midline incision 3 cm in length is made in the posterior fourchette and extended 6 cm into vaginal mucosa, submucosa, and pubococcygeus muscle (**Box 4**).[5,6] For the median episiotomy, the incision extends until the anal sphincter diaphragm. For the mediolateral approach, the incision is directed downward and outward in the direction of the lateral aspect of the anal sphincter either way left or right, and then extended to the lowermost perineal muscles, the pubococcygeus and bulbocavernosus, including the posterior vaginal fourchette, vaginal mucosa, and submucosa.[5]

Box 3
Indications for selective episiotomy

Preterm labor

Breech delivery

Shoulder dystocia

Rigid perineal muscle

Fetal distress/late decelerations

Perineal tear imminent

Fetal macrosomatia

Occipitoposterior presentation

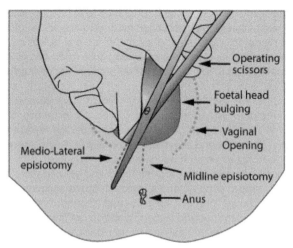

Fig. 7. Episiotomy modalities. (*From* Wikipedia contributors. Medio-laterial episiotomy. Wikipedia, The Free Encyclopedia. Available at: http://en.wikipedia.org/wiki/File:Medio-lateral-episiotomy.gif.)

Repair

The recommended time for repair of the episiotomy is after infant and placenta delivery. The cervix and vaginal canal should be closely inspected to assess for other causes of bleeding. Bleeding from a vaginal or cervix laceration should be corrected before repair of the episiotomy.[5] Hemostasis should be achieved before suturing, with gauze used to pack the vaginal canal. Ligation of vessels is recommended if necessary for hemostasis. The episiotomy can then be repaired.[16] The authorities recommend 2-0 or 3-0 absorbable sutures (eg, chromic gut or polyglycolic acid).[6] The risk of infection is diminished if the site is adequately prepared and cleaned before the incision is made.

POTENTIAL DELIVERY COMPLICATIONS
Obstetric Vaginal Lacerations

Perineal injuries after birth are a major health problem that affects thousands of women and require special attention. A thorough genital examination is needed to identify this injury and avoid its complications. As many as 91% of women report perineal pain, dyspareunia, sexual dysfunction, or bladder or bowel function disturbances 8 weeks after delivery. More than 60% women experience perineal injury after spontaneous vaginal delivery, and approximately 1000 women per day require perineal repair after vaginal birth.[17]

Maternal factors that may contribute to the extent of trauma during childbirth are ethnicity, age, primiparity, fetal weight greater than 4 kg, prolonged second stage of

Box 4
Equipment for episiotomy
Lidocaine 1% or 2%
Mayo scissors or blade
2-0 or 3-0 absorbable suture

labor, instrumental delivery, direct occipitoposterior fetal head position, and precipitate delivery. Perineal injuries may occur spontaneously during vaginal birth or from surgical incision made to increase the diameter of the vulva outlet to facilitate delivery.[18] These injuries are classified according to extent, allowing differentiation of those to the external anal sphincter, internal anal sphincter, and anal epithelium (**Table 2**).[18]

A complete and careful genital examination should be performed to identify the extent of injury. A rectal examination must be completed to assess for anal sphincter integrity. Third- and fourth-degree perineal injuries must be repaired by an experienced gynecologist under general anesthesia, whereas first- and second-degree perineal injuries can be repaired under local anesthesia.

Repair of the perineum requires good lightning and visualization, proper surgical instruments (**Box 5**), proper suture material, and adequate analgesia.[19] Some studies recommend the nonsuturing practice for first- and second-degree perineal injuries. The Royal College of Obstetrician and Gynecologist do not favor this practice because it is associated with poorer wound healing and no significant differences in short-term discomfort (level of evidence A).[18]

First-degree injuries are repaired with an absorbable synthetic material (Vicryl) using a continuous subcuticular technique. Vicryl is associated with less perineal pain, analgesic use, dehiscence, and resuturing compared with catgut sutures (level of evidence A).[18]

Second-degree injuries require approximation of the vaginal tissues, perineal muscles, and skin. An anchoring suture is placed 1 cm above the apex of the laceration. The vaginal mucosa and underlying rectovaginal fascia are closed using a running unlocked 3-0 Vicryl suture. The sutures must include the rectovaginal fascia. The running suture is carried to the hymenal ring and tied proximal to it. The muscles of the perineal body are identified and approximated with transverse interrupted 3-0 Vicryl sutures. A single interrupted 3-0 Vicryl suture is then placed through the bulbocavernosus muscle. When the perineal muscles are repaired anatomically, the overlying skin is closed with 4-0 Vicryl suture in a continuous subcuticular fashion.[19]

When the wound is contaminated with stools, second- or third-generation cephalosporin may be given before the procedure is started.[19] A rectal examination should be performed after the procedure to ensure that suture material was not accidentally inserted through the rectal mucosa.

Common pitfalls

The common pitfalls of vaginal laceration repair include (1) poor genital examination, which leads to missed anal sphincter injuries, and (2) use of catgut sutures, which leads to increased perineal pain, dyspareunia, and wound dehiscence.

Table 2 Perineal injury classification	
First-degree	Involving the perineal and vaginal skin
Second-degree	Perineal skin and muscle involvement, intact anal sphincter
Third-degree	Perineal skin, muscle, and anal sphincter are torn a. <50% of the EAS is torn b. >50% of the EAS, intact IAS c. Both EAS and IAS are torn, intact anal mucosa
Fourth-degree	Perineal skin, muscles, anal sphincter, and anal mucosa torn

Abbreviations: EAS, external anal sphincter; IAS, internal anal sphincter.

Box 5
Equipment for perineal repair
Sterile gloves
Sterile drapes
Irrigation solution
Needle holder
Forceps with teeth
Allis clamp
Suture scissors
3-0 Vicryl on a CT-1 needle
4-0 Vicryl on an SH needle

Breech Presentation

Breech is the most common fetal malpresentation.[20] Breech delivery accounts for approximately 3% to 4% of deliveries and is associated with increased perinatal morbidity and mortality.[8,20–23]

Breech presentation can be classified as frank, complete, or incomplete (**Fig. 8**). In frank breech, the fetal legs are flexed at the hips and the knees are extended. In complete breech the legs are flexed at the hips and one or both knees are flexed. Incomplete breech differs in that one or both hips are not flexed, resulting in both feet and knees being in the lowest part of the birth canal.[8,20] Frank breech accounts for most cases.[21]

Breech delivery is often encountered in the delivery of premature infants.[4,6] It is also associated with congenital and uterine anomalies, prolapsed cord, placenta previa, and multiple gestations.[6,8]

The 3 methods of breech delivery are spontaneous, partial, and total breech. During spontaneous breech delivery, expulsion of the fetus occurs spontaneously without any intervention other than supporting the neonate after delivery.[6,20] Incomplete breech delivery refers to spontaneous delivery of the fetus to the level of the umbilicus with subsequent assisted delivery of the remainder of the body.[6,8,20] Total breech delivery refers to extraction of the entire body of the fetus by the physician.[6,8,20]

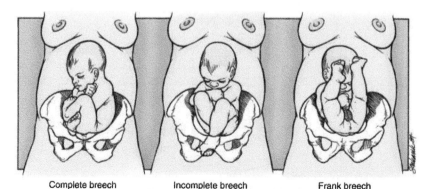

Complete breech   Incomplete breech   Frank breech

Fig. 8. Different breech presentations. (*From* Lanni SM, Seeds JW. Malpresentations and shoulder dystocia. In: Gabbe SG, ed. Obstetrics: Normal and Problem Pregnancies. Philadelphia, Elsevier Churchill Livingstone, 2007; with permission.)

Hannah and colleagues[24,25] determined that elective cesarean section was safer for the delivery of a breech presentation compared with vaginal delivery. Although, cesarean section might be considered the standard of care,[6] the emergency medicine physician should be able to perform breech delivery techniques in case of imminent breech delivery.

Management

Once a breech presentation is recognized, immediate consultation with an obstetrician, anesthesiologist, and neonatologist should occur. If the breech delivery is progressing spontaneously, it is better for the physician to wait expectantly until the delivery of the fetal umbilicus.[4] A premature intervention can result in higher maternal and fetal morbidity.[6] Efforts should be made to transfer the patient to a labor and delivery unit if time allows and the fetal umbilicus has been delivered yet.[6]

If spontaneous breech delivery is unlikely, the physician must assist the delivery. With the patient in the lithotomy position, episiotomy should be performed (as discussed previously) unless there is considerable perineum relaxation.[8] As the breech distends the perineum, the posterior hip should be delivered, commonly from the 6 o'clock position. This is followed by the anterior hip and external rotation to a sacrum anterior position (**Fig. 9**). To deliver the legs, the clinician should splint the medial aspect of each thigh by placing the fingers parallel to each femur, and then apply pressure laterally with the goal of sweeping each leg away from the midline (**Fig. 10**). Once the legs are delivered, the fetal bony pelvis should be grasped with both hands using a towel to prevent slippage of the fetus. This is accomplished by placing the fingers over the anterior superior iliac crest with the thumbs resting over the sacrum.[6] Careful placement of the fingers over the bony pelvis will prevent injury to the fetal abdominal soft tissue. Gentle rotational downward traction should be applied in conjunction with maternal bearing down efforts. To deliver the scapula, a 90° rotation is applied to the fetal pelvis, placing the fetal sacrum into the transverse position. A counterclockwise 180° rotation can then be applied to deliver the opposite scapula. Attempts to deliver the shoulder and arms should not occur until one of the axilla becomes visible.[8]

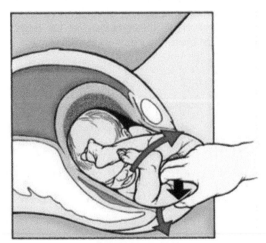

Fig. 9. In breech delivery, extraction of the hip should be attempted by pulling downward and rotating the hips. (*From* Lanni SM, Seeds JW. Malpresentations and shoulder dystocia. In: Gabbe SG, ed. Obstetrics: Normal and Problem Pregnancies. Philadelphia, Elsevier Churchill Livingstone, 2007; with permission.)

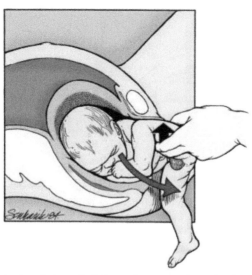

Fig. 10. Delivery of the legs in breech delivery. (*From* Lanni SM, Seeds JW. Malpresentations and shoulder dystocia. In: Gabbe SG, ed. Obstetrics: Normal and Problem Pregnancies. Philadelphia, Elsevier Churchill Livingstone, 2007; with permission.)

The shoulders can be delivered by 2 methods. With the scapulas visible, the first method is performed by rotating the trunk so that the anterior shoulder and arm appear at the vulva. Once at the vulva, the anterior shoulder and arm can be delivered with relative ease. Next, the body of the fetus is rotated in the reverse direction to deliver the other shoulder and arm.[6] If trunk rotation is unsuccessful and neither shoulder nor arm is free, the posterior shoulder must be delivered first (see **Fig. 10**). For this second method, the clinician will grasp both feet in one hand and apply upward traction over the mother's groin. With the clinician's free hand, leverage is applied to the posterior shoulder, which should become free over the mother's perineum, followed by the arm and hand. The anterior shoulder, arm, and hand are delivered by downward traction of the fetal body. If the arm and hand do not spontaneously deliver after the shoulder, upward traction of the fetal body is continued while 2 fingers of the other hand are used to locate the fetal posterior humerus to the level of the elbow. Once identified, and while using the fingers to splint the humerus, the posterior arm can be delivered by sweeping it downward (**Fig. 11**). The anterior arm is delivered with downward movement of the fetal body. If this is not sufficient, the anterior arm is splinted using 2 fingers and is delivered by sweeping it down over the thorax.

To deliver the head, the Mauriceau maneuver is performed (**Fig. 12**). With the fetal body resting on the clinician's hand and forearm, the index and middle finger are placed over the fetal maxilla to flex the head.[5] The index and middle finger of the other hand are placed on each side of the neck to grasp the shoulders and downward traction is applied until the suboccipital region appears under the pubic symphysis. The fetal body is then elevated upward toward the maternal abdomen, with the rest of the fetal head successfully being delivered. As the head is delivered, suprapubic pressure applied by an assistant is helpful (**Fig. 13**).

Postpartum Hemorrhage

Although controversial because of blood loss underestimation, postpartum hemorrhage can be defined as loss of more than 500 mL of maternal blood during vaginal

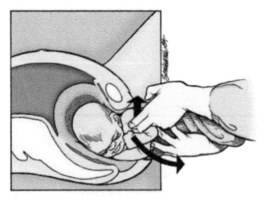

Fig. 11. Delivery of the shoulders in breech delivery. (*From* Lanni SM, Seeds JW. Malpresentations and shoulder dystocia. In: Gabbe SG, ed. Obstetrics: Normal and Problem Pregnancies. Philadelphia, Elsevier Churchill Livingstone, 2007; with permission.)

delivery.[6,8,21] In an urgent setting, in which multiple tasks are occurring simultaneously, the emergency physician should give special attention to the amount of maternal blood loss after delivery. Bleeding may be subtle but constant, and if unnoticed can become life-threatening.

Risk factors for postpartum hemorrhage include prior postpartum hemorrhage, uterus overdistention (multiple fetuses, macrosomia, polyhydramnios), prolonged labor, and coagulopathy among others.[6,8] The differential diagnosis includes uterine atony, genital tract lacerations (cervix or vagina), retained products of conception, uterine inversion, uterine rupture, and coagulopathies.[6,8,21]

The management of postpartum hemorrhage is based on identification of the cause. First, however, the emergency physician should consult an obstetrician and anesthesiologist. Adequate hemodynamic evaluation and initiation of volume-expander fluids and blood products should occur in cases of cardiovascular compromise.

Uterine Atony

Uterine atony is considered the most common cause of early postpartum hemorrhage.[6,8,21,24,26] A hypotonic uterus may result from uterine overdistention, tocolysis,

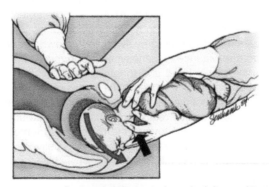

Fig. 12. Mauriceau maneuver for head delivery in breech delivery. (*From* Lanni SM, Seeds JW. Malpresentations and shoulder dystocia. In: Gabbe SG, ed. Obstetrics: Normal and Problem Pregnancies. Philadelphia, Elsevier Churchill Livingstone, 2007; with permission.)

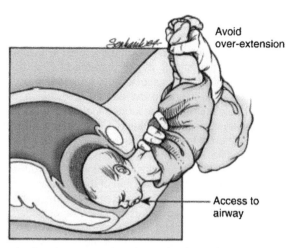

Avoid
over-extension

Access to
airway

Fig. 13. Delivery the head to open the airway for immediate nasopharynx suction and oxygen supplementation. (*From* Lanni SM, Seeds JW. Malpresentations and shoulder dystocia. In: Gabbe SG, ed. Obstetrics: Normal and Problem Pregnancies. Philadelphia, Elsevier Churchill Livingstone, 2007; with permission.)

and prolonged labor.[8,21] The diagnosis is confirmed by evidence of a soft, boggy uterus in the setting of excessive vaginal bleeding after delivery. Once identified, uterotonic agents must be started with concurrent suprapubic transabdominal uterine massage.[6,8,21] Among the uterotonic agents, oxytocin is the first-line agent. An intravenous infusion can be prepared by adding 10 to 40 units of oxytocin to 1000 mL of crystalloid, with the infusion rate titrated to achieve uterine contraction.[6,8,21,24] If intravenous access is not available, 10 units of oxytocin can be administered intramuscularly.[6,8,21,24] If oxytocin fails to improve the hemorrhage, second-line agents such as methylergonovine can be used at an intramuscular dose of 0.2 mg.[8,24] This ergot derivative should be used with caution in hypertensive and preeclamptic patients because of its effects in raising blood pressure.[8,21] Other second-line agents to be considered are prostaglandins, such as carboprost (derivative of 15-methyl prostaglandin F_2-alpha) administered intramuscularly at an initial dose of 0.25 mg. Dose may be repeated every 15 minutes, but should not exceed 8 doses.[8] Because of the bronchoconstrictive and vasoconstrictive effects, carboprost should be avoided in patients with asthma and hypertension.[8]

If hemorrhage persists despite these measures, a 2-handed uterine compression massage may be performed.[6,8,21] For this technique, 1 hand should apply pressure to the posterior aspect of the uterine fundus through the abdominal wall, while the other is made into a fist, introduced into the vagina, and firm pressure applied to the anterior aspect of the uterus.[6,8,21] If this technique fails to stop the bleeding, alternative causes of hemorrhage should be sought. A thorough inspection of the genital tract may reveal lacerations, and manual examination of the uterine cavity may show retained segments of placenta. Lacerations can be initially managed with direct pressure and the use of nonabsorbable sutures for control of bleeding.[6] Further management of the laceration is better left to the expertise of an obstetrician. Postpartum hemorrhage that continues despite these techniques and measures indicates the need for more invasive procedures, such as embolization or surgery.[27]

Uterine Inversion

Uterine inversion usually occurs after forceful traction of the umbilical cord during delivery of the placenta.[6,8,28] Although uncommon, uterine inversion can be life-threatening and may lead the shock if left untreated.[8] The patient commonly complains of severe abdominal pain associated with excessive vaginal bleeding. Physical examination varies according to the degree of inversion, but generally will reveal absence of a palpable uterus on transabdominal examination and visualization of a protruding mass during vaginal examination. Once patient stabilization has been initiated, immediate reposition of the uterus must occur. For reposition, the clinician's hand is placed into the vagina with the palm of the hand grasping the uterus and the fingertips placed at the uterocervical junction.[6,8,28] Digital upward pressure should be applied to the edges of the uterus in the direction of the umbilicus.[6,8,21] If unsuccessful, tocolytics such as terbutaline, ritrodrine, and magnesium sulfide can be used to relax the uterus to facilitate uterine reposition.[8,29] Once repositioned, manual uterine pressure should continue while tocolytics are stopped and oxytocin started.[8,21] General anesthesia and surgery may be required if these measures fail.[6]

Shoulder Dystocia

Shoulder dystocia refers to the inability to deliver the fetal shoulders after delivery of the fetal head in the vertex presentation (**Fig. 14**). Most commonly, the anterior fetal shoulder becomes impacted in the pubic symphysis. Shoulder dystocia is considered a true obstetric emergency because of the potential traumatic and hypoxic events on the fetus. According to the ACOG, shoulder dystocia occurs in approximately 0.6% to 1.4% of vaginal deliveries.[8] Risk factors for shoulder dystocia include fetal macrosomia, postterm pregnancy, and diabetes among others.[16,30]

Management

General measures that should not be overlooked are emptying of the patient's bladder, consideration of episiotomy, and placing the patient in the lithotomy position. Although some of the different techniques to relieve shoulder dystocia can be undertaken simultaneously, no universal consensus exists on a particular order. The most common initial techniques performed after calling for help are the McRoberts maneuver and suprapubic pressure. These techniques are initially preferred because

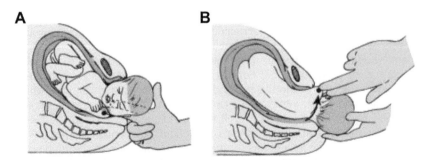

Fig. 14. Shoulder dystocia maneuver: Rubin and reverse Woods screw. (*A*) place two fingers in the posterior vaginal to identify the posterior fetal shoulder. (*B*) a 180 ° rotational force is applied then the posterior shoulder is more oblique in position resulting in adduction and oblique position that allow the delivery. (*From* Probst BD. Emergency childbirth. In: Roberts JR, Hedges JR, eds. Clinical Procedures in Emergency Medicine, 5th ed. Philadelphia: Elsevier 2009; with permission.)

they are noninvasive and can be performed with relative ease. The McRoberts maneuver consists of placing the mother in the extreme lithotomy position with the hips completely flexed, allowing the knees to fall on the mothers chest, the so-called knee–chest position.[6,31] This maneuver causes straightening of the sacrum in relation with the lumbar spine, which slides the pubic symphysis cephalad over the fetal shoulder. If the McRoberts maneuver fails to disengage the fetal shoulder, suprapubic pressure can apply by an assistant while the patient remains in the extreme lithotomy position. Some studies have shown that delivery of the posterior shoulder results in resolution of shoulder dystocia.[5] Delivery of the posterior shoulder is performed by placing a sterile gloved hand into the posterior aspect of the vagina and localizing the posterior shoulder of the fetus (**Fig. 15**). Once the posterior shoulder is identified, the clinician should slide a hand down the fetus arm until reaching the elbow. Pressure can then be applied on the antecubital fossa to cause flexion of the fetus forearm. If forearm flexion does not occur, the clinician can gently grasp the forearm and attempt to flex it. The forearm should be flexed over the fetus chest and delivered over the mother's perineum, allowing delivery of the anterior shoulder under the pubic symphysis. Another maneuver that can be performed is known as the Rubin or reverse Woods corkscrew maneuver (see **Fig. 14**).[6] To perform this maneuver, the clinician introduces 2 fingers posteriorly into the vagina to identify the posterior aspect of the posterior shoulder. A 180° rotational force is then applied, causing anterior movement of the posterior shoulder into a more oblique position within the pelvic outlet. The resulting adduction and oblique position of the shoulders may cause complete delivery of the fetus. If the shoulder dystocia persists despite attempting all of the described techniques, the clinician may attempt the Zavanelli maneuver to replace the fetal head into the uterine cavity with subsequent cesarean delivery.

Umbilical Cord Prolapse

Umbilical cord prolapse (UCP) transforms an emergency delivery in a real emergency. UCP complicates labor in approximately 0.5% of deliveries.[6] The most accepted presentation of this condition is when the fetal presenting part does not fill enough

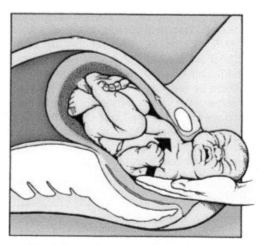

Fig. 15. Shoulder dystocia delivery. (*From* Lanni SM, Seeds JW. Malpresentations and shoulder dystocia. In: Gabbe SG, ed. Obstetrics: Normal and Problem Pregnancies. Philadelphia, Elsevier Churchill Livingstone, 2007; with permission.)

of the lower uterine segment during active labor. Low birth weight, multiparity, fetal malpresentation are the most common risks factors related to UCP. Some studies suggest that premature rupture of membranes (amniotomy) and polyhydramnios increase the risk of UCP.[32]

When a pregnant patient arrives at the emergency department, a history and physical examination should be performed. The history may not be contributory to the diagnosis of UCP. To diagnose UCP, careful pelvic examination should be performed with sterile gloves. If a pulsatile structure can be felt once the examiner reaches the oz, UCP can be diagnosed.

Once UCP is diagnosed, the preferred management is emergent cesarean section.[4,21] While the operating room is being prepared, some maneuvers may be performed. First, the examiner who diagnosed the UCP should keep a finger inside the cervix to continue lifting the presenting part and minimize cord compression. With this maneuver some authors recommend filling the bladder with 500 to 700 mL of saline to maintain cord decompression, after which the examiner can remove the hand from the vagina very carefully. The mother should be placed in knee–chest position and encouraged not to push, cough, or move in any way that will increase the intra-abdominal pressure.

The prognosis is based on the time of compression. If more than 10 minutes elapses from the door to cesarean section, the prognosis decreases and more fetal complications might be expected.[33,34] The emergency physician should be prepared to resuscitate the newborn.

When surgery cannot be performed promptly, funic reduction can be performed. This maneuver involves manual replacement of the cord into the uterus, but immediate vaginal delivery should be attempted.

Umbilical Cord Entanglement

The incidence of true umbilical cords knots is 0.3% to 2.1%. The umbilical cord can tangle by itself or during pregnancy with fetal movements. Long umbilical cords are associated with entanglement. Some authors remark that a higher incidence occurs during early pregnancy rather than late, suggesting that it is part of normal pregnancy.[35] Usually it is diagnosed during labor when the presenting part has an umbilical cord loop.[36] Fetal heart rate (FHR) monitoring is a valuable tool for evaluation in this setting. Variable or prolonged decelerations are the most common finding of cord entanglement during FHR monitoring. This variable deceleration is related to increased incidence of fetal distress in labor, low APGAR scores, neonatal intensive care unit admission, and nuchal cord involvement, as reported by some studies.[37]

The entanglement should be reduced promptly during delivery to preserve blood flow and oxygenation. Some of the loops disentangle without manipulation. If spontaneous disentanglement does not occur, the loops should be slipped over the extremities or forward over the head (see **Fig. 6**). In some instances the loops are too tight to disentangle, and the physician should be aware and prepared to cut the cord and immediately deliver the fetus to avoid hypoxia.[21]

PERIMORTEM CESAREAN SECTION

Perimortem cesarean section, one of the oldest and most dramatic emergency surgical procedures, has long been used as an attempt to preserve the life of the fetus.[38]

Since the 1980s, some case reports have shown that the mother could recover after perimortem cesarean section.[39] Thus, emergency physician must be familiar and comfortable with this procedure.

Indications

Survival of the infant is directly related to the elapsed time from death of the mother to delivery, the maturity of the fetus, the performance of cardiopulmonary resuscitation (CPR) on the mother, and the availability of neonatal intensive care facilities. Although, the lower limit of fetal viability varies among institutions, in general, performing the procedure before the point of fetal viability at approximately 24 weeks is not indicated. If the duration of gestation is not known from the history, fetal maturity may be quickly estimated by calculating gestational age based on the date of the mother's last normal menstrual period or measuring the height of the uterine fundus.[7] Between 18 and 30 weeks' gestation, the age of the fetus in weeks will correspond to the distance in centimeters from the uterine fundus to the symphysis pubis (eg, at 28 weeks' gestation the fundus is approximately 28 cm above the symphysis pubis or halfway between the umbilicus and the costal margin). Criteria for intervention should be established prospectively at each institution and be in accordance with the institution's general neonatal policies.

The potential for infant survival decreases and the chance of neurologic damage increases as the time from maternal death (cessation of circulation) to cesarean section increases (**Fig. 16**). Because even in optimal conditions CPR results in a cardiac output of 30% to 40% of normal output and placental perfusion may be severely compromised, every attempt should be made to begin cesarean delivery within 4 minutes of the cardiopulmonary arrest, completing the procedure within 5 minutes of arrest.[40] Fetal prognosis is generally better after the sudden death of a previously healthy mother than after the death of a mother with a prolonged and debilitating illness.

CPR should be initiated immediately on cardiac arrest of the mother and be continued until after the infant is delivered. The pregnant state produces certain physiologic changes that adversely affect the adequacy of standard CPR.[41] Vena cava occlusion by the gravid uterus hampers venous return and thus compromises maternal cardiac output. A decreased functional residual capacity of the lungs may impede ventilation. An assistant may attempt manual displacement of the uterus away from the inferior vena cava. However, perimortem cesarean delivery in itself may be the most important variable in a successful maternal resuscitation.

Legal and ethical considerations

Because no standard of care exists for emergency clinicians performing a perimortem cesarean delivery, each case must be individualized. Limited resources often place the clinician in the difficult position of deciding whether to continue efforts to resuscitate the mother or to attempt to deliver the fetus in a difficult situation in less-than-ideal conditions. In the absence of obstetric backup immediately at hand, it is reasonable for the emergency clinician to proceed with delivering the child if the mother cannot be resuscitated. Prolonged attempts to resuscitate the mother are unlikely to benefit either the mother or the fetus.[5]

Technique

The most experienced person, preferably an obstetrician, should perform perimortem cesarean section. But, in the emergency setting, the emergency physician should be prepared to do so. When possible, a neonatologist should be in attendance; however, arrival should not delay the procedure. CPR on the mother should be initiated at cardiac arrest and continued throughout the procedure. Although, it is helpful if fetal heart tones are present premortem, time should not be wasted searching for them or attempting to evaluate fetal viability with abdominal ultrasonography.

Because neonatal survival is enhanced as the time from maternal death to delivery decreases (although the irreversible nature of maternal cardiac arrest becomes more

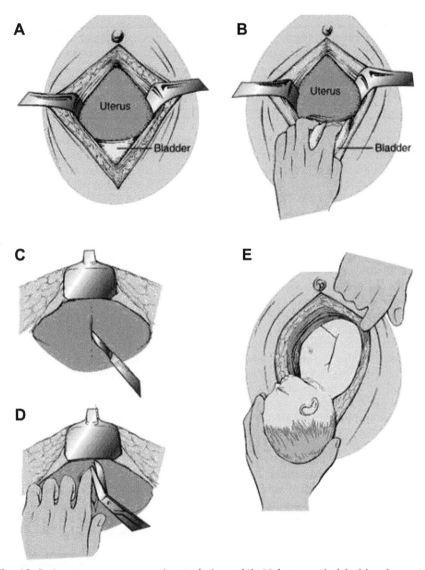

Fig. 16. Perimortem cesarean section technique. (*A*), Make a vertical incision in ventral aspect of the abdomen. (*B*) place retractors and identify the bladder, place a bladder retractor. (*C*) make a vertical incision with the scalpel in the uterus. (*D*) with a scissors to extend the incision inferiorly. (*E*) extract the fetus head, suction the pharynx and deliver the fetus completely. (*From* Pearlman M, Tintinally JE. Emergency care of the woman. New York: McGraw-Hill 1998; with permission).

apparent as resuscitative efforts progress), the decision to perform a perimortem cesarean section may be one of the most difficult an emergency clinician must makes.[41] When time matters, the emergency physician should be familiar with the minimum equipment necessary to perform this procedure (**Box 6**).

Rapid extraction of the infant while avoiding fetal and maternal injury is the goal of the procedure. Hence, time should not be wasted preparing a sterile operating

Box 6
Equipment for perimortem cesarean delivery
Retractors
Clamps
Vascular clamps or hemostats
Neonatal resuscitation kit: neonatal air bag, intubation tray, suction bulb
Warmer
Curved scissors
Blades #10
Blood gas syringe
Sutures

field or transporting the patient to an operating suite outside the emergency department.[42]

Using a large (eg, No. 10) scalpel, a midline vertical incision should be made through the abdominal wall extending from the symphysis pubis to the umbilicus and carried through all abdominal layers to the peritoneal cavity. In most gravid women, the hyperpigmented linea nigra is apparent and may serve as a guide for the incision (see **Fig. 12**).[21] If available, retractors should be placed in the abdominal wound and drawn laterally to expose the anterior surface of the uterus. The bladder should be reflected inferiorly; if it is full, it may be aspirated to evacuate it and permit better access to the uterus. While avoiding injury to fetal parts, a small (≈ 5 cm) vertical incision should be made through the lower uterine segment until amniotic fluid is obtained or until the uterine cavity is clearly entered. The index and middle fingers should then be inserted into the incision and used to lift the uterine wall away from the fetus.[21,41] Bandage scissors should be used to extend the incision vertically to the fundus until a wide exposure is obtained. The infant should then be delivered gently, the mouth and nose suctioned, and the umbilical cord clamped and cut. Because the incision is high in the uterus, the infant's head may not be readily accessible to the clinician, in which case the infant's feet should be grasped that the infant delivered using maneuvers similar to those for a breech delivery.[6] Neonatal resuscitation should be performed as necessary. The incision should be repaired if spontaneous recovery of circulation is achieved by the mother.[7]

Potential complications

Bladder injury is common. Therefore, if a full bladder obstructs the view of the uterus, it should be decompressed with a puncture incision and deflated with either pressure or suction. Bladder repair may be performed later if the mother recovers spontaneous circulation. Other complications include bowel injury, fetal laceration and injuries, neonatal neurologic deficits or demise, maternal bleeding and infection, and maternal mortality.[6] Cases of maternal survival have been reported, hence the importance of checking maternal pulses, performing continuous CPR, and relieving aortocaval compression by the uterus to improve maternal hemodynamics.[5]

GYNECOLOGIC PROCEDURES
Bartholin Abscess

Bartholin glands are a pair of glands localized in the labia minora in the 4 and 8 o'clock positions. Each gland secretes mucus into the Bartholin ducts, a 2.5-cm duct that emerges into the vestibule at either site of the vagina to aid in lubrication. Generally, these glands are nonpalpable, except in the presence of obstruction or infection.[43]

Bartholin abscesses are common in women 20 to 29 years of age and may present as a protruding painful vaginal mass. Women usually complain of vulvar pain that worsens with sitting, walking, or intercourse.

For many years, Bartholin abscesses were thought to be the result of sexually transmitted diseases (STDs). Today, Bartholin gland abscesses are widely known to be polymicrobial in origin, with anaerobes the most common pathogens.[44] In women with risks factors for STDs, colonization with Neisseria gonorrhea and Chlamydia trachomatis should be highly considered.[45]

Incision and drainage is a simple procedure that provides immediate relief in symptomatic patients (**Boxes 7** and **8**).[46] A Worth catheter, a small rubber catheter with an inflatable balloon tip, is left in place for continuous drainage for approximately 6 to 8 weeks. If it is not available, an 8-French Foley catheter may be used. Patients must be informed that abscess may recur after incision and drainage (**Fig. 17**), and they should be referred for follow-up in 48 hours with a gynecologist. Oral analgesics should be prescribed. Sitz baths 3 times daily may aid with drainage. If any signs of cellulitis are present, a broad-spectrum antibiotic should be started. In patients at high risk for STDs, coverage should be provided, with cephalexin and metronidazole appropriate treatment choices.[46]

Some complications are associated with this procedure. For some patients the procedure can be very painful despite adequate local anesthesia, and adjunctive pain medications or procedural sedation should be considered. Another complication is when the catheter falls out because of a large incision. Instead of a very large incision, a 5-mm incision should be made so that the catheter will stay in place.

GENITAL TRAUMA
Vulvar Hematoma

Nonobstetric vulvar hematomas are essentially a rare condition. They are often the result of straddle injuries, traumatic sexual intercourse, or physical assault. Obstetric vulvar hematomas are more common than nonobstetric vulvar hematoma with an incidence of 1:300 to 1:1500 deliveries.[47] Nulliparity, preeclampsia, episiotomy, multiple gestations, and operative vaginal deliveries have been associated with an increased incidence of hematoma formation in the obstetric population.[48]

Box 7
Equipment for Bartholin abscess

Sterile gloves

Iodine solution

Lidocaine 1% or 2%

Sterile gauzes

Small needle holder

Small hemostat forceps

No. 11 scalpel

5-mL syringe for lidocaine injection

3-mL syringe for inflating balloon

Word catheter

Box 8
Technique for incision and drainage of Bartholin abscesses

1. Clean the affected area with iodine solution.

2. Apply anesthesia with lidocaine 1% or 2%.

3. Make a small elliptical, vertical incision along the vaginal mucosal surface.

4. Apply gentle pressure.

5. Insert a small hemostat and break any adhesions.

6. Insert tip of word catheter, inflate balloon with saline solution.

The female genitalia is highly vascular, with loose subcutaneous tissues. The vascular supply of the female perineum is derived from the branches of the internal pudendal artery. The accompanying perineal veins are valveless and have free anastomoses with the intrapelvic venous plexuses. Massive vulvar hematomas can form because the loose connective tissue affords little resistance until the mass is large enough to cause tamponade of the bleeding vessels.[48] Although bleeding is most commonly of venous origin, some reported cases have involved the internal iliac artery, in which embolization was required.[47]

A thorough physical examination of the genitalia and abdomen should be performed to rule out any intra-abdominal injury. The examiner must perform a complete vulvar, vaginal, and rectal examination to assess the size and extension of the hematoma. Abdominal ultrasound and/or abdominopelvic CT may be ordered to assess for extension into the peritoneum.

Conservative and surgical management are the treatment options for vulvar hematoma. Conservative management consists of external compression and ice pack for 24 hours. Because local swelling may be sufficient to impair voluntary voiding, a Foley catheter should be inserted and left it in place. Adequate analgesia is an essential part of the treatment. Narcotics and nonsteroidal anti-inflammatory drugs are equally recommended. Patients who are treated conservatively should be followed up with frequent examination and serial cell blood cell count.

If a vulvar hematoma is continuing to expand despite external pressure or is presenting acutely with a size greater than 10 cm, or the patient is presenting with shock and/or anemia, prompt evacuation of the hematoma is mandatory. To avoid the risk of wound infection, this procedure should be performed in a sterile room. A large incision is made, followed by ligation of bleeding vessels and packing to secure hemostasis. Drainage should be left in place. Hematoma evacuation can be a very painful and uncomfortable procedure; procedural sedation or general anesthesia should be considered. For emergency physicians, a safe approach is to make a small elliptical incision and place a Worth catheter for continuous drainage (see Bartholin abscess section for Worth catheter placement instructions). Sitz baths are recommended to aid with drainage.

Infection, anemia, and shock are the most common complications of conservative management. In a retrospective review, Propst and colleagues[49] found that 4 of 10 nonobstetric vulvar hematomas required intravenous antibiotics and subsequent operative procedure. In another retrospective review, Benrubi and colleagues[50] reported increases in intravenous antibiotics, transfusion, readmission, subsequent operative procedures, and length of hospitalization in patients managed conservatively.

Common pitfalls

Poor physical examination of genitalia may cause the extension of the hematoma to be missed.

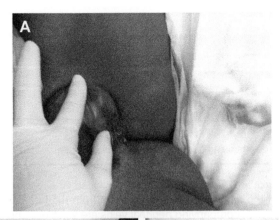

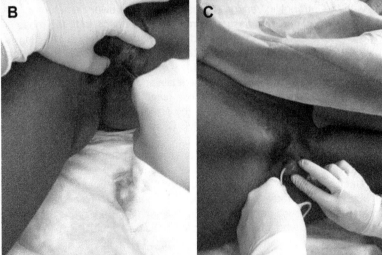

Fig. 17. Bartholin abscess drainage. (*A*) Identify the mucosal border of the vulva and make 5-mm incision. (*B*) Open the incision with the hemostat. (*C*) After drainage occur place a Worth catheter or indwelling Foley catheter # 8 French. (*Courtesy of* Dr Mercado, UPR Hospital Carolina, PR.)

Vulvar and Vaginal Laceration

Vulvar trauma can cause significant bleeding because the area is highly vascular. Straddle injuries and consensual and nonconsensual coitus are the most common causes of vulvar lacerations. Most lacerations are superficial and can be left open if no active bleeding is identified.

Nonobstetric vaginal lacerations can range from minor simple lacerations to life-threatening events. Most cases resolve without medical intervention, but severe lacerations may require emergent surgical repair. Lacerations are usually 3 to 5 cm long and are commonly localized in the posterior fornix.[50]

The most common mechanism of nonobstetric vaginal injury is consensual coitus. Other common factors are first coitus, disproportion of male and female genitalia, female in dorsal decubitus position, hyperflexion of the thighs and setting intercourse may result in vaginal laceration as well.[51] Among other factors are tissue friability, foreign bodies, previous surgeries, atrophic vagina in postmenopausal women, rough or nonconsensual coitus, and pelvic radiation therapy.

In pediatric and adolescent population, hymenal disruption at the 3 to 9 o'clock positions should raise concern about sexual abuse.[52] A detailed history and physical examination should be performed to rule out sexual abuse. Normal-appearing genitalia is not evidence enough to exclude the possibility of abuse.

Physical examination is an important tool in diagnosis and management. A thorough examination of the external and internal genitalia should be performed. If excessive bleeding obscures examination, the vagina should be packed with sterile gauze and the patient taken to the operating room for evaluation and bleeding control. Urethral catheterization must be performed to assess for bladder and urethral injury. Digital rectal examination should be performed to determine sphincter tone, assess mucosal integrity, and evaluate for posterior vaginal injuries.

Lacerations that are superficial, clean, and less than 6 hours old can be closed with a fine absorbable suture. Deeper lacerations should be explored for foreign bodies and the patient assessed for rectal, urethral, or periclitoral injuries. Wounds located near the urethra or clitoris may cause severe postrepair pain. If no significant bleeding is identified, these injuries may be left to heal by secondary intention. Infected wounds should not be closed. Wound debridement is encouraged. Wounds should be packed with saline-moistened gauzes and allowed to close by secondary intention. Vulvar lacerations are very painful, and urinary retention can be a complication. In these

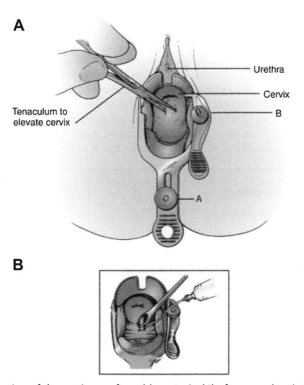

Fig. 18. Preparation of the cervix area for culdocentesis. (*A*) after speculum introduction the cervix is identified, fix the speculum and with a tenaculum elevate the cervix. (*B*) the posterior cervix area exposed. (*Adapted from* Webb MJ. Culdocentesis. Journal of the American College of Emergency Physicians 1978;7:452; with permission.)

cases, a Foley catheter should be inserted and left in place. Patients should have a follow-up examination with a gynecologist.

Patients presenting with signs and symptoms of shock should immediately be resuscitated with isotonic fluids. A complete blood cell count and a type and cross for 2 units of packed red blood cells should be ordered. These patients need emergent gynecologist consult for pelvic examination under general anesthesia.

Any patient presenting with vaginal bleeding and abdominal pain should be evaluated for injuries extending into the peritoneal cavity. Upright abdominal radiographs may show free air under the diaphragm. Abdominopelvic CT may show injury to hollow or solid organs and/or bone.

Superficial vaginal lacerations limited to the mucosal and submucosal tissues can be approximated with a fine absorbable suture under local anesthesia. Catgut may increase postrepair pain. Deep or complicated vaginal lacerations are best repaired in an operating room under general anesthesia. The proximity of the bladder, small bowel, rectum, ureters, and uterine vessels place them at high risk of injury during the procedure. Laparoscopy or exploratory laparotomy may be needed for assessment of a deep vaginal laceration that extends into the peritoneal cavity. A gynecologist or general surgeon should repair injuries extending into the rectum.

Prophylactic antibiotics are not usually required. In sexual abuse victims, prophylaxis for STDs is adequate.

In general, adequate and extensive physical examination should be performed to avoid missing deep vaginal lacerations or rectal injuries. The physician should be careful in choosing the appropriate sutures to avoid poor cosmetic results.

Culdocentesis

Culdocentesis is a procedure performed in women to assess for the presence of intra-abdominal fluid. It requires peritoneal fluid to be aspirated transvaginally from the rectouterine pouch to reveal the nature of the fluid. The procedure can help the physician assess for a certain number of conditions, such as ruptured viscous (ectopic pregnancy, or corpus luteum cyst) and pelvic inflammatory disease, abdominal infections, intra-abdominal injuries to liver and spleen and ruptured aortic aneurysms.[6,53] Although, the sensitivity and specificity of culdocentesis are low compared with ultrasonography

---

Box 9
Equipment for culdocentesis

Adjustable examination table

Bivalve vaginal speculum

Uterine cervical tenaculum

19-guage butterfly needle or 18-guage spinal needle

25-guage needle (local anesthesia)

Ring sponge forceps

Syringes (20 mL)

Surgical preparation solution

Sterile water, cotton balls, 4 × 4 gauzes

Lidocaine (1%) with epinephrine

Culture media or test tube without anticoagulation

Written/verbal consent

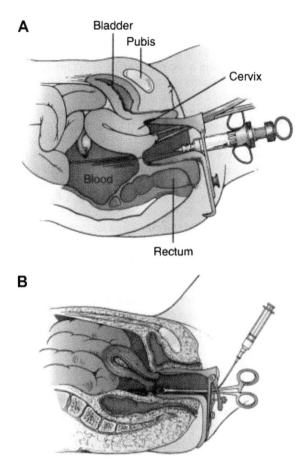

A

Bladder

Pubis

Cervix

Blood

Rectum

B

Fig. 19. Puncture area for the culdocentesis. (*A*) the needle should penetrate 2 to 2.5 cm to avoid perforate a bowel. (*B*), gentle suctionis then applied with the syringe as the needle is withdrawn. (*Adapted from* Webb MJ. Culdocentesis. Journal of the American College of Emergency Physicians 1978;7:452; with permission).

(66% and 80% respectively),[54] this procedure could be beneficial when ultrasound is not available or in patients too unstable to leave the emergency department.[5,6]

Before performing a culdocentesis, a bimanual examination is recommended to assess for possible contraindications. Contraindications include an uncooperative patient, a pelvic mass detected on bimanual pelvic examination, a nonmobile retroverted uterus, and coagulopathies. Pelvic masses include tubo-ovarian abscesses, appendiceal abscesses, ovarian masses, and pelvic kidneys. The major risk with the procedure is rupturing an unsuspected tubo-ovarian abscess into the peritoneal cavity, which can be avoided with careful bimanual examination.[6]

Culdocentesis is an invasive procedure that requires written/verbal consent by the patient. Once obtained, the patient is placed in the lithotomy position with the head slightly elevated to allow intraperitoneal fluid to settle in the rectouterine pouch. A bimanual examination should be performed to rule out presence of a pelvic mass. Examination with a vaginal speculum is performed and the lithotomy position is maintained for the procedure. The posterior tip of the cervix is grasped with a uterine cervical tenaculum and used to elevate the cervix (**Fig. 18**). This maneuver exposes the puncture site and stabilizes the posterior wall during the procedure. After this is achieved, the vaginal wall in the area of the rectouterine pouch should be cleaned with surgical preparation and a small amount of sterile water. Local anesthesia may be administered at this point using a separate 25- to 27-gauge needle.[6] Both needles used for local anesthesia and culdocentesis (spinal needle) should be attached to a 20-mL syringe for better control (**Box 9**). Once anesthesia is obtained, the spinal needle is introduced parallel to the lower blade of the speculum. Using 2 to 3 mL of sterile saline in the syringe may help expel tissue, which can clog the needle, and also helps confirm that the needle tip is in place. The needle should penetrate a total of 2 to 2.5 cm into the midline (**Fig. 19**). Gentle suction is then applied with the syringe as the needle is withdrawn. If no fluid is aspirated, the needle should be reintroduced and directed only slightly to the left or right of the midline.[5] Directing it too far laterally may result in puncture of mesenteric or pelvic vessels. The aspirated fluid may be old, nonclotting blood, bright red blood, pus, exudates, or serous depending on the cause of the intraperitoneal fluid. Other fluid than blood should be submitted for cytology and bacterial culture.

The most serious complication is rupture of a tubo-ovarian abscess. Among others are perforation of bowel and uterine wall and bleeding from the puncture site in patients with clotting disorders. Bowel and uterine wall punctures are common, and occasionally air or fecal matter can be aspirated, confirming inadvertent puncture of the rectum. Even though this could be disconcerting, it is seldom of serious clinical concern and requires no immediate change in therapy. Although common, bowel and uterine wall punctures usually do not result in serious morbidity requiring immediate therapy.[6]

SUMMARY

Emergency department visits for obstetric and gynecologic complaints continue to increase, and therefore emergency physicians must be proficient in diagnosing and managing these common conditions, which include emergent delivery and potential complications. In addition, the successful management of many gynecologic conditions depends on a good differential diagnosis to minimize morbidity and mortality.

REFERENCES

1. American College of Obstetricians and Gynecologists practice Bulletin. Dystocia and augmentation of labor. Clinical management guidelines for obstetricians-gynecologists. No 49. Washington, DC: American College of Obstetricians and Gynecologists; 2003.
2. Norwitz ER, Robinson JN, Repke JT. Labor and delivery. In: Gabbe SG, Niebyl JR, Simpson JL, editors. Obstetrics: normal and problem pregnancies. 3rd edition. New York: Churchill Livingstone; 2003. p. 353.
3. Kilpatrick SJ, Laros RK. Characteristics of normal labor. Obstet Gynecol 1989; 74(1):85–7.
4. Tintinalli J E, Stapczynski S, Cline DM, et al. Tintinalli's emergency medicine: a comprehensive study guide. 7th edition. New York: McGraw-Hill; 2011.
5. Benrubi GI. Handbook of obstetric and gynecologic emergencies. 2nd edition. Lippincott Williams and Wilkins; 2001.
6. Roberts JR, Hedges JR. Clinical procedure in emergency medicine. 5th edition. Saunders Elsevier; 2010.
7. Stallard TC, Burns B. Emergency delivery and perimortem C-section. Emerg Med Clin North Am 2003;21:679–93.
8. Cunningham FG, Leveno KJ, Gilstrap LC, et al. Normal labor and delivery. Williams obstetrics. 22nd edition. McGraw-Hill; 2005.

9. Gibbs CE. Obstetrics-an overview. In: Pauerstein CJ, editor. Clinical obstetrics. 1st edition. New York: John Wiley; 1987. p. 871.

10. American College of Obstetricians and Gynecologists (ACOG). Episiotomy. Washington, DC: American College of Obstetricians and Gynecologists (ACOG); 2006.

11. Landy HJ, Laughon SK, Bailit JL, et al. Characteristics associated with severe perineal and cervical lacerations during vaginal delivery. Obstet Gynecol 2011; 117(3):627–35.

12. Räisänen S, Vehviläinen-Julkunen K, Gissler M, et al. High episiotomy rate protects from obstetric anal sphincter ruptures: a birth register-study on delivery intervention policies in Finland. Scand J Public Health 2011;39(5):457–63.

13. Weber AM, Meyn L. Episiotomy use in the United States, 1979–1997. Obstet Gynecol 2002;100(6):1177–82.

14. American College of Obstetricians-Gynecologists. ACOG Practice Bulletin. Episiotomy. Clinical Management Guidelines for Obstetrician-Gynecologists. Number 71, April 2006. Obstet Gynecol 2006;107(4):956–62.

15. Frankman EA, Wang L, Bunker CH, et al. Episiotomy in the United States: has anything changed? Am J Obstet Gynecol 2009;200(5):573.e1–7.

16. DeCherney A, Nathan P, Martini P, et al. Measurement of the thickness of the urethrovaginal space in women with or without vaginal orgasm. J Sex Med 2008;5(3):610–8.

17. Fernando RJ. Risk factors and management of obstetric perineal injury. Obstetric, Gynecology and Reproductive Medicine August 2007;17(8):238–43.

18. Roos AM, Thakar R, Sultan AH. Outcome of primary repair of obstetric anal sphincter injuries (OASIS): does grade of tear matter? Ultrasound Obstet Gynecol 2010;36:368–74.

19. Leeman L, Spearman M, Rogers R. Repair of obstetric perineal lacerations. Am Fam Physician 2003;68(8):1585–90.

20. Givens ML, Westermyer R. Term incomplete breech delivery in an ambulance: a case report. J Emerg Med 2005;28(3):301–3.

21. Desai S, Henderson O, Mallon WK. Labor and delivery and their complications. In: Marx JA, Hockberger RS, Walls RM, et al, editors. Marx: Rosen's emergency medicine. 7th edition. Elsevier; 2010. p. 2327–47.

22. Molkenboer FM, Vencken PM, Sonnemans LG, et al. Conservative management in breech deliveries leads to similar results compared with cephalic deliveries. J Matern Fetal Neonatal Med 2007;20(8):599–603.

23. Simms A, Woods A. Fetal malpresentation. Curr Obstet Gynecol 2004;14(4):231–8.

24. Daskalakis G, Anastasakis E, Papantoniou N, et al. Cesarean vs. vaginal birth for term breech presentation in 2 different study period. Int J Gynaecol Obstet 2007; 96(3):162–6.

25. Anderson JM, Etches D. Prevention and management of postpartum hemorrhage. Am Fam Physician 2007;75(6):875–82.

26. Breathnach F, Geary M. Uterine atony: definition, prevention, nonsurgical management, and uterine tamponade. Semin Perinatol 2009;33(2):82–7.

27. Schmitz T, Tararbit K, Dupont C, et al. Prostaglandin E2 analogue sulprostone for treatment of atonic postpartum hemorrhage. Obstet Gynecol 2011;118(2 Pt 1):257–65.

28. Wendel PJ, Cox SM. Emergent obstetrics management of uterine inversion. Obstet Gynecol Clin North Am 1995;22(2):261–74.

29. Gray H. Anatomy of the human body. Philadelphia: Lea & Febiger; 1918.

30. Danakas GT, Pietrantoni M. Practical guide to the care of the gynecologic/obstetric patient. St Louis (MO): Mosby; 1997.

31. Gurewitsch ED, Kim EL, Yang JH, et al. Comparing Mc Robert's and Rubin's maneuvers for initial management of shoulder dystocia: an objective evaluation. Am J Obstet Gynecol 2005;192(1):153–60.

32. Dilbaz B, Ozturkoglu E, Dilbaz S, et al. Risk factors and perinatal outcomes associated with umbilical cord prolapse. Arch Gynecol Obstet 2006;274:104–7.
33. Kahana B, Sheiner E, Levy A, et al. Umbilical cord prolapse and perinatal outcomes. Int J Gynaecol Obstet 2004;84(2):127.
34. Lin MG. Umbilical cord prolapse. Obstet Gynecol Surv 2006;61(4):269–77.
35. Amer S, Kidron D, Aviram R, et al. High incidence of cord entanglement during early pregnancy detected by three dimensional sonography. Am J Perinatol 2009;26(5):379–82.
36. Gembrush U, Baschat A. True knot of the umbilical cord: transient constrictive effect to umbilical venous blood flow demonstrated by Doppler sonography. Ultrasound Obstet Gynecol 1996;8:53–6.
37. Anyaegbunam A, Brustman L, Divon M, et al. The significance of antepartum variable decelerations. Am J Obstet Gynecol 1986;155(4):707–10.
38. Ritter JW. Postmortem cesarean section. JAMA 1961;175:715–6.
39. DePace NL, Betesh JS, Kotler MN. 'Postmortem' cesarean section with recovery of both mother and offspring. JAMA 1982;248(8):971–3.
40. Katz VL, Dotters DJ, Droegemueller W. Perimortem cesarean delivery. Obstet Gynecol 1986;68:571.
41. American Heart Association. 2005 American Heart Association Guidelines for Cardiopulmonary Resuscitation and Emergency Cardiovascular Care. Part 10.8: cardiac arrest associated to pregnancy. Circulation 2005;112:IV-15–153.
42. Dillon WP, Lee RV, Tronolone MJ, et al. Life support and maternal brain death during during pregnancy. JAMA 1982;248:1089.
43. Krantz KE. Anatomy of the female reproductive system. In: Decherney AH, Nathan L, Goodwin TM, et al, editors. Current diagnosis & treatment: obstetrics & gynecology. 10th edition. McGraw-Hill; 2007. p. 21.
44. Azzan BB. Bartholin's cyst and abscess. A review of treatment of 53 cases. Br J Clin Pract 1978;3294:101–2.
45. Omole F, Simmons BJ, Hacker Y. Management of Bartholin's duct cyst and gland abscess. Am Fam Physician 2003;68(1):135–40.
46. Pundir J, Auld BJ. A review of the management of diseases of the Bartholin's gland. J Obstet Gynaecol 2008;28(2):161–5.
47. Frioux SM, Blinman T, Christian CW. Vaginal lacerations from consensual intercourse in adolescents. Child Abuse Negl 2011;35:69–73.
48. Egan E, Dundee P, Lawrentschuck N. Vulvar hematoma secondary to spontaneous rupture of the internal iliac artery: clinical review. Am J Obstet Gynecol 2009;200:e17–8.
49. Propst AM, Thorp JM Jr. Traumatic vulvar hematomas: conservative versus surgical management. South Med J 1998;91(2):144–6.
50. Benrubi G, Numan C, Nuss RC, et al. Vulvar and vaginal hematomas: a retrospective study of conservative versus operative management. South Med J 1987;80: 991–4.
51. Sloin MM, Karimian M, Ilbeigi P. Non obstetric lacerations of the vagina. J Am Osteopath Ass May 2006;106(5):271–3.
52. Okur I, Yildirim AM, Kose R. Severe haematoma of the vulva and defloration caused by goring. Eur J Obstet Gynecol Reprod Biol 2004;119:250–2.
53. Romero R, Copel JA, Kadar N, et al. Value of culdocentesis in the diagnosis of ectopic pregnancy. Obstet Gynecol 1985;65:519–22.
54. Chen PC, Sickler GK, Dubinski TJ, et al. Sonographic detection of echogenic fluid and correlation with culdocentesis in the evaluation of ectopic pregnancy. ARJ Am J Roentgenol 1998;170(5):1299–302.

Critical Urologic Skills and Procedures in the Emergency Department

Maria R. Ramos-Fernandez, MD*, Roberto Medero-Colon, MD, Lorraine Mendez-Carreno, MD

KEYWORDS

- Urologic procedures • Urethral catheterization • Manual testicular detorsion
- Dorsal penile nerve block

KEY POINTS

- Emergency physicians must be familiar with urologic emergencies; they should be dexterous performing urologic procedures to maintain function while avoiding complications.
- Among critical skills and procedures performed by emergency practitioners are urethral and suprapubic catheterization, manual testicular detorsion, dorsal penile nerve block, cavernosal aspiration, dorsal slit, and paraphimosis reduction.
- Depending on the urologic condition, emergent consultation and/or close follow-up with a urologist are highly encouraged to assure proper patient care and satisfaction.

URETHRAL CATHETERIZATION

Acute urinary retention (AUR) is a common urologic condition that often presents to an emergency department (ED) as a sudden inability to pass urine accompanying with lower abdominal pain.[1] It increases in incidence with age and most often occurs in men over the age of 60 years.[1-3] Generally, the causes of AUR can be classified into 3 categories. The first category relates to any event that increases the resistance

Disclosures: Dr Ramos-Fernandez has funding from Grant Number R25 RR17589 from the National Center for Research Resources (NCRR)/ National Institute on Minority Health and Health Disparities (NIMHD), a component of the National Institutes of Health (NIH). The written content and expressions are solely the responsibility of the authors and do not necessarily represent the official views of the NIH.
Disclosures: None (R.M-C., L.M-C.).
Department of Emergency Medicine, University of Puerto Rico School of Medicine, 65th Infantry Avenue, Km 3.8, Carolina, PR 00985, USA
* Corresponding author.
E-mail address: maria.ramos5@upr.edu

Emerg Med Clin N Am 31 (2013) 237–260
http://dx.doi.org/10.1016/j.emc.2012.09.007
0733-8627/13/$ – see front matter © 2013 Elsevier Inc. All rights reserved.

emed.theclinics.com

to the urine flow, including, for example, benign prostatic hyperplasia (BPH), urethral stricture, or detrusor sphincter dysfunction. Second, AUR may result from an interruption of either the sensory innervation of the bladder wall or the motor supply of the detrusor muscle. It is most commonly seen in spinal cord injuries, progressive neurologic diseases, diabetic neuropathy, and cerebrovascular accidents.[1,2,4] The third mechanism relates to any situation that either permits or causes the bladder to overdistend.[1] Overdistension of the bladder is most commonly encountered by the pharmacologic use of opiates, anticholinergic administration, and the generalized increase in α-adrenergic activity that exists after surgery.[1]

The initial management of AUR of urine is prompt relief of retention and pain by catheterization of the bladder.[1,5–7] There are no uniform guidelines for bladder decompression but most urologists prefer urethral catheterization for the initial management of AUR.[8]

Box 1 summarizes the most common indications for urethral catheterization in the ED.

As in any other procedure performed in the ED, urethral catheterization has several contraindications; among them are exposure to a recent urologic surgery, pelvic or abdominal trauma, and blood in urethral meatus or perineal hematoma. Patients with mentioned conditions should not have urethral catheterization as initial procedure for bladder decompression.[8]

The equipment is available as a commercial nonreusable kit. **Box 2** lists the content of the catheterization tray.

Urethral catheterization must be done using sterile technique, always taking into consideration that male and female patients have special anatomic landmarks. After careful exposure, use an antiseptic solution soaked into cotton balls to cleanse the exposed meatus and surrounding tissues. Cleaning should be done in circular motion starting on the urethral meatus and proceeding outward.[2,9]

In uncircumcised men, total control of the penile foreskin is paramount to ensuring success. Retract the available foreskin to its fullest extent proximal to the glans penis.[2,9] The appropriately sized catheter previously lubricated with jelly should be gently passed into the urethra and upward into the bladder. An appropriate initial Foley size is a 14F to 18F Foley catheter. Inject male or female urethra with 5 mL to 7 mL of 2% viscous lidocaine or other similar anesthetic lubricant to help urethral distention and anesthesia. After passing the catheter, slowly inflate the balloon with 10 mL of tap water. Obvious resistance or patient discomfort on balloon inflation should signal potential erroneous urethral positioning and mandates re-evaluation.[4] After successful catheter passage and Foley balloon inflation, slowly withdraw the catheter until the approximation of the balloon with the bladder neck precludes further withdrawal.[1,2,9] After catheterization, reduce the penile foreskin to its normal anatomic position to

---

Box 1
Indications for urethral catheterization
AUR
Hydronephrosis
Continuous bladder irrigation
Neurogenic bladder
Bedridden patients

Box 2
Equipment in catheterization tray

Foley catheter: straight tip, Coudé tip, 3-way irrigation catheter

Sterile gloves

14F Foley catheter

10-mL normal saline prefilled syringe

Collection bag

Cotton balls

Povidone-iodine solution

Lubricant jelly

Water

Sterile drape

prevent the development of iatrogenic paraphimosis. Then connect the catheter to either a sterile leg bag or a closed-system bedside drainage bag. In cases when patient disposition is discharged with an indwelling catheter, it can initially be connected to a leg bag, which is then comfortably fastened to the lower thigh and upper calf. Patients and families must be instructed regarding proper care of the catheter and drainage device.[4,5]

If obstruction does not allow passage of a flexible catheter, possible causes of obstruction should be taken in to consideration to fix the problem. Patient urethral meatus may be constricted due to trauma or prior transurethral procedure. The scar may prevent admission of a normal-sized catheter. In this case, the obstruction may be bypassed by downsizing the catheter to a 10F to 12F Foley.[2,4,10] In the absence of prior instrumentation, the more common cause of obstruction is an enlarged prostate. In this case, a larger catheter (20 or 22 gauge) with a firm Coudé tip may be needed and may require urologic consultation.[2] The procedure to place the Coudé uses the same technique as the Foley except that the catheter used is a Coudé. The Coudé catheter is placed into the meatus of the penis with the curved tip pointing up, cephalad, and is advanced with gentle but continuous pressure past the resistance point, typically in the region of an enlarged prostate (**Fig. 1**).[2,6]

A common complication of urinary catheterization is the development of a urinary tract infection (UTI). Patients with catheters for more than 10 days are at higher risk for infection.[2] Infection from the urethra and the bladder might spread to cause epididymitis, pyelonephritis, and bacteremia. Other rare complications of long-term

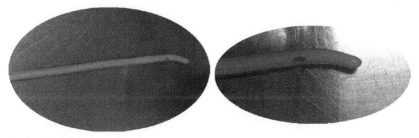

Fig. 1. Coudé foley.

indwelling urethral catheterization include bladder stones, recurring bladder spasm, periurethral abscesses, urethral stricture, bladder perforation, and urethral erosion.[2,11] Complications that occur during the act of catheterization include false passages in any area of the urethra, urethral catheter retention, and paraphimosis.[2,11] **Box 3** list the complications associated with urethral catheterization.

SUPRAPUBIC CATHETERIZATION

Suprapubic catheterization is indicated in patients who require a urethral catheter, but it cannot be passed or is contraindicated.[2,5] Difficulties with urethral instrumentation require a suprapubic catheterization to prevent further urethral injury.[6,12] **Box 4** summarizes the indications for suprapubic catheterization.

Suprapubic catheter placement is contraindicated in an empty bladder.[2,5] There must be sufficient urine to allow the needle to penetrate the bladder dome without exiting through the base and also displace the bowel away from the surface of the bladder. Ultrasound should be used to define bladder anatomy.[2,5] Blind suprapubic catheterization should be avoided in patients with previous abdominal surgery or previous pelvic irradiation that may have developed adhesions and scaring. Ultrasound guidance is indicated when adhesions are a possibility from prior abdominal surgery.[4,5] Major bleeding disorders are a relative contraindication and should be considered on a case-by-case basis (**Box 5**).[2,6]

Suprapubic catheterization is performed under local anesthesia and using sterile technique. Patients are placed in supine position.[2,5] The bladder should be palpated and identified the insertion site, which is midline and 4 cm to 5 cm above the pubic bone.

A preliminary bladder ultrasound examination should be performed by an emergency physician to confirm and visualize bladder limits, lower abdominal contents, and midportion of the bladder where catheterization is to occur (**Fig. 2**).[2,5] Local anesthesia should be used at the insertion site, using 5 mL of 1% lidocaine by raising a wheal and then injecting the local tissue toward the bladder with the 22-gauge spinal needle at an angle aiming 20° to 30° caudal from midline (toward patient legs).[1,2] While the needle is advanced and lidocaine is injected, intermittent stopping

| Box 3 |
Complications with urethral catheterization
Nosocomial UTI
Epididymitis
Pyelonephritis
Bacteremia
Bladder spasm
Periurethral abscess
Bladder perforation
Urethral erosion
Urethral stricture
Urethral catheter retention
Paraphimosis

| **Box 4** |
| **Indications for suprapubic catheterization** |
| Urethral catheterization is contraindicated |
| Suspected urethral trauma |
| BPH |
| Bladder neck mass |

and withdrawing to assess for urine return should be performed. All suprapubic catheter units are placed with a similar approach until this stage. The following steps describe the placement of the Cook Medical Peel-Away Sheath.[9,11] As soon as the bladder has been located, remove the syringe from the needle and advance a guide wire through the needle into the bladder. Withdraw the needle, leaving only the guide wire traversing the anterior abdominal wall and positioned inside the bladder. Small vertical skin 4-mm incision should be made with no. 11 or no. 15 blade to facilitate the Peel-Away Sheath and indwelling fascial dilator insertion through abdominal wall in to the bladder.[1,2,5] The physician's nondominant hand should be placed on the lower abdominal wall, and the unit should be stabilized between the thumb and index fingers. The dominant hand should be used to advance the unit. An ultrasound probe should be placed lateral to the incision, at all times, with a diagonal valgus orientation within a sterile glove to visualize and direct the procedure.[1,5] Remove the guide wire and fascial dilator, leaving only the Peel-Away Sheath inside the bladder. Then pass a Foley balloon catheter through the indwelling intravesical sheath.[2,4,5] Aspirate urine to confirm proper placement. Inflate the Foley balloon with a minimum of 10-mL solution. Withdraw the Peel-Away Sheath leaving only the indwelling suprapubic Foley catheter. Withdraw the catheter slowly until the inflated balloon approximates the cystostomy site. Connect the catheter to a drainage bag, and then dress the wound with 4 × 4 gauze pads to complete the procedure.[4] Catheter should be taped or stitched to the skin. All patients who undergo suprapubic tube placement should be referred to a urologist for correction of the underlying disease as well as routine cystostomy tube care.[2,5]

Suprapubic catheters carry an increased risk for complications associated with its placement. Serious complications involve perforation of the intraperitoneal contents (bowel perforation, ureteral injury, or large vessel injury) and drains of bladder contents into the peritoneal cavity. Through-and-through bladder penetration with associated rectal, vaginal, or uterine injury has been reported.[2,4,5] Infection may occur at the suprapubic insertion site or anywhere along the course of the catheter. Hematuria is rarely more than a transient problem. Other complications include deeper tissue

| **Box 5** |
| **Equipment for suprapubic catheterization** |
| Shaver (to remove hair from suprapubic area) |
| Lidocaine 1% (5 mL) |
| Scalpel with no. 11 blade |
| Skin tape of nylon 3.0 suture (to secure catheter) |
| Trocar-type cystostomy tube (Cystocath) |

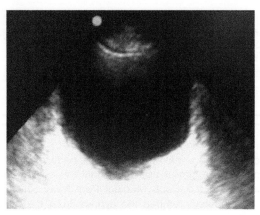

Fig. 2. Sonographic view needed for suprapubic catheterization.

infections that may result from extravasated infected urine or from a superficial infection spreading along the tube. Also common are catheter obstruction by kinking or from blood and inadvertent tube removal.[2,5,10]

Frequently, patients can be managed as outpatients after bladder decompression. Surgery remains the ultimate management of AUR and is considered the gold standard.[1,6,9,12] General recommendation is to wait 30 days or more after an episode of AUR.[7,10] Emergency surgery for relief of prostatic obstruction is infrequently directed and carries an increased danger over elective surgery.[7,13] Hospital admission is indicated for patients with urosepsis, obstruction related to malignancy, spinal cord compression, or failure to recent urologic procedure.[7,13]

TESTICULAR DETORSION

Acute scrotal pain with or without swelling and erythema in a male child, adolescent, or adult should always be treated as an emergent condition.[14,15] Most of the conditions that cause the signs and symptoms (listed previously) are not emergent but of vital importance are the prompt diagnosis and treatment of torsion of the spermatic cord to avoid permanent ischemic damage to the testicle.[14–17] Torsion of the testicle results from twisting of the spermatic cord in its own axis, which compromises testicular blood supply.[15,18,19] There is a 4-hour to 8-hour window before significant ischemic damage occurs.[15,18,19] The classic clinical presentation of testicular torsion is the sudden onset of severe, unilateral pain, often with nausea and vomiting. It often occurs several hours after vigorous physical activity or minor testicular trauma.[16,19,20]

A typical finding on physical examination is an asymmetrically high-riding testis on the affected side, with the long axis of the testis oriented transversely, or the epididymis may be located anteriorly.[14,15] Cremasteric reflex should be assessed by lightly pinching the skin of the superior thigh while observing the ipsilateral testis.[14,15] A normal response, contraction with elevation of the testis, is usually not present in patients with testicular torsion. Other less-specific findings of testicular torsion include the Prehn sign, generalized testicular tenderness, testicular swelling, and erythema. The Prehn sign[14,15] is a description of how elevation of affected scrotum relieves pain in patients with epidimytis and aggravates, or has no effect on, patients with testicular torsion. The Prehn sign is not a reliable physical finding to distinguish between torsion and epididymitis.[14,15]

The diagnosis of testicular torsion should be based on clinical suspicion, but there are adjunctive diagnostic studies that may aid in determining the etiology of testicular pain, such as color-flow Doppler ultrasound.[17,21] Management for a suspected testicular torsion is immediate surgical repair (**Figs. 3** and **4**).[17]

All patients with suspected testicular torsion should be immediately consulted to a urologist service. Manual detorsion should be attempted while awaiting patient transport to the operating room.[17,22]

Manual detorsion objective is to regenerate blood flow to the affected testis but it should never delay operative intervention. Manual detorsion is not recommended if duration of torsion is more than 6 hours.[17,22]

Patients should be placed in supine position with the hips and knees flexed and the thighs apart (lithotomy position). This position allows the physician easy access and prevents patients from withdrawing during the procedure. Analgesia or sedation use during manual detorsion is controversial.

Most torsions are in medial direction; therefore, clinicians should detorse testes from medial to the lateral side, rotating outward toward the thigh (open book rotation).[17] Patients must be as comfortable as possible in lithotomy position.[17] Some experts recommend that physicians should be positioned in front of the patient while others endorse that clinicians should be standing at the side of the bed (right side if the clinician is right handed or vice versa).[17] Manual detorsion starts as a book would be opened. Detorsion of the patient's right testis is done in a counterclockwise fashion while the patient's left testis is detorsed in a clockwise fashion.[17] If pain is partially relieved, continue with another rotation; the degree of torsion my range from 180° to 1080°.[17] If detorsion is too difficult or makes the pain worse, the emergency physician must attempt to detorse the testis in the opposite direction (**Fig. 5**).[17]

Manual detorsion has no complications[17,23] but the procedure may be difficult due to acute pain during manipulation.

Successful detorsion is suggested by relief of pain, resolution of the transverse lie of the testis to a longitudinal orientation, lower position of the testis in the scrotum, and return of normal arterial pulsations detected with a Doppler stethoscope[22,23] Surgical exploration is necessary even after clinically successful manual detorsion. Manual detorsion is not a substitute for definitive surgical exploration.[22,23]

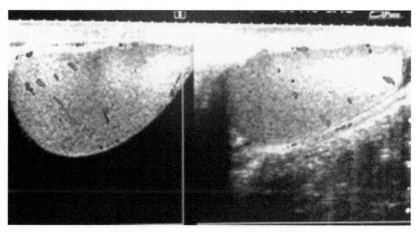

Fig. 3. Testicular ultrasound with bilateral color flow. (*A*) Right testicle. (*B*) Left testicle.

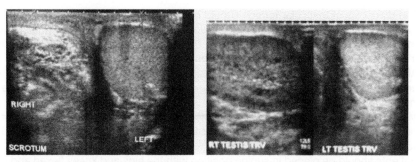

Fig. 4. Testicular ultrasound with right testicular torsion and normal left testicle.

DORSAL PENILE NERVE BLOCK

The penis receives its innervation by the pudendal nerve (S2–S4).[24,25] This nerve divides into the right and left dorsal nerves of the penis; it travels under the pubis symphysis and enters just below the Buck fascia to provide sensory innervation to the penis.[24,25]

Many causes of penile pain may be managed with a dorsal nerve block. The procedure is indicated for circumcision, phimosis reduction, paraphimosis reduction, penile laceration repairs, and release of entrapped penile skin from zippers.[24–26] Small children may require the use of conscious sedation.[24]

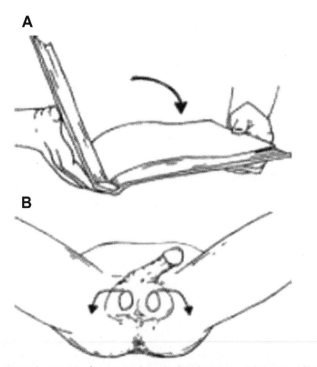

Fig. 5. (*A*) Open Book rotation for manual testicular detorsion (*B*) Rotate affected testicle away from midline. This is a counterclockwise rotation for right testicle and a clockwise rotation for the left testicle.

Box 6
Equipment for dorsal penile nerve block
Povidone-iodine solution
4 × 4 Sterile gauze
Local anesthetic without epinephrine
5-mL syringe
16-Gauge and 27-gauge needles
Sterile drapes

The procedure is contraindicated if testicular torsion is suspected or there is evidence of skin infection at the site of injection (**Box 6**).[27]

Patients should be placed in the supine position with genitals exposed. Gross debris should be cleansed and copious amounts of povidone-iodine solution applied to the penis and scrotum using a soaked 4 × 4 gauze. The glans and shaft of the penis should be cleaned at least twice using a circular motion. The sterile field is created by placing sterile drapes between the scrotum and shaft, above the shaft, and on both sides of the shaft.

The following steps are involved in the technique and much has remained unchanged since the original description of the procedure by Kirya and colleagues[27] in 1978 (**Fig. 6**). The dorsal penile nerves should be blocked as proximately to the base of the penis as possible. A 27-gauge needle is used to create a small wheal at the 2 o'clock and 10 o'clock positions of the base of the penis.[28] Then, the needle is slowly inserted through the center of each wheal, advancing the needle approximately 0.5 cm or until loss of resistance is felt, at which point the needle is within Buck fascia. At this point, the syringe is aspirated to ensure that needle is not within a blood vessel. Anesthetic (2 mL) is injected on each side. When dealing with

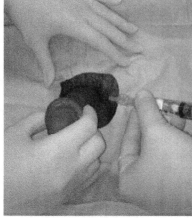
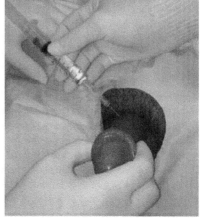

2 o'clock injection   10 o'clock injection

Fig. 6. Dorsal penile nerve block.

children and neonates (<10 kg), 0.2 mL to 0.4 mL of 1% lidocaine is injected on each side using a 30-gauge needle. No more than 4.5 mg/kg of lidocaine should be injected.[29]

Complications associated with dorsal penile block include bleeding and hematoma formation, which can be controlled with local pressure.[30,31] Inadequate anesthesia should prompt an attempt with a different nerve block.

CAVERNOSAL ASPIRATION

Priapism is manifested by a persisting erection caused by disturbances in the mechanism controlling penile detumescence and the maintenance of penile flaccidity.[32] It is usually painful, unrelated to sexual stimulation, and not relieved by ejaculation. It is associated with high incidence of impotence regardless of treatment.[32] Most studies identify priapism as an erection lasting at least 4 hours.[32]

Anatomically, it involves the corpora cavernosa only, sparing the corpus spongiosum and the glans.[32–35] Priapism results from a derangement of the penile hemodynamics, affecting the arterial component or the veno-occlusive mechanism.[33] This mechanism explains the 2 types of priapism—high-flow and low-flow types. High-flow priapism commonly follows an episode of trauma to the perineum or the genitalia, resulting in increased flow through the arteries.[32,34,35] High-flow priapism does not represent an emergency situation; it resolves spontaneously in up to 62% of untreated cases.[32,34,35] In low-flow or ischemic priapism, there is an abnormality in the veno-occlusive mechanism, resulting in venous stasis and accumulation of deoxygenated blood within the cavernous tissue.[34,35] Oxygenation of the erectile tissues is compromised and risk of future erectile dysfunction secondary to ischemia and subsequent fibrosis is high if not treated expeditiously.[35]

The diagnosis of priapism is generally clinical.[36] Visual inspection reveals an erect penis, and the erection has been present for more than 2 to 4 hours in the absence of sexual excitation.[36] Cavernosa blood gas analysis and Doppler ultrasonography may be performed to differentiate between ischemic and nonischemic types of priapism.[32,36,37] The Doppler can also detect cavernous arterial fistula, pseudoaneurysm, or other anatomic abnormalities.[32,36–38]

Prompt intervention is warranted in all cases of low-flow priapism to prevent long-term erectile dysfunction.[32] Emergency clinicians should identify reversible causes of priapism and in conjunction with urologist consultation initiate specific corrective therapy.[32] Every patient should receive narcotic analgesia regardless of the cause.[32] Some studies recommend empiric terbutaline, 0.25 mg to 0.5 mg subcutaneously for every patient presenting to the ED with low-flow priapism.[39] Recent studies favor starting with corpora cavernosa aspiration, with a nonheparinized syringe, as first-line treatment, with a success rate of approximately 30%.[39] Aspiration can be combined with flushing the cavernosa using normal saline to clear the sludged blood.[40] If this fails, instillation of a vasoconstrictive agent, such as phenylephrine, should be used until complete detumescence is achieved.[41,42] If urologic consultation is unavailable or delayed, the emergency physician should initiate therapeutic corporal aspiration.[39]

Despite widespread administration of pharmacologic substances in the treatment of priapism, there is still a call for surgical intervention if all attempts of conservative treatment fail.[32,41] Nonischemic priapism is not an urgent condition and may resolve spontaneously.[41] If priapism does not respond to pharmaceutical treatment, it can be treated with penile injection and aspiration.[32,36] This procedure entails drainage of blood from the erect penis and instillation of vasoactive medication. Alternatively, irrigation with a dilute vasoactive solution is also effective.

Box 7
Equipment for priapism and cavernosal aspiration and irrigation

Cardiac monitor with blood pressure monitoring capability

Sterile gloves, sterile basin (for collection of drained blood), and sterile drapes.

Antiseptic solution

Gauze squares

Local anesthetic: 1% lidocaine without epinephrine (penile block)

Syringes: one 1 mL (local anesthetic), two 20 mL or 30 mL

Needles: 19 gauge or 21 gauge (for aspiration, butterfly, or straight for aspiration), 27 gauge (penile block)

Irrigation fluid:

    Phenylephrine, 10 mg/500 mL of saline

    Norepinephrine, 1 mg/500 mL of saline

    Epinephrine, 0.5 mg/500 mL of saline

Contraindications for cavernosal aspiration are high-flow priapism, overlying cellulitis, and uncontrolled bleeding disorder.[32,36,43,44] **Box 7** lists the equipment needed for priapism and cavernosal aspiration and irrigation.

Patients should be placed in the supine position.[39] Systemic analgesia should be applied before beginning the procedure. In certain patients, such as children, conscious sedation should be added. An injection of 1% plain lidocaine at the base of the penis for a dorsal penile nerve block or placement of a circumferential penile block is highly recommended.[39,41] Patients should be connected to a cardiac monitor with frequent blood pressure measurements. After induction of conscious sedation with intravenous midazolam or other sedatives, the penis, scrotum, and lower abdomen should be cleaned and prepared with the antiseptic solution and allowed to dry. Apply sterile drapes to area.[32,39,41]

Using left hand thumb and index finger, grasp penis shaft.[39] Insert a 19-gauge butterfly needle into the lateral midshaft of the penis at the 3-o'clock or 9-o'clock position, directing the needle straight toward the center of the corpora. Any side of penis could be punctured because there is communication of blood flow (bilateral anastomoses) between both sides.[39] The end of the tubing could be placed in a sterile basin, because blood is likely to spontaneously drain from the corpora. Nevertheless, most of the time butterfly or straight needles are attached to a 20-mL or 30-mL syringes for active aspiration.[39,41] Too much suction should not be applied because this often stops the aspiration; it should not exceed 20 mL to 30 mL of corporal blood. A common mistake is to use too much suction with a large syringe.[39] Aspiration should continue until aspiration of dark blood ceases and bright red arterial blood returns or complete detumescence is obtained and persists.[39] Once blood has been drained and the penis has softened, inject 1 mL to 2 mL of the 10-μg/mL phenylephrine solution into the midshaft of each corpora using the same needle that was used for blood aspiration. The injection may be repeated to a maximal dose of 1 mg (1000 μg).[32,39]

In cases of prolonged priapism or recurrent cases, active irrigation of the old blood might be required. A 21-gauge butterfly needle should be inserted into the proximal penis on the same side of the penis as the aspiration needle.[41] Different irrigating solutions have been suggested, but none has proved superiority. Clinicians suggest 20 mL to 30 mL of a phenylephrine/normal saline solution (10 mg of phenylephrine in 500 mL of normal saline) as the exchange for 20 mL to 30 mL of aspirated corporal blood.[39] A norepinephrine solution also may be used. Some clinicians add heparin to the solution but value has been unproved.[39] Failure to maintain detumescence requires immediate urology evaluation. All other patients require discontinuation of the causal agent and follow-up with a urologist 24 hours after the procedure.[43] Vasoactive substance can be absorbed systemically and produce potential side effects, such as arrhythmias, hypertension, and headache.[44] The use of vasoactive agents is contraindicated in patients with severe hypertension, dysrhythmias, and monoamine oxidase inhibitor use.[44] Patients need to be connected to cardiac monitor and blood pressure monitor at all times, if patients have comorbid conditions. Impotence is a complication after priapism, regardless of the cause or the promptness of therapeutic intervention.[43,44] Patients must be advised verbally and in writing of this possible complication.[2,6,9] Hematoma and infection can occur, even with correctly performed aspiration (**Fig. 7**).[44]

DORSAL SLIT

Phimosis is the inability to retract and expose the glans.[45] Up to 10% of boys have physiologic phimosis at 3 years of age, and a larger percentage of children have only partially retractable foreskins. One to 5% have nonretractable foreskins by age 16 years.[45] Most healthy adult men should not have phimosis; the presence should raise the suspicion of balanitis, balanoposthitis, diabetes mellitus, or malignancy (**Fig. 8**).[46,47]

The indications for performing a dorsal slit include relieving urinary retention in patients with phimosis in whom a urethral catheter cannot be blindly inserted.[48] There are no absolute contraindications to the procedure but it should be avoided in patients with bleeding disorders, who are taking anticoagulants, who have infected foreskin, or who are immunocompromised (**Box 8**).[49,50]

Using a 5-mL syringe with a 27-gauge needle, a small wheal of local anesthetic is created in the 12-o'clock position of the dorsal midline penis. The needle needs to be advanced through the center of the wheal, injecting subcutaneously. This method does not provide anesthesia to the ventral aspect of the penis and foreskin.

In order to perform the dorsal slit, patients should be placed in the supine position with genitals exposed. The genitalia should be cleaned with copious amounts of povidone-iodine solution using soaked 4 × 4 gauze at least twice. The sterile field is created by placing sterile drapes between the scrotum and shaft, above the shaft,

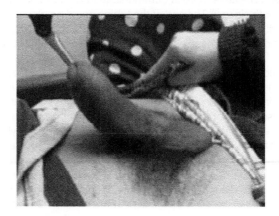

Fig. 7. Priapism.

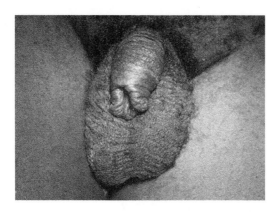

Fig. 8. Phimosis.

and on both sides of the shaft. Then, the bottom of the jaw of a straight hemostat should be inserted between the foreskin and the glans penis at the 12-o'clock position and the hemostat advanced until its tip reaches the coronal sulcus. The hemostat needs to be swiped to break any adhesions between the foreskin and the glans; the tip of the hemostat should be palpated and cause a tenting of the foreskin at the coronal sulcus. Once placement is confirmed, the hemostat is closed to allow it to crush the foreskin for 2 to 3 minutes. Then, the hemostat should be removed and, with a straight scissors, the crushed foreskin cut. The area should be covered with dry sterile gauze; then, the phimotic foreskin should be removed using a manual technique. Using an absorbable 3-0 or 4-0 suture, the edges of the foreskin are approximated leaving a gap in the 12-o'clock position. Finally, the foreskin is reduced to a natural position covering the glans and topical antibacterial ointment should be applied to the penile skin. The most common complication associated with dorsal slit is bleeding.[51–53] Patients should be observed

Box 8
Equipment
Povidone-iodine solution
4 × 4 Sterile gauze
Local anesthetic without epinephrine
5-mL syringe
18-Gauge and 27-gauge needles
Sterile drapes
Straight hemostats or straight Kelly clamps
Straight scissors or no. 15 scalpel
Needle driver
Absorbable sutures 3-0 or 4-0
Petroleum gauze
Topical antibiotic ointment

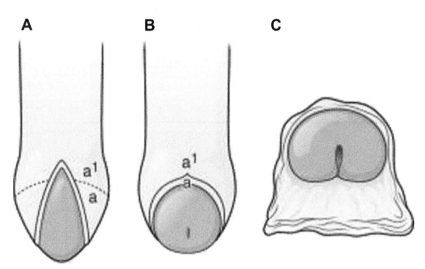

Fig. 9. Phimosis dorsal slit.

in the ED for at least 30 minutes and urgent follow-up with a urologist within 1 to 2 days should be arranged before discharge (**Fig. 9**).

PARAPHIMOSIS REDUCTION

Paraphimosis is the inability to reduce a swollen and proximately positioned foreskin over the glans penis.[54,55] Retracted foreskin obstructs lymphatic drainage of the distal penis, causing edema of the retracted foreskin; venous obstruction followed by arterial flow may develop within hours to days. If not corrected in a timely fashion, penile necrosis, infraction of the glans, or gangrene can occur, followed by autoamputation.[56,57] The incidence of paraphimosis in the United States and elsewhere is unknown. It can occur at any age but is most common in children and older people (**Fig. 10**).[54]

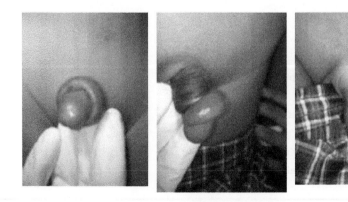

Pediatric patient with paraphimosis

Frontal View   Lateral View   Reduced paraphimosis

Fig. 10. Pediatric paraphymosis.

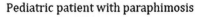

Patients with phimosis who forcibly retract the foreskin past the glans penis or caretakers who forget to replace the foreskin after retraction can cause paraphimosis. Also reported in the literature, as an associated risk factor for the development of paraphimosis, is penile piercing; there are case reports that described coital paraphimosis leading to penile necrosis.[52,53]

The clinical presentation most commonly seen is penile pain and swelling. Patients may also present with urinary retention. Although this is a late finding, it requires immediate reduction. Diagnosis of paraphimosis is clinically based on history and physical findings (**Fig. 11**).

All patients with paraphimosis require emergent reduction. Contraindications to the procedure include the presence of necrotic tissue or ulcerated foreskin or penis.[56,57]

Equipment and materials needed for the performance of manual paraphimosis reduction are summarized in **Box 9**.

Before the performance of the procedure, patients should be placed in the supine position with genitals exposed. An anesthetic cream should be applied to the glans and foreskin. Then, the area should be cleansed at least twice, with copious amounts of povidone-iodine solution, using a soaked 4 × 4 gauze. After placing sterile drapes between the scrotum and shaft creates a sterile field, reassessment of the anesthetic effect should be evaluated. If adequate anesthetic has not been achieved, a nerve block should be performed. Paraphimosis is a painful condition; consider parenteral analgesia and/or procedural sedation with analgesia.

Steady manual compression over the glans penis and edematous foreskin should be applied, squeezing distally to proximally, and maintained for 5 to 10 minutes. Thumbs should be positioned on both sides of the urethral meatus and the index

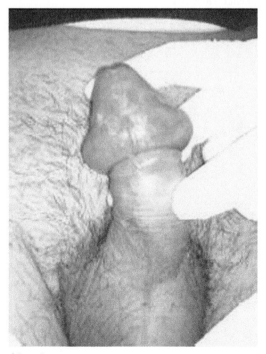

Fig. 11. Adult paraphimosis.

> **Box 9**
> **Equipment for manual paraphimosis reduction**
>
> Topical anesthetic cream (eutectic mixture of local anesthetics [EMLA])
>
> 4 × 4 Sterile gauze
>
> Povidone-iodine solution
>
> Sterile drapes
>
> Sterile gloves
>
> Local anesthetic solution without epinephrine
>
> 10-mL syringe
>
> Needles, 18-gauge and 27-gauge
>
> Crushed ice

and middle fingers proximal to the phimotic ring; continuous traction moves the phimotic ring distally over the glans.[57]

Successful reduction should look like a normal uncircumcised penis. Patients should feel relief of pain; pressure and residual swelling should resolve in a few days. If manual reduction technique fails, a dorsal slit is indicated.[58]

Patients should be observed for recovery from anesthesia, adequate hemostasis, and ability to urinate. They could be discharge home with instructions to follow-up with a urologist within 1 to 2 days (**Fig. 12**).

MANAGEMENT OF PENILE FRACTURE

A fractured penis occurs when there is a traumatic rupture of the corpus cavernosum. Sudden blunt trauma or abrupt lateral bending of the penis in an erect state can break the markedly thinned and stiff tunica albuginea.[59]

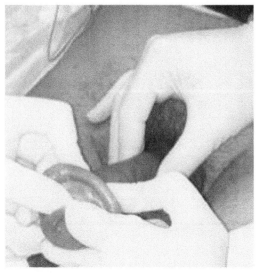

Fig. 12. Adult paraphimosis reduction.

History and physical examination findings provide the diagnosis. Patients often report penile injury coincident with sexual intercourse, often accompanied by a popping or cracking sound with immediate detumescence. The normal penile appearance is obliterated because of significant deformity, swelling, and ecchymosis, producing the eggplant deformity.[60,61] Approximately 30% of men with penile fractures present with blood at the meatus.[62] Whenever urethral injury is suspected, a retrograde urethrography is required. The ability to void, however, does not exclude injury.

The treatment of penile fractures is immediate surgical intervention. Fluid resuscitation and stabilization of patients should be the focus in the ED. If surgical therapy must be delayed, initial medical therapy consists of cold compresses, pressure dressings and anti-inflammatory medications, followed by definitive surgical therapy.[59–63]

All patients must understand that erectile dysfunction, abnormal penile curvature, painful erections, and formation of fibrotic plaques are all possible outcomes that are a result of the nature of the injury. With prompt diagnosis and expedient surgical management, however, outcomes remain excellent and complications are minimal.[63]

Postsurgical management includes pain medications and oral antibiotics. Patients may be discharged home 1 to 3 days after the surgery (**Fig. 13**).

MANAGEMENT OF COMMON UROLOGIC PROCEDURES

Emergency medicine providers must be proficient while managing the complications of urologic procedures completed by a urologist. **Table 1** lists the most common procedures performed by urologists as well as the associated complications and ED management.

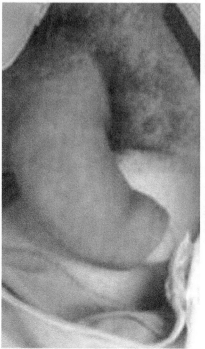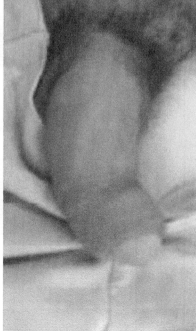

Fig. 13. Penile fracture.

Table 1
Common complications of urologic procedures

Procedure	Notes	Complications	ED Management	Disposition
ESWL	Preferred treatment modality for renal and ureteric calculi[64,65]	1. Rare but there are reports of visceral and thoracic injuries[66-68] 2. Subcapsular hematoma and hematuria is reported from 1% to 20% of patients[69-75] 3. Fever and UTI are commonly reported[76,77]	Consider U/A, type and screen, renal function test, and CBC Administer IV fluids, antiemetic, narcotic for pain, and prophylaxis antibiotics for all[77]	Urologist ED evaluation vs close outpatient follow-up in 24-48 h
Vasectomy	Most commonly performed urologic surgical procedure[78,79]	1. Most common complication is scrotal hematoma formation (2%)[80,81] 2. Wound infection, UTI, epididymitis 3. Rare complications include Fournier gangrene and sperm granulomas[81-84]	Scrotal elevation and support. NSAIDs for pain[78,84-90]	Urology follow-up in 2-3 d Long-term follow-up recommended because some patients developed chronic testicular pain[78,85-88]
AUS complications	Device of choice for patients with moderate to severe urinary incontinence[91-95]	1. Urinary retention is a common complication 2. Postoperative AUS infection	1. Place urinary catheter after cuff deactivation[96-108] 2. Start antibiotic and consult for admission[109]	Urologist ED evaluation for AUS evaluation and removal consideration[91,109-111]

Abbreviations: AUS, artificial urinary sphincter; CBC, complete blood cell count; ESWL, extracorporeal shock wave lithotripsy; NSAID, nonsteroidal anti-inflammatory drug; U/A, urinalysis.

SUMMARY

Emergency physicians must be proficient in the acute management of urologic conditions, especially those that require performing procedures. Most urologic conditions and injuries are initially evaluated in the ED. Several urologic disorders can be evaluated as an outpatient consultation with an urologist; however, a subset of conditions, such as testicular torsion, priapism, and paraphimosis, require immediate identification and expedited intervention and proficiency in the execution of urologic procedures to avoid complications and functional impairment. Early recognition of procedural complications to improve outcomes in these urologic conditions is of utmost importance.

REFERENCES

1. Thomas K, Chow K, Kirby RS, et al. Acute urinary retention: a review of the etiology and management. Prostate Cancer Prostatic Dis 2004;7:32–7.
2. Vilke GM, Ufberg JW, Harrigan RA, et al. Evaluation and treatment of acute urinary retention. J Emerg Med 2008;35(2):193–8.
3. Jacobsen SJ, Jaconsen DJ, Girman CJ, et al. Natural history of prostatism: risk factors for acute urinary retention. J Urol 1997;158:481.
4. Nyman MA, Schwenk NM, Silverstein MD, et al. Management of urinary retention: rapid versus gradual decompression and risk of complications. Mayo Clin Proc 1997;72:951.
5. Hargreave TB, McNeill SA. Sustained-release alfuzosin and trial without catheter after acute urinary retention: a prospective, placebo-controlled trial. Br J Urol 1999;84:622–7.
6. McNeill AS, Rizvi S, Byrne DJ, et al. Long term follow up following presentation with first episode of acute urinary retention. J Urol 2000;163:559–62.
7. Wasson JH, Reda DJ, Bruskewitz RC, et al. A comparison of transurethral surgery with watchful waiting for moderate symptoms of benign prostatic hyperplasia. N Engl J Med 1995;332:75–9.
8. Desgrandchamps F, De la Taille A, Doublet JD, et al. The management of acute urinary retention in France: a cross-sectional survey in 2618 men with benign prostatic hyperplasia. BJU Int 2006;97:727.
9. Horgan AF, Prasad B, Waldron DJ, et al. Acute urinary retention. Comparison of supra-pubic and urethral catheterisation. Br J Urol 1992;70:149–51.
10. Kessler CS, Bauml J. Non-traumatic urologic emergencies in men: a clinical review. West J Emerg Med 2009;10(4):281–7.
11. Aguilera PA, Choi T, Durham BAI, et al. Ultrasound-guided suprapubic cystostomy catheter placement in the emergency department. J Emerg Med 2004; 26(3):319–21.
12. Mc Connell JD, Bruskewitz R, Walsh P, et al. The effect of finasteride on the risk of acute urinary retention and the need for surgical treatment among men with benign prostatic enlargement. N Engl J Med 1998;338:557–63.
13. Patel MI, et al. The optimal form of urinary drainage after acute retention of urine. BJU Int 2001;88:26.
14. Beni-Israel T, Goldman M, Bar Chaim S, et al. Clinical predictors for testicular torsion as seen in the pediatric ED. Am J Emerg Med 2010;28(7):786–9.
15. Gatti JM, Patrick Murphy J. Current management of the acute scrotum. Semin Pediatr Surg 2007;16(1):58–63.
16. Hayn MH, Herz DB, Bellinger MF, et al. Intermittent torsion of the spermatic cord portends an increased risk of acute testicular infarction. J Urol 2008;180(Suppl 4): 1729–32.

17. Sessions AE, Rabinowitz R, Hulbert WC, et al. Testicular torsion: direction, degree, duration and disinformation. J Urol 2003;169(2):663. Department of Urology, University of Rochester School of Medicine, Rochester, New York.

18. Cattolica EV. Preoperative manual detorsion of the torsed spermatic cord. J Urol 1985;133:803.

19. Karmazyn B, et al. Clinical and sonographic criteria of acute scrotum in children: a retrospective study of 172 boys. Pediatr Radiol 2005;35(3):302–10.

20. Cummings JM, Boullier JA, Sekhon D, et al. Adult testicular torsion. J Urol 2002; 167:2109.

21. Sparano A, Acampora C, Scaglione M, et al. Using color power Doppler ultrasound imaging to diagnose the acute scrotum. A pictorial essay. Emerg Radiol 2008;15(5):289–94.

22. Ransler CW 3rd, Allen TD. Torsion of the spermatic cord. Urol Clin North Am 1992;9:245.

23. Jefferson RH, Perez LM, Joseph DB. Critical analysis of the clinical presentation of acute scrotum: a 9-year experience at a single institution. J Urol 1997;158:1198.

24. Telgarsky B, Karovic D, Wassermann O, et al. Penile block in children, our first experience. Bratisl Lek Listy 2006;107(8):320–2.

25. Soh CR, Ng SB, Lim SL. Dorsal nerve block. Paediatr Anaesth 2003;13(4): 329–33.

26. Taddio A, Pollock N, Gilbert-MacLeod C, et al. Combined analgesia and local anesthesia to minimize pain during circumcision. Arch Pediatr Adolesc Med 2000;154(6):620–3.

27. Kirya C, Werthmann MW. Neonatal circumcision and penile dorsal nerve block: a painless procedure. J Pediatr 1978;92:988–1000.

28. Lehr VT, Cepeda E, Frattarelli DA, et al. Lidocaine 4% cream compared with lidocaine 2.5% or dorsal penile block for circumscision. Am J Perinatol 2005; 22(5):231–7.

29. Choi WY, Irwin MG, Hui TW, et al. EMLA cream versus dorsal penile nerve block for postcircumcision analegsia in children. Anesth Analg 2003;96(2):396–9.

30. Emsen IM. Catastrophic complication of the circumcision that carried out with local anesthesia contained adrenaline. J Trauma 2006;60(5):1150.

31. Abaci A, Makay B, Unsal E, et al. An unusual complication of dorsal penile nerve block for circumscision. Paediatr Anaesth 2006;16(10):1094–5.

32. Cherian J, Rao AR, Thwaini A, et al. Medical and surgical management of priapism. Postgrad Med J 2006;82:89.

33. Medina CA. Clitoral priapism: a rare condition presenting as a cause of vulvar pain. Obstet Gynecol 2002;100:1089.

34. Eland IA, van der Lei J, Stricker BH, et al. Incidence of priapism in the general population. Urology 2001;57:970.

35. Broderick GA, Gordon D, Hypolite J, et al. Anoxia and corporal smooth muscle dysfunction: a model for ischemic priapism. J Urol 1994;151:259.

36. Harmon WJ, Nehra A. Priapism: diagnosis and management. Mayo Clin Proc 1997;72(4):350–5. Department of Urology, Mayo Clinic Rochester.

37. Champion HC, Bivalacqua TJ, Takimoto E, et al. Phosphodiesterase-5A dysregulation in penile erectile tissue is a mechanism of priapism. Proc Natl Acad Sci U S A 2005;102:1661.

38. Kim NN, Kim JJ, Hypolite J, et al. Altered contractility of rabbit penile corpus cavernosum smooth muscle by hypoxia. J Urol 1996;155:772.

39. Roberts. Clinical procedures in emergency medicine. 5th edition. Chapter 55. Urologic procedures. Elsevier; 2009.

40. Minevich E. Genitourinary emergencies in children. Minerva Pediatr 2009;61(1): 53–65.
41. Van der horst C, et al. Priapism—etiology, pathophysiology and management. Int Braz J Urol 2003;29(5):391–400.
42. Coward RM, Carson CC. Tadalafil in the treatment of erectile dysfunction. Ther Clin Risk Manag 2008;4:1315.
43. Mantadakis E, Ewalt DH, Cavender JD. Outpatient penile aspiration and epinephrine irrigation for young patients with sickle cell anemia and prolonged priapism. Blood 2000;95(1):78–82. Division of Hematology-Oncology, Department of Pediatrics, The University of Texas Southwestern Medical Center at Dallas.
44. Volkmer BG, Nesslauer T, Kraemer SC, et al. Prepubertal high flow priapism: incidence, diagnosis and treatment. J Urol 2001;166:1018.
45. McGregor TB, Pike JG, Leonard MP. Pathologic and physiologic phimosis: approach to the phimotic foreskin. Can Fam Physician 2007;53(3):445–8.
46. Bromage SJ, Crump A, Pearce I. Phimosis as a presenting feature of diabetes. BJU Int 2008;10(30):338–40.
47. Tsen HF, Morgenstern H, Mack T, et al. Risk factors for penile cancers: results of a population-based case-control study in Los Angeles County (United States). Cancer Causes Control 2001;12(3):267–77.
48. Thiruchelvam N, Nayak P, Mostafid H. Emergency dorsal slit for balanitis with retention. J R Soc Med 2004;97(4):205–6.
49. Borsellino A, Spagnoli A, Vallasciani S, et al. Surgical approach to concealed penis: technical refinements and outcomes. Urology 2007;69(6):1195–8.
50. Chu CC, Chen YH, Diau GY, et al. Preputial flaps to correct buried penis. Pediatr Surg Int 2007;23(11):1119–21.
51. Chloe JM. Paraphimosis: current treatment options. Am Fam Physician 2000; 62(12):2623–6.
52. Koenig LM, Carnes M. Body piercing medical concerns with cutting-edge fashion. J Gen Intern Med 1999;14(6):379–85.
53. Raman SR, Kate V, Ananthakrishnan N. Coital paraphimosis causing penile necrosis. Emerg Med J 2008;25:454.
54. William JC, Morrison PM, Richardson JR. Paraphimosis in elderly men. Am J Emerg Med 1995;13(3):351–3.
55. Rangarajan M, Jayakar SM. Paraphimosis revisited: is chronic paraphimosis a predominantly third world condition? Trop Doct 2008;38(1):40.
56. McCollough M, Sharieff GQ. Abdominal surgical emergencies in infants and young children. Emerg Med Clin North Am 2003;21:909.
57. Mackway-Jones K, Teece S. Best evidence topic reports. Ice, pins or sugar to reduce paraphimosis. Emerg Med J 2004;21(1):77–8.
58. Little B, White M. Treatment options for paraphimosis. Int J Clin Pract 2005; 59(5):591–3.
59. Agarwal MM, Singh SK, Sharma DK, et al. Fracture of the penis: a radiological or clinical diagnosis? A case series and literature review. Can J Urol 2009;16(2): 4568–75.
60. Miller S, McAninch JW. Penile fracture and soft tissue injury. In: McAninch JW, editor. Traumatic and reconstructive urology. Philadelphia: W.B. Saunders; 1996. p. 693–8.
61. Ferhany AF, Angermeier KW, Montague DK. Review of Cleveland Clinic experience with penile fracture. Urology 2003;61:1259.
62. Roy M, Matin M, Alam M, et al. Fracture of the penis with urethral rupture. Mymensingh Med J 2008;17(1):70–3.

63. Sack GS, Garraway I, Reznichek R, et al. Current treatment options for penile fractures. Rev Urol 2004;6(3):114–20.
64. Evan AP, Willis LR, Connors B, et al. Shock wave lithotripsy–induced renal injury. Am J Kidney Dis 1991;17:445–50.
65. Evan AP, Willis LR, Lingeman JE, et al. Renal trauma and the risk of long-term complications in shock wave lithotripsy. Nephron 1998;78:1–8.
66. Ruiz Marcellan FJ, Ibarz Servio L. Evaluation of renal damage in extracorporeal lithotripsy by shock waves. Eur Urol 1986;12:73–5.
67. Chaussy C, Schmiedt E. Extracorporeal shock wave lithotripsy (ESWL) for kidney stones: an alternative to surgery? Urol Radiol 1984;6:80–7.
68. Krambeck AE, Rohlinger AL, Lohse CM, et al. Long term effects of shock wave lithotripsy for nephrolithiasis: a nineteen year study. J Endourol 2005; 19(Suppl):A33.
69. Piper NY, Dalrymple N, Bishoff JT. Incidence of renal hematoma formation after ESWL using the new Dornier Doli-S lithotriptor. J Urol 2001;165:377.
70. Dhar NB, Thornton J, Karafa MT, et al. A multivariate analysis of risk factors associated with subcapsular hematoma formation following electromagnetic shock wave lithotripsy. J Urol 2004;172(Pt 1):2271–4.
71. Knapp PM, Kulb TB, Lingeman JE, et al. Extracorporeal shock wave lithotripsy–induced perirenal hematomas. J Urol 1988;139:700–3.
72. Peterson JC, Finlayson B. Effects of ESWL on blood pressure. In: Gravenstein JS, Peter K, editors. Extracorporeal shock wave lithotripsy for renal stone disease: technical and clinical aspects. Boston: Butterworths; 1986.
73. Williams CM, Kaude JV, Newman RC, et al. Extracorporeal shock-wave lithotripsy: long-term complications. AJR Am J Roentgenol 1988;150:311–5.
74. Orestano F, Caronia N, Gallo G, et al. Functional aspects of the kidney after shock wave lithotripsy. In: Lingeman JE, Newman DM, editors. Shock wave lithotripsy 2: urinary and biliary lithotripsy. New York: Plenum Press; 1989. p. 15–7.
75. Brito CG, Lingeman JE, Newman DM. Long-term follow-up of renal function in ESWL treated patients with a solitary kidney. J Urol 1990;143(Suppl):299.
76. Chaussy C, Fuchs G. Current state and future developments of noninvasive treatment of human urinary stones with extracorporeal shock wave lithotripsy. J Urol 1989;141(Pt 2):782–9.
77. Doran O, Foley B. Acute complications following extracorporeal shock-wave lithotripsy for renal and ureteric calculi. Emerg Med Australas 2008;20:105–11.
78. Awsare NS, Krishnam J, Boustead GB, et al. Complications of vasectomy. Ann R Coll Surg Engl 2005;87(6):406–10.
79. Kendrick J, Gonzales B, Huber DH, et al. Complications of vasectomies in the United States. J Fam Pract 1987;25:245–8.
80. Pant PR, Sharma J, Subba S, et al. Scrotal haematoma: the most common complication of no-scalpel vasectomy. Kathmandu Univ Med J (KUMJ) 2007; 5(2):279–80.
81. Romero Perez P, Merenciano Cortina FJ, Rafie Mazketli W, et al. Vasectomy: study of 300 interventions. Review of the national literature and of its complications. Actas Urol Esp 2004;28(3):175–214.
82. Tandon S, Sabanegh E Jr. Chronic pain after vasectomy: a diagnostic and treatment dilemma. BJU Int 2008;102(2):166–9.
83. Selikowitz S, Schned AR. A late post-vasectomy syndrome. J Urol 1985;134: 494.
84. Viddeleer AC, Lycklama A, Nijeholt GA. Lethal Fournier's gangrene following vasectomy. J Urol 1992;147:1613–4.

85. Nangia AK, Myles JL, Thomas AJ. Vasectomy reversal for the postvasectomy pain syndrome: a clinical and histological evaluation. J Urol 2000;164:1939–42.

86. Davis BE, Noble MJ, Wigel JW, et al. Analysis and management of chronic testicular pain. J Urol 1990;143:936–9.

87. Schuman LM, Coulson AH, Mandel JS, et al. Health status of American men— a study of post-vasectomy sequelae. J Clin Epidemiol 1993;46:697–958.

88. Barone MA, Hutchinson PL, Johnson CH, et al. Vasectomy in the United States, 2002. J Urol 2006;176(1):232–6.

89. Adams CE, et al. Risks and complications of vasectomy. Urol Clin North Am 2009;36:331–6.

90. Kuznetsov DD, Kim HL, Patel RV, et al. Comparison of artificial urinary sphincter and collagen for the treatment of postprostatectomy incontinence. Urology 2000;56:600–3.

91. Montague DK, Angermeier KW. Postprostatectomy urinary incontinence: the case for artificial urinary sphincter implantation. Urology 2000;55:2–4.

92. Dalkin BL, Wessells H, Cui H. A national survey of urinary and health related quality of life outcomes in men with an artificial urinary sphincter for post-radical prostatectomy incontinence. J Urol 2003;169:237–9.

93. Elliott DS, Barrett DM. Mayo Clinic long-term analysis of the functional durability of the AMS 800 artificial urinary sphincter: a review of 323 cases. J Urol 1998; 159:1206–8.

94. Gundian JC, Barrett DM, Parulkar BG. Mayo Clinic experience with use of the AMS800 artificial urinary sphincter for urinary incontinence following radical prostatectomy. J Urol 1989;142:1459–61.

95. Marks JL, Light JK. Management of urinary incontinence after prostatectomy with the artificial urinary sphincter. J Urol 1989;142:302–4.

96. Kowalczyk JJ, Nelson R, Mulcahy JJ. Successful reinsertion of the artificial urinary sphincter after removal for erosion or infection. Urology 1996;48:906–8.

97. Bell BB, Mulcahy JJ. Management of cuff erosion of the double cuff artificial urinary sphincter. J Urol 2000;163:85–6.

98. Bryan DE, Mulcahy JJ, Simmons GR. Salvage procedure for infected noneroded artificial urinary sphincters. J Urol 2002;168:2464–6.

99. Mulcahy JJ, Brant MD, Ludlow JK. Management of infected penile implants. Tech Urol 1995;1:115–9.

100. Furlow WL, Barrett DM. The artificial urinary sphincter: experience with the AS 800 pump-control assembly for single-stage primary deactivation and activation—a preliminary report. Mayo Clin Proc 1985;60:255–8.

101. Motley RC, Barrett DM. Artificial urinary sphincter cuff erosion. Experience with reimplantation in 38 patients. Urology 1990;35:215–8.

102. Raj GV, Peterson AC, Webster GD. Outcomes following erosions of the artificial urinary sphincter. J Urol 2006;175:2186–90.

103. Debell M, Wessells H. Recurrent bulbar urethral stricture in the region of an artificial urinary sphincter. J Urol 2001;166:1006–7.

104. Westney OL, Del Terzo MA, McGuire EJ. Balloon dilation of posterior urethral stricture secondary to radiation and cryotherapy in a patient with a functional artificial urethral sphincter. J Endourol 1992;13:585–6.

105. Anger JT, Raj GV, Delvecchio FC, et al. Anastomotic contracture and incontinence after radical prostatectomy: a graded approach to management. J Urol 2005;173:1143–6.

106. Magera JS Jr, Elliot DS. Artificial urinary sphincter infection: causative organisms in a contemporary series. J Urol 2008;180(6):2475–8.

107. Venn SN, Greenwell TJ, Mundy AR, et al. The long-term outcome of artificial urinary sphincters. J Urol 2000;164(3 Pt 1):702–6.
108. Maillet F, Buzelin JM, Bouchot O, et al. Management of artificial urinary sphincter dysfunction. Eur Urol 2004;46(2):241–5.
109. Wolf JS Jr, Bennett CJ, Dmochowski RR, et al. Best practice policy statement on urologic surgery antimicrobial prophylaxis. J Urol 2008;179:1379–90.
110. Litwiller SE, Kim KB, Fone PD, et al. Post-prostatectomy incontinence and the artificial urinary sphincter: a long-term study of patient satisfaction and criteria for success. J Urol 1996;156:1975–80.
111. Montague DK. The artificial urinary sphincter (AS 800): experience in 166 consecutive patients. J Urol 1992;147:380–2.

Critical Orthopedic Skills and Procedures

Stuart E. Boss, MD*, Amit Mehta, MD, Charles Maddow, MD,
Samuel D. Luber, MD, MPH

KEYWORDS

- Dislocation • Reduction • Arthrocentesis • Splint • Fracture
- Compartment pressure • Immobilize

KEY POINTS

- Arthrocentesis is both a diagnostic and therapeutic tool, and knowledge of technique and various approaches will aid the emergency physician in rapidly evaluating a joint effusion.
- Synovial fluid analysis provides important information about the etiology of a monoarticular arthritis, and being able interpret the analysis to distinguish between inflammatory, noninflammatory, and septic processes is a critical skill.
- Fractures are commonly seen in patients who sustain an acute traumatic injury, and Emergency Department treatment usually consists of fracture reduction, pain control, and immobilization.
- Joint dislocations are extremely painful injuries that require prompt evaluation with a thorough neurovascular examination, and timely reduction not only decreases time to patient comfort but also yields better long-term clinical outcomes.
- Joint dislocations are typically the result of high-energy trauma, and reduction techniques are multiple and varied. One should understand different techniques, yet be cognizant of potential complications, which include neurovascular injury, fracture, and inability to reduce.
- Acute limb compartment syndrome is a limb-threatening entity, and the emergency physician should maintain a high index of suspicion for the development of this condition in any patient with extremity trauma.

ARTHROCENTESIS

Arthrocentesis is the aspiration of synovial fluid from a joint capsule (**Figs. 1–4**). It is a safe and simple procedure that may be indicated in the presence of a joint effusion for either diagnostic or therapeutic purposes. As a diagnostic procedure, the fluid obtained by arthrocentesis may provide clues as to the specific conditions or injuries

Disclosures: None to report.
Department of Emergency Medicine, The University of Texas Medical School at Houston, 6431 Fannin, JJL 431, Houston, TX 77030, USA
* Corresponding author.
E-mail address: stuartboss@gmail.com

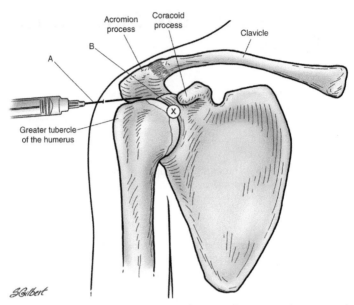

Fig. 1. Shoulder joint arthrocentesis. A, Lateral approach; B, Anterior approach. The site of needle insertion is represented by an X. (Used with permission from Reichman EF, Simon RR: Emergency Medicine Procedures, McGraw-Hill, 2004, copyright Eric F. Reichman.)

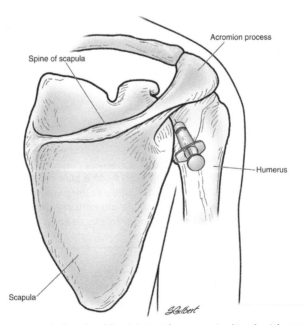

Fig. 2. Posterior approach for shoulder joint arthrocentesis. (Used with permission from Reichman EF, Simon RR: Emergency Medicine Procedures, McGraw-Hill, 2004, copyright Eric F. Reichman.)

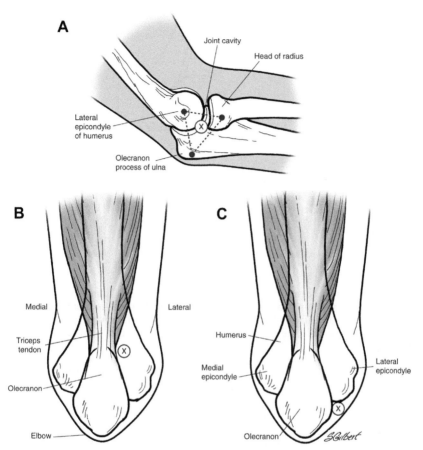

Fig. 3. Elbow joint arthrocentesis. The site of needle insertion is represented by an X. A, Lateral approach; B, Posterior approach; C, Posterolateral approach. (Used with permission from Reichman EF, Simon RR: Emergency Medicine Procedures, McGraw-Hill, 2004, copyright Eric F. Reichman.)

leading to a joint effusion. Diagnostic arthrocentesis should be performed when the cause of a joint effusion is not clear based on history and physical examination, and must be performed when the differential diagnosis includes septic arthritis.[1] As a therapeutic procedure, arthrocentesis can provide pain relief and improve acute mobility by decompressing a tense joint effusion. It also provides a means for injecting analgesic and therapeutic drugs into a joint.[2] Injection of local anesthetic solutions can relieve pain, as well as improve the quality and reliability of the physical examination. Because of their anti-inflammatory and analgesic properties, corticosteroid solutions injected into the joint offer more durable comfort and range of motion for patients with chronic or recurrent arthritis (**Box 1**).[1,3–6]

In most cases of traumatic arthritis, the patient can easily recall the traumatic event, and the resultant injury is acute and obvious to the examiner. However, in cases where the trauma might be remote or minimal, an arthrocentesis can be used to determine if an effusion is a result of trauma. If the synovial fluid is grossly bloody or contains a large number of red blood cells, this likely represents an intra-articular injury to either the

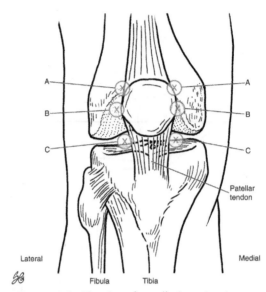

Fig. 4. Knee joint arthrocentesis. The site of needle insertion is represented by an X. A, Medial and lateral suprapatellar approach; B, Medial and lateral parapatellar approach; C, Medial and lateral infrapatellar approach. (Used with permission from Reichman EF, Simon RR: Emergency Medicine Procedures, McGraw-Hill, 2004, copyright Eric F. Reichman.)

bone or other structures. In addition, evaluation of the synovial fluid for fat globules can be performed, which if positive confirms the presence of an intra-articular fracture versus a disruption of an intra-articular ligament.[1]

The therapeutic benefits of arthrocentesis include decreasing pain and increasing joint range of motion by the removal of synovial fluid or blood as well as the injection of therapeutic agents. For patients who have hemophilia and are predisposed to developing acute hemarthroses, an arthrocentesis can be performed to aspirate a significant amount of blood from the joint space, once the appropriate clotting factor is replaced.[3]

Box 1
Indications for arthrocentesis

Evaluate monoarticular arthritis

Evaluate traumatic arthritis

Identify the cause of an effusion

Rule out joint infection

Diagnose inflammatory versus noninflammatory disorders

Identify intra-articular fracture or disruption of intra-articular structures

Identify crystal-induced arthritis

Relieve pain caused by a tense effusion or acute hemarthrosis by aspiration of fluid

Inject therapeutic agents

Data from Refs.[3,7,8]

Contraindications

Arthrocentesis should not be performed through sites of overlying skin or soft-tissue infection because of the risk of introducing infectious organisms into the joint capsule. In the presence of such infection, an uninvolved entry site should be selected. If all potential entry sites over a patient's joint are affected, arthrocentesis is generally thought to be contraindicated. Likewise, bacteremia and sepsis are considered relative contraindications out of concern for hematogenous introduction of infectious organisms. However, given the substantial morbidity of septic arthritis, some advise diagnostic arthrocentesis if this condition is suspected.[8,9] If performed under such conditions, these investigators suggest that arthrocentesis should be followed by admission for 24 hours of intravenous antibiotic administration.

Although proposed as a relative contraindication to arthrocentesis, few data exist regarding the safety of arthrocentesis in patients receiving anticoagulant therapy.[3] One study, involving 32 arthrocentesis procedures, demonstrated that patients with international normalized ratios as high as 4.5 experienced no joint or soft-tissue hemorrhage.[10] When performing this procedure on anticoagulated patients, it has been suggested to use a smaller-gauge needle and that special care be taken not to strike articular surfaces when directing the needle (**Box 2**).[1]

Patient Preparation

The joint should first be examined for any overlying superficial lesions, wounds, or signs of infection such as erythema, warmth, and tenderness, and any such areas should be avoided.

Patient positioning will depend on which joint is to be aspirated. Once the patient is positioned, the necessary bony landmarks should be identified. If a large effusion is present, it may be difficult to palpate and identify these landmarks, in which case it may be useful to compare the patient's affected joint with their contralateral, "normal" joint. Ultrasound-guided arthrocentesis has been evaluated, with mixed results. Some evidence demonstrates improved success, greater synovial fluid yield, and less procedural pain[11]; however, other investigators have not found this to be the case.[12]

Once the proper landmarks are identified, the skin over the entry site should be cleansed thoroughly with either povidone-iodine or a chlorhexidine-based solution.

Box 2
Equipment for arthrocentesis

Sterile gloves

Sterile drapes

10 × 10-cm gauze

Povidone-iodine solution or chlorhexidine topical solution

1% lidocaine solution for local anesthesia

One 3- to 10-mL syringe for local anesthetic

One Small-bore needle (25- or 27-gauge) to inject local anesthetic

One 10- to 60-mL syringe to collect aspirated synovial fluid

One 18- to 22-gauge needle to aspirate synovial fluid

Specimen tubes for laboratory analysis of synovial fluid

Culture tubes or media

Next, the joint should be covered with a sterile drape to create a sterile field for the procedure.

Adequate anesthesia may be obtained by injecting lidocaine (with or without epinephrine), first as a superficial wheal at the puncture site, then by infiltrating deeper into the subcutaneous tissues. One should avoid injecting local anesthetic into the joint space at this stage, as doing so may interfere with laboratory analysis of the synovial fluid.[1]

General Technique

The needle should be attached to the syringe before penetrating the skin to avoid sudden and painful movements of the needle in the joint cavity. Stretch the skin over the needle insertion site, and insert the needle through the skin and into the joint space. Aspirating with the syringe, the needle should be advanced until synovial fluid is returned. If the articular surface is encountered, an occurrence that generally produces significant pain, the needle should be slightly withdrawn and advanced at a different angle away from the joint surface. Once synovial fluid is encountered, aspiration should continue until no more fluid can be withdrawn. Once the synovial fluid has been collected, the needle should be withdrawn and the puncture site dressed.[1]

Joint-Specific Techniques

Shoulder arthrocentesis	
Anterior Approach	
Positioning	The patient may be sitting upright or supine. The arm should be flexed 90° at the elbow, adducted, and internally rotated so that the forearm is resting against the abdomen.
Landmarks	Palpate the coracoid process of the scapula below the lateral third of the clavicle. Then palpate the groove between the coracoid process and the humeral head. This landmark will serve as the needle entry site.
Needle insertion	Insert the needle perpendicular to the skin, into the aforementioned groove. The needle should be aimed directly posterior and should be advanced until a loss of resistance is encountered signaling that the needle is in the joint cavity.
Comments	In regard of all the approaches for a shoulder arthrocentesis, this is the simplest but most painful. A rare but serious complication is damage to the brachial plexus or axillary vessels with the needle.
Posterior Approach	
Positioning	With the patient sitting upright, place the palm of the hand of the patient's affected shoulder on the anterior surface of the opposite shoulder, with the arm and forearm held against the chest.
Landmarks	Identify the spine of the scapula and follow it laterally to the acromion process. The posterior border of the acromion process will be the landmark for needle insertion.
Needle insertion	As the clinician, place the nondominant thumb on the posterior border of the acromion process and the nondominant index finger on the coracoid process. Insert the needle 1–2 cm below the thumb, parallel to the floor, and directed to the tip of the index finger. The needle should be aimed approximately 30° medially.

(continued on next page)

Shoulder arthrocentesis (*continued*)	
Comments	With this approach, the needle avoids the tendons of the rotator cuff, the joint capsule is more easily penetrated because it is thinner than compared with the anterior aspect, and there are no neurovascular structures that can be injured.
Lateral Approach	
Positioning	The patient should be seated upright with the affected arm hanging by the side.
Landmarks	Identify the acromion process of the scapula and locate the groove just inferior to the lateral aspect of the acromion process. This groove lies between the acromion process and the greater tubercle of the humerus.
Needle insertion	Insert the needle into the midpoint of the groove, directing it medially and slightly posteriorly.
Comments	The subacromial bursa is just below the deltoid muscle and does not communicate with the shoulder joint. The needle must be inserted at least 2.5–3 cm to ensure insertion into the joint capsule and to avoid aspirating fluid from the subacromial bursa.

Elbow arthrocentesis	
Lateral Approach	
Positioning	Have the patient sit upright with the affected elbow flexed 45° and with the hand pronated; this will widen the joint space and help the clinician avoid any neurovascular structures during the procedure.
Landmarks	Identify the depression between the lateral epicondyle of the humerus, the radial head, and the tip of the olecranon process of the ulna. It will be located proximal to the radial head in the area where no bony structures can be palpated. Having the patient flex the elbow 45° and pronate the hand will widen the cavity and should help with identifying the needle insertion site.
Needle insertion	Insert the needle perpendicular to the skin into the depression.
Comments	This is the preferred approach because it avoids tendons and neurovascular structures.
Posterior Approach	
Positioning	With the patient seated upright, flex the elbow 90° with the hand supinated.
Landmarks	Find the top of the olecranon process and the triceps muscle insertion into the olecranon. The needle will be inserted at the point just proximal to the top of the olecranon and just lateral to the triceps insertion point.
Needle insertion	Insert the needle perpendicular to the skin and parallel to the radial shaft at the palpated indentation.
Comments	Because the radial nerve can be damaged, this approach should be used in patients in whom the lateral approach cannot be used.
Posterolateral Approach	
Positioning	With the patient sitting upright, flex the elbow 90° with the hand supinated.
Landmarks	Palpate the indentation just lateral to the olecranon process and just distal to the lateral epicondyle.
Needle insertion	Insert the needle perpendicular to the skin and parallel to the radial shaft at the palpated indentation.
Comments	Can be used as an alternative approach to the lateral approach.

Knee arthrocentesis	
Suprapatellar Approach	
Positioning	The patient should be placed supine with the affected knee fully extended.
Landmarks	Palpate the midpoint of the lateral or medial aspect of the superior portion of the patella. Either aspect may be used as the landmark to guide needle insertion.
Needle insertion	Insert the needle through one of the aforementioned landmarks and direct it between the posterior surface of the patella and the intercondylar femoral notch.
Comments	With this approach, the needle will enter the suprapatellar bursa, which is a direct continuation of the synovial cavity. This approach will avoid potential damage to the articular cartilage and avoids important neurovascular structures.
Parapatellar Approach	
Positioning	The patient should be placed supine with knee fully extended.
Landmarks	Identify the midpoint of either the lateral or medial border of the patella.
Needle insertion	Insert the needle just below the midpoint of patellar borders mentioned earlier and direct it perpendicular to the long axis of the leg. The needle should be aimed toward the intercondylar femoral notch.
Comments	The medial parapatellar approach is the easiest site for knee arthrocentesis.
Infrapatellar Approach	
Positioning	The patient should be seated upright with the affected knee flexed 90°, hanging off the edge of the stretcher.
Landmarks	Identify the inferior border of the patella and the patellar tendon.
Needle insertion	Insert the needle below the inferior border of patella along the level of the joint line. The needle can be inserted medial or lateral to the patellar tendon. Aim the needle toward the intercondylar notch of the femur and perpendicular to the long axis of the leg.
Comments	The risk of injuring the articular cartilage is minimal but there exists the risk of piercing the patellar tendon.

Complications

Arthrocentesis is a relatively safe procedure. Infection of a sterile joint can occur when the needle used for the procedure pierces through infected skin or subcutaneous tissue. Performing this procedure under rigorous sterile technique can minimize the risk of infection, with the incidence of infection approximately 1 in 10,000 arthrocenteses.[7]

Significant bleeding with subsequent hemarthrosis is extremely rare, and any external bleeding can usually be controlled with direct pressure over the needle insertion site. In patients with a bleeding diathesis or who are on anticoagulants, arthrocentesis can be safely performed.

Synovial Fluid Analysis

The synovial fluid should be grossly inspected for color, clarity, viscosity, and the presence of blood or inclusions (eg, fat globules) that indicate fracture. Normal synovial fluid is straw colored, clear enough to read newsprint through, and will not clot. The clarity of the synovial fluid roughly predicts the leukocyte count in the specimen, as an elevated synovial fluid leukocyte count results in a more opaque specimen.

Regardless of general appearance, samples of the fluid obtained should always have laboratory analysis of cell count with differential, Gram stain, culture, and crystal analysis to help determine the etiology of the patient's condition. The total leukocyte count is used to help differentiate between an inflammatory, noninflammatory, or septic process. In general, a leukocyte count greater than 100,000 indicates an infectious process, a leukocyte count between 2000 and 100,000 indicates an inflammatory process, and a leukocyte count less than 2000 is considered within normal limits.[5] However, significant overlap exists within these cutoffs.[13] A moderate white blood cell count does not exclude an infectious process,[14] as lower white blood cell counts may be seen early in the course of an infectious process or in a partially treated septic arthritis, whereas higher counts can be seen in rheumatoid arthritis or crystal-induced arthropathies.[13] As a result, the clinician must not rely solely on the total leukocyte count to establish a diagnosis.[15,16]

Crystal analysis is best performed using polarized microscopy. Analysis involves microscopic examination of the shape, size, and birefringence of any crystals identified. Monosodium urate crystals are commonly seen in gout and are needle-shaped, 2 to 10 μm in length, and negatively birefringent. Calcium pyrophosphate crystals are seen in pseudogout and appear as rods, rhomboids, plates, or needle-like forms. These crystals are weakly positively birefringent under polarized microscopy.[3]

FRACTURE MANAGEMENT

Fractures typically result from acute trauma, although overuse syndromes and underlying pathology may be the cause in certain cases. In most cases, acute pain and deformity prompts the visit to the Emergency Department (ED). Plain radiography is sufficient in the majority of cases, but special imaging techniques such as computed tomography (CT), magnetic resonance imaging (MRI), and radionucleotide bone scanning may be useful in some instances. The keys to management of acute fractures in the ED are pain control, fracture reduction, and immobilization.

Essential components of the musculoskeletal physical examination include a detailed neurovascular examination and inspection of the overlying skin to determine whether the fracture is open or closed. Deformity or bony tenderness suggestive of fracture should prompt plain radiography of the injured area. All radiographic series should include a minimum of 2 views taken at right angles to each other.

Fractures should be reduced and splinted as quickly as possible to minimize pain, blood loss, and injury to surrounding structures.[17] The goal of reduction is to reestablish anatomic alignment, providing the best chance of healing effectively, as the local hematoma creates a medium for eventual callus formation, which then bridges together the two ends of the fractured bone. Every effort should be made to attain this goal, as it helps to limit the downstream complications of delayed union, malunion, and nonunion. It is not always possible to achieve satisfactory alignment via closed reduction in the ED, and some fractures may require operative reduction.

Indications

The emergency physician (EP) should be well-versed in splint application techniques and in splint selection for various injuries (**Tables 1**). All fractured extremities and dislocated joints that have been reduced should be splinted. Other musculoskeletal injuries such as sprains and strains may also benefit from splint immobilization, as may tendon repairs and certain lacerations over or near joints, to prevent wound dehiscence.

Table 1	
Common orthopedic injuries and splints	
Injury	**Preferred Splint**
Distal phalanx fracture of the hand	Finger protector splint
Boxer's fracture	Ulnar gutter splint
Metacarpal fracture	Radial or ulnar gutter splint
Scaphoid fracture	Thumb spica splint
Carpal fracture	Dorsal splint of the forearm
Radius and ulna fracture	Sugar-tong splint
Elbow dislocation	Posterior long arm (elbow) splint
Supracondylar fracture of the humerus	Posterior long arm (elbow) splint
Proximal humerus fracture	Coaptation splint, sling, and swathe
Shoulder dislocation	Shoulder immobilizer or sling and swathe
Metatarsal fracture	Posterior short leg (posterior ankle) splint
Ankle sprain	Posterior short leg (posterior ankle) splint
Ankle dislocation	Trilaminar ankle splint
Distal tibia/fibula fracture	Trilaminar ankle splint
Knee dislocation	Knee immobilizer or knee splint
Patellar dislocation	Knee immobilizer or knee splint

Contraindications

There are no absolute contraindications to splint application, and splinting may offer distinct advantages over circumferential casting. Among these is the risk of lower compartment syndrome by splinting, rather than casting of an acute injury. In addition, extremity injuries that require frequent wound care may benefit from standard or modified splinting as a means of stabilization. For example, a splint could be fashioned so that easy removal is possible and/or access to the wound is available through a "window" in the splint.[18]

Patient Preparation

After the injury is identified a thorough physical examination should be performed, including a meticulous neurovascular assessment and inspection for associated wounds that may require attention or that may complicate the injury. The patient should always be optimally positioned to allow the most efficient and effective application of the splint, as well as to obtain appropriate pain control during the procedure.

General Splinting Techniques

The general components of a properly constructed splint include cotton padding, plaster or fiberglass splinting material, and an elastic bandage to hold the splint in place (**Box 3**; **Figs. 5–9**). First, apply the cotton padding. The goal is to provide sufficient protection from the overlying splinting material. The padding may be wrapped in 1 to 2 layers around the affected limb. Use 3 to 4 layers at bony prominences and at the proximal and distal ends of the splint so as to adequately distribute stresses.[19] Alternatively, padding may be layered to fit the length of the casting material, to form a "sandwich splint." Using enough padding is crucial. Pressure sores are a common splint complication and may develop rapidly if the proper amount of padding is not applied underneath the splint. However, too much padding may result in inadequate immobilization. Splinting material should be measured and cut with

Box 3
Equipment for splinting

Water source and sink

Padding material (cotton roll)

Splinting material (fiberglass, plaster)

Elastic bandages

Adhesive tape

Metal clips

sufficient length to cross and immobilize the joints proximal and distal to the injury. Wetting the material is required before application; this induces an exothermic reaction, forming crystals that cross-link through the gauze matrix, and take form, approximating the mineralized matrix of bone. Excess water should be wrung out before splint application, and the splint applied in the desired position and shape. Exposed fiberglass strands may cause painful abrasions or lacerations once they harden, so care must be taken to ensure that no fiberglass comes into direct contact with the skin. Once the splint is in the desired shape and position, it should be secured in place with an elastic bandage wrapped around the splinted extremity. Each wrap of the elastic bandage should overlap the next layer by 50% until the splint is secured. Some further molding of the splint into the desired form may be necessary. The splint should be smoothed and molded with the palm of the hand rather than the fingers to avoid creating indented areas that could result in pressure against the surface of the limb, which may lead to ulceration. The hardening process should be complete in several minutes, depending on the temperature of the water: because crystal

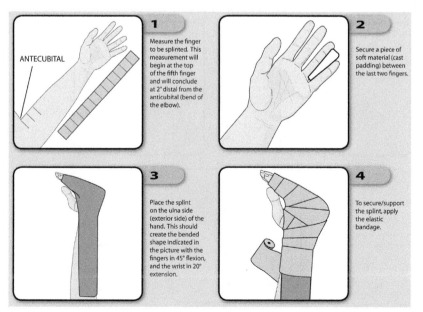

Fig. 5. Ulnar Gutter Splint. (*Courtesy of* EzySplint, DeFuniak Springs, FL; with permission.)

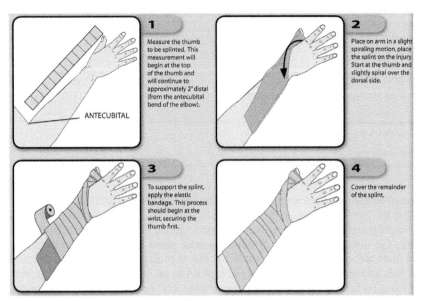

Fig. 6. Thumb Spica Splint. (*Courtesy of* EzySplint, DeFuniak Springs, FL; with permission.)

formation is an exothermic reaction, the warmer the water used to wet the material, the faster it will set (**Box 4**).

JOINT DISLOCATIONS
Indications

Dislocated joints should be reduced as rapidly as feasible, not only to relieve pain and anxiety but also because earlier reduction is believed to lead to better long-term

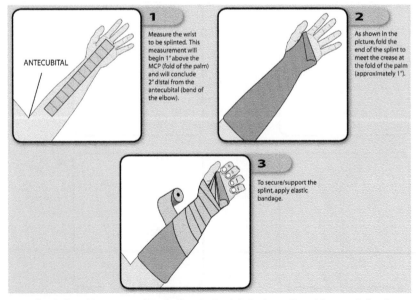

Fig. 7. Volar Splint. (*Courtesy of* EzySplint, DeFuniak Springs, FL; with permission.)

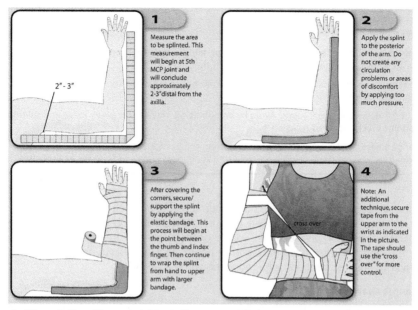

Fig. 8. Elbow Splint. (*Courtesy of* EzySplint, DeFuniak Springs, FL; with permission.)

functional outcomes.[20] If vascular or neurologic deficits are present, immediate reduction is indicated so as to limit the time-dependent and potentially devastating consequences of nerve damage and avascular necrosis.[21]

Contraindications

There are no absolute contraindications to reducing a dislocated joint, although attention to more critical conditions and resuscitation should always come first. Relative

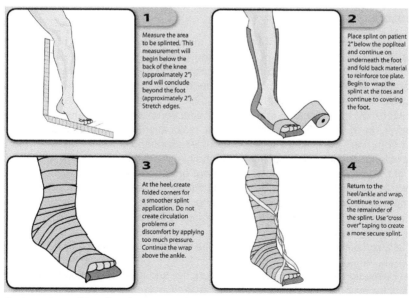

Fig. 9. Posterior Ankle Splint. (*Courtesy of* EzySplint, DeFuniak Springs, FL; with permission.)

Box 4
Complications of splinting

Pressure sores: Avoid by providing sufficient padding over bony prominences and areas of stress and using the palm of the hand to mold the splint.

Inadequate immobilization: Avoid by taking care not to lay down too much padding. Overpadding allows for more mobility.

Joint stiffness of adjacent joints: Avoid by immobilizing only the necessary joints and splinting the joint in a position of function.

Compartment syndrome: Avoid by not wrapping the extremity too tightly with the elastic bandage as well as performing a postsplinting functional and neurovascular assessment.

---

contraindications are few and include interposition of osteochondral fragments in the joint, or the presence of an open fracture-dislocation with immediate orthopedic surgical intervention available, in which case surgery is the definitive therapy.[22] Even in such circumstances, however, if neurovascular deficits are present, the EP should nonetheless proceed with reduction without delay.

Patient Preparation

After a joint dislocation has been identified, a thorough physical examination of the affected extremity should be performed and the urgency of reduction determined. Next, the clinician should prepare by selecting the particular reduction technique, providing adequate analgesia, determining whether procedural sedation will be required, recruiting appropriate assistants and personnel, and gathering necessary materials, including those for postprocedural immobilization. Preprocedural and/or postprocedural radiography may also be necessary to characterize the injury or confirm success. After the joint has been reduced and appropriately immobilized, a repeat neurovascular examination should be performed.

SHOULDER DISLOCATION

The glenohumeral joint is one of the most mobile joints in the human body.[23] While capable of substantial range of motion and flexibility, the shoulder's mobility also makes it prone to injury, particularly dislocation. The shoulder is the most commonly dislocated large joint; the annual incidence of shoulder dislocations is 17 per 100,000,[24] accounting for approximately 50% of all large joint dislocations.[25] The shoulder may be dislocated in 3 different directions: anterior, posterior, or inferior; however, in 95% to 97% of all shoulder dislocations, anterior dislocation is the most common type.[24] Most anterior shoulder dislocations are reducible in the ED, but posterior and inferior dislocations can be highly unstable injuries. After ED reduction of these rare kinds of dislocation, urgent orthopedic consultation should be obtained to discuss the possibility of early follow-up versus hospital admission for prompt operative intervention.[24] In glenohumeral dislocations, the brachial plexus and axillary nerve and artery are at risk for injury. Fortunately, these injuries are rare and patients usually have good functional recovery.[26]

Muscle relaxation is crucial for a successful reduction, as this not only decreases the time requirement for reduction but also minimizes the patient's pain during the procedure. Relaxation may be achieved with adjunctive sedative medications, with intravenous, intramuscular, and/or intra-articular analgesic agents, as well as by procedural sedation. Intra-articular local anesthetic injection has received recent support, demonstrating similar procedural success rates and shorter recovery times when compared with procedural sedation with benzodiazepines and narcotics.[27]

Common Shoulder Dislocations and Reduction Techniques

Anterior dislocation

Hennepin technique Depicted in **Figs. 10** and **11**, this technique is a popular method of reduction and is accomplished with the patient supine or at a 45° angle on a stretcher. This technique often requires procedural sedation. The provider should gently externally rotate the arm with the elbow flexed at 90° until the arm approaches the coronal plane.[28] If the humeral head has not already been relocated, the arm may then be abducted until reduction of the humeral head occurs. Full abduction, signaled by the ability of the patient's hand to cross over the head and touch the contralateral ear, may be required for successful reduction.[29] A palpable "clunk" is typically noted as the humeral head relocates.

Stimson technique (shoulder) The Stimson technique shares the advantages of requiring neither procedural sedation nor constant vigilance by the EP. With the patient prone on a stretcher and a pillow supporting the affected shoulder, allow the arm to dangle off the side of the stretcher toward the ground. Apply a strap to the distal forearm and attach 10 to 15 lb (4.5–7 kg) of weight to the strap. The constant arm traction tires the spastic shoulder musculature, after which the humeral head will relocate, usually within 20 to 30 minutes. If reduction is not achieved spontaneously after 30 minutes, the provider may grasp the forearm and externally rotate and then internally rotate the arm while gently applying traction to complete the reduction.[30]

Traction/countertraction technique (shoulder) This technique generally requires procedural sedation and an assistant. With the patient supine, wrap a sheet around the axilla and torso of the affected extremity. As the assistant holds on tightly to the ends of the sheet to provide countertraction, grasp the distal forearm of the patient with both hands and steadily apply traction with the patient's arm abducted at a 45° angle (**Fig. 12**). Slight external rotation may be used to promote reduction, and relocation should occur within several minutes.

Traction with lateral traction technique More commonly used as an alternative technique in difficult reductions, this technique is slightly different to the traction/

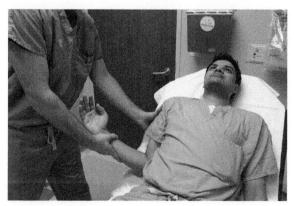

Fig. 10. The Hennepin technique. The provider begins the reduction by externally rotating the arm.

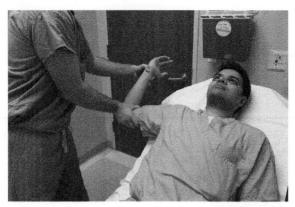

Fig. 11. The Hennepin technique. After external rotation the arm is abducted until the humeral head relocates.

countertraction method. An additional force is used and requires another assistant. When using this technique for shoulder reduction, one should apply traction and direct the first assistant to exert countertraction as previously described. The second assistant should then wrap a sheet around the affected humerus and gradually exert lateral traction in a direction perpendicular to the examiner's in-line traction until relocation occurs.

Scapular manipulation technique Rather than using humeral head manipulation to effect reduction, this technique uses glenoid fossa repositioning.[31] Like the Stimson technique, this method generally does not require procedural sedation. As with the Stimson technique, the patient is placed prone on a stretcher with a pillow situated under the affected shoulder and the arm hanging over the side. Next, palpate the borders of the scapula and stabilize the superior portion with one hand. The thumb should be positioned along the superolateral aspect of the scapula. With the other hand or thumb, palpate the inferior tip of the scapula and direct pressure medially

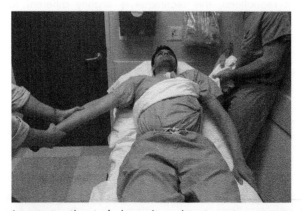

Fig. 12. Traction/countertraction technique. An assistant exerts countertraction while the provider applies steady traction until reduction occurs. This technique should not be used for shoulder dislocations associated with significant fractures, as it may lead to displacement of fracture fragments.

and superiorly. This maneuver is also very useful as an adjunct to the standard Stimson technique. Reduction should occur within 1 to 3 minutes.[29]

Posterior dislocation

Similar to the traction/countertraction technique described for anterior dislocations, a sheet should be placed around the axilla and torso of the affected arm with the patient in the supine position before reduction. As an assistant provides countertraction by pulling the sheet looped around the patient, grasp the forearm of the affected extremity and apply steady traction in-line with the humerus and simultaneously adduct and internally rotate the arm.[29] For this difficult reduction a second assistant may be required, who should be instructed to apply posterior pressure on the humeral head in an attempt to slide it over the glenoid rim and reduce the shoulder.

Inferior dislocation (luxatio erecta)

With the patient supine, wrap a sheet around the clavicle of the affected extremity with the loose ends directed toward the opposite hip. As an assistant exerts countertraction by pulling on the loose ends of the sheet one must grasp the forearm, apply steady traction in line with the humerus, and slowly adduct the arm until it reaches the patient's side. A noteworthy barrier to reduction is the classically described "buttonhole" deformity that has been observed in cases of inferior shoulder dislocation. Although not common, buttonholing describes the situation whereby the humeral head protrudes through a defect in the inferior glenohumeral capsule[32]; this may render the joint locked and irreducible, mandating open reduction in the operating room.

ELBOW DISLOCATION

The elbow is the second most commonly dislocated joint.[25] The articulations between the humerus, ulna, and radius as well as 4 ligamentous structures (medial collateral ligament, lateral collateral ligament, annular ligament, and the anterior capsule) provide the stability of the elbow joint. In particular, the medial collateral ligament appears to be the foundation of elbow joint stability.[33] The relationship of these components allow for movements of flexion, extension, pronation, and supination. Five types of elbow dislocation can occur: anterior, posterior, medial, lateral, and divergent. The classification terminology is based on the relationship of the ulna and radius relative to the humerus (ie, in a posterior elbow dislocation the ulna and radius are displaced posteriorly to the distal humerus). Posterior dislocations comprise the great majority of elbow dislocations (>90%) with all other types being uncommon; of importance, 10% to 20% have associated fractures.[34] The divergent type is extremely rare and is separate from other types of dislocations, as not only are the radiohumeral and ulnohumeral articulations disrupted, but there is dissociation of the proximal radius and ulna via tearing of the annular ligament and interosseus membrane. Several important neurovascular structures course through the elbow region and are at particular risk for injury. These structures include the median, ulnar, and radial nerves, and the brachial artery. Neurovascular deficits are an indication for emergent reduction, but certainly any elbow dislocation should be reduced expeditiously because prolonged dislocation can increase joint effusions and hemarthroses, potentially creating an environment that leads to an inability to reduce. Simple elbow dislocations, which are successfully reduced, have a good prognosis and can be effectively managed with immobilization, orthopedic follow-up, and early range of motion. However, complex dislocations, those dislocations that have an associated fracture, have a poorer prognosis and often require surgical treatment owing to the instability of the joint.[35]

Common Elbow Dislocations and Reduction Techniques

Posterior dislocation

Stimson technique (elbow) Position the patient prone on the stretcher with the affected extremity hanging off the side. The antecubital fossa of the affected elbow should meet the edge of the stretcher. Place towels or sheets under the shoulder and humerus for padding. Suspend 10 to 15 lb (4.5–7 kg) of weight from the wrist. This weight will provide constant traction on the forearm, and the dislocation should reduce within 20 minutes.

Traction/countertraction technique (elbow) With the patient sitting upright or at a 45° angle and the affected elbow held in slight flexion, the provider should firmly grasp the mid-humerus with the nondominant hand. This action will stabilize the upper arm and provide countertraction. Next, with the dominant hand the provider should firmly grasp the distal forearm and provide steady in-line traction to effect reduction, which is noted by a sudden release in resistance and a palpable clunk (**Fig. 13**).

Anterior dislocation

With the patient sitting upright or at a 45° angle and the affected elbow held in slight flexion, an assistant should firmly grasp the mid-humerus to provide stabilization and countertraction. Then the provider should grasp the distal forearm with the dominant hand and provide steady in-line traction. Simultaneously the provider should use his or her other hand to apply downward and backward pressure to the proximal forearm until reduction occurs.

Medial and lateral dislocations

Medial and lateral elbow dislocations are extraordinarily uncommon and can usually be reduced using a traction/countertraction technique similar to that used for posterior dislocations. However, it is advised that reduction of these types of dislocations be completed in conjunction with orthopedic consultation, because of the severity of concomitant injuries to the elbow that are likely present.

HIP DISLOCATION

The hip is the major weight-bearing joint of the human body. Because it is a true ball-and-socket joint, and because it is reinforced by strong ligaments, a fibrous ring, and

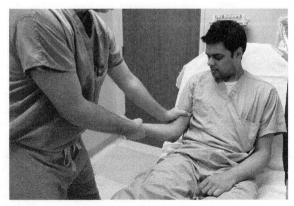

Fig. 13. Traction/countertraction technique for the elbow.

the tendons of large muscles, it is an incredibly strong and secure joint. Therefore large forces are required to dislocate this joint, and a hip dislocation constitutes a true orthopedic emergency. High-speed motor vehicle crashes and falls are common mechanisms of injury. Dislocations may be posterior, anterior, or central based on the relationship of the femoral head to the acetabulum. Posterior dislocations are the most common type and account for 90% or more of all hip dislocations.[36] Central-type dislocations are rare and occur when the femoral head is dislocated superiorly to the acetabulum, although remaining in the same coronal plane. Because of the large amount of energy required to dislocate a hip, patients frequently have other injuries. Up to 88% of patients with hip dislocations have associated fractures (eg, fractures of the acetabulum and femoral head), and 95% have injuries to other areas of the body.[37,38] Fracture-dislocations may be highly unstable or irreducible, and may require open reduction in the operating room.

Late complications of hip dislocation include avascular necrosis, arthritis, and sciatic nerve palsy.[39] Avascular necrosis of the femoral head is a particularly devastating complication. The majority of the blood supply to the femoral head is via the lateral ascending cervical arteries, and flow through these vessels may easily be compromised in the event of hip dislocation. Although there is no evidence for a definitive time frame for which reduction should occur to avoid avascular necrosis, it is commonly agreed that a delay of 6 hours may result in this debilitating problem.[36,37]

Common Hip Dislocations and Reduction Techniques

Posterior dislocation
Allis maneuver This reduction method is the most commonly used reduction technique.[40] With the patient supine an assistant should stabilize the pelvis by directing force posteriorly to the ipsilateral anterior superior iliac spine. The provider should then flex the affected hip and knee to 90°, grasp the knee with both hands, and apply progressively increasing traction anteriorly to the femur (**Fig. 14**). Simultaneous gentle lateral to medial rotation of the femur should be used to effect reduction.

Bigelow maneuver With the patient in the supine position, an assistant should apply force posteriorly to the ipsilateral anterior superior iliac spine. With the patient's affected knee and hip flexed to 90°, the provider should grasp the ankle of the affected

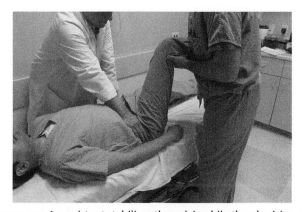

Fig. 14. Allis maneuver. An assistant stabilizes the pelvis while the physician provides steady anterior traction to the femur.

limb with one hand and lever his or her opposite elbow behind the knee. Progressive distal traction should be applied to the femur, then hip extension and external rotation is used to effect reduction (**Fig. 15**).

Whistler/Rochester/Tulsa technique With the advantage being able to perform this reduction technique without the requirement of an assistant, the provider performs this with the patient supine and the unaffected leg flexed to 130° at the knee. The provider places one arm under the knee of the affected leg and then grasps the unaffected knee with the palm. With the other hand the provider grasps the ankle of the affected leg. The affected knee is then elevated by raising the shoulder, using the arm for leverage to apply distal traction to the femur.[40] Lastly, with the hand that is holding the affected ankle, the leg is externally rotated to complete the reduction.

Anterior dislocation
Reduction techniques described for posterior dislocations should be attempted. If irreducible, emergent orthopedic consultation is warranted.

KNEE DISLOCATION

Dislocations of the knee are rare, and gross deformity of the knee is readily noted. Dislocations are commonly the result of high-energy impacts from auto-pedestrian accidents and motor vehicle crashes, although obese patients may sustain this injury with seemingly minor trauma.[41] The stability of the knee can be attributed to strong support provided by the anterior and posterior cruciate ligaments, medial and lateral collateral ligaments, and the joint capsule. Inevitably, injuries to multiple ligamentous structures accompany a dislocation.

The 5 types of knee dislocations are anterior, posterior, medial, lateral, and rotatory, and are described based on the relationship of the tibia to the femur. Anterior-type dislocations are the most common and result from an acute hyperextension of the knee. Medial, lateral, and rotatory types are uncommonly seen. As a knee dislocation is a true orthopedic emergency, it requires the EP to respond in a timely fashion. Reduction should be performed as quickly as possible. Careful attention must be paid to ensure the vascular integrity of the popliteal artery in the event of dislocation. As the popliteal artery courses posterior to the knee it is anchored to surrounding soft

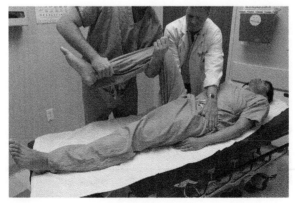

Fig. 15. Bigelow maneuver. An assistant stabilizes the pelvis while the physician levers his elbow behind the patient's knee and applies steady traction anteriorly.

tissues both proximally and distally, which make it particularly vulnerable to injury. Approximately 20% of patients with a knee dislocation also have a popliteal artery injury.[37] This rate is even higher, 30 to 40%, in patients with anterior knee dislocations.[42] CT angiography has become a widely used modality for assessment of vascular damage, and has started to supplant traditional angiography as the preferred method.[37] In addition, nerve injury is a familiar complication of knee dislocations. The peroneal nerve is the most frequently injured nerve and is found in 10% to 35% of patients with knee dislocations.[43] The EP should evaluate both its sensory components (sensation to lateral calf, dorsum of foot, and first dorsal web space) and its motor components (ankle eversion, dorsiflexion, and great toe extension) before and after reduction. In most cases, inpatient admission for frequent neurovascular checks and monitoring for delayed hard signs of arterial injury are advised.

Common Knee Dislocations and Reduction Techniques

Anterior dislocation
One assistant should grasp the tibia distally and apply steady in-line, longitudinal traction. A second assistant should simultaneously grasp the distal femur and provide countertraction. The provider should then grasp the proximal tibia and apply a posteriorly directed force until the knee reduces (**Fig. 16**). Take caution to avoid hyperextension of the knee. Reduction usually occurs without much difficulty.

Posterior dislocation
One assistant should grasp the tibia distally and apply steady in-line, longitudinal traction. A second assistant should simultaneously grasp the distal femur and provide countertraction. The provider should then grasp the proximal tibia and apply an anteriorly directed force until the knee reduces.

Lateral dislocation
This reduction technique is similar to that for anterior and posterior knee dislocations. With assistants providing traction and countertraction, the provider exerts a medially directed force to the proximal tibia until it reduces and slides back into normal alignment.

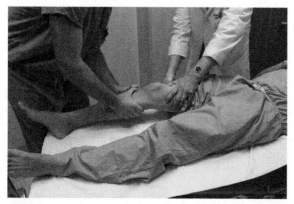

Fig. 16. Anterior knee dislocation reduction. Depicted here using 2 operators instead of 3, the assistant stabilizes the distal femur while the physician grasps the proximal tibia with both hands and exerts force posteriorly.

Medial dislocation
This reduction technique is similar to that for anterior and posterior knee dislocations. With assistants providing traction and countertraction, the physician exerts a laterally directed force to the proximal tibia until it reduces and slides back into normal alignment.

ANKLE DISLOCATION

The ankle comprises the tibia, fibula, and talus. It is a strong modified saddle joint, supported by multiple ligamentous connections between the proximal bones of the foot and malleoli. The strength of this joint is necessary, as it must provide stability while large amounts of forces are translated through it during everyday activities. Walking, running, or jumping may require the ankle to bear more than several times the body's weight. These great stresses certainly make the ankle more susceptible to injury, as sprains, fractures, and dislocations are common ED injuries. Dislocations occur when the talus is extruded outside of the mortise created by the distal tibia and fibula. Because of the significant force that it takes to dislocate an ankle, the patient will frequently have associated fractures as surrounding ligaments stretch and avulse portions of the malleoli. Ankle dislocations can be posterior, anterior, lateral, or superior, and are described based on the relationship of the talus to the tibia. Lateral dislocations are the most common type and are always associated with a fracture of either the distal fibula or the malleoli.[30] Superior dislocations are rare and are caused by substantial axial loading, which results in diastasis of the tibiofibular joint.[37] As the EP assesses these severe injuries it is of paramount importance to note the neurovascular examination of the distal extremity. Extensive soft-tissue edema can make palpation of the dorsalis pedis and posterior tibial pulses difficult. It is advantageous in these cases to use a Doppler ultrasound to rapidly evaluate vascular integrity. Reduction of an ankle dislocation is an exceedingly painful procedure for the awake patient and almost always necessitates the use of procedural sedation for a satisfactory result.

Common Ankle Dislocations and Reduction Techniques

Posterior dislocation
With the patient supine and the knee flexed, the provider should grasp the hindfoot with one hand and the forefoot with the other hand, then apply steady distal traction and plantarflex the foot while one assistant grasps the calf and provides countertraction. Next, the provider should dorsiflex the foot while maintaining distal traction. Simultaneously a second assistant grasps the distal tibia and exerts force posteriorly until the talus reduces.

Anterior dislocation
With the patient supine and the knee flexed, the provider should grasp the hindfoot with one hand and the forefoot with the other hand, then apply steady distal traction and dorsiflex the foot while one assistant grasps the calf and provides countertraction. A second assistant then grasps the distal tibia and exerts an anteriorly directed force. While maintaining dorsiflexion and distal traction, the provider then simultaneously exerts a posteriorly directed force on the foot until reduction occurs.

Lateral dislocation
With the patient supine and the knee flexed, the provider should grasp the hindfoot with one hand and the forefoot with the other hand, then apply distal traction while an assistant grasps the calf and provides countertraction. Then the provider

simultaneously dorsiflexes and medially rotates the foot while maintaining steady traction to effect reduction (**Box 5**).

ACUTE LIMB COMPARTMENT SYNDROME

Acute limb compartment syndrome (ALCS) is a condition whereby the pressure within 1 or more limb compartments prevents perfusion of the intracompartmental tissues, leading to ischemia and, in a matter of hours, necrosis and permanent damage.[44,45] Without early diagnosis and treatment, ALCS may result in disabling contractures, lost sensation, amputation, renal failure, or even death.[45,46]

A limb compartment consists of compressible tissues, bound by an inelastic sheath of fascia and bone.[47] Limb perfusion occurs across the tissue arteriovenous gradient ($P_{arterial} - P_{venous}$), where $P_{arterial}$ is a function of diastolic blood pressure and P_{venous} is a function of intracompartmental pressure (ICP).[48] Perfusion depends on the lower arteriolar, rather than the systemic, arterial pressures. The normal ICP in adults is 0 to 10 mm Hg; in children, it is 13 to 16 mm Hg.[49]

The sine qua non of ALCS is increased ICP, sufficient to decrease limb perfusion to less than the metabolic needs of tissues within a compartment.[48,50] The numerous causes of ALCS increase ICP by either decreasing the volume of a compartment by compression and/or increasing the contents of a compartment. Constrictive bandages and casts are the most common causes of decreased compartment volume, but other causes include intravenous fluid extravasation, compression by prolonged lying on a limb, extracompartmental hemorrhage or hematoma, prolonged tourniquet time, excessive traction, and burns.[48,51,52] Common causes of increased intracompartmental contents include fractures, spontaneous or traumatic muscular hemorrhage or hematoma, excessive exercise, seizures, tetany, and reperfusion.[52] Fractures are by far the most common cause, responsible for 70% of all ALCS cases; isolated soft-tissue injury represents 23%. Tibial fractures are the most common, involved in 40% of ALCS cases, followed by forearm fractures, which cause 18% of adult ALCS cases.[45] In terms of ICP and ALCS, there is no difference between open and closed fractures,[46] and reduced fractures have a higher risk of ALCS then do fractures that have not been reduced.[51]

Box 5
Complications and pitfalls of joint reductions

Inability to reduce. Although the great majority of patients present to the ED soon after an injury occurs, some patients with joint dislocations may present many hours or even days after the injury. Such may especially be the case in elderly patients who have been unable to call for help because of an incapacitating injury. Such delays in care allow severe muscle spasm and edema to develop, making reduction of the dislocated joint considerably more difficult. If this occurs, open reduction in the operating room may be required. Other special situations that may also lend toward an inability to reduce include injuries associated with significant fractures or extreme ligamentous instability; interposed fracture fragments or soft tissue may also render a joint irreducible.

Neurovascular injury. This injury may occur as a result of the injury or as a complication of the reduction. Orthopedic consultation should be sought immediately if this occurs.

Fractures. Great forces may be required to reduce a dislocation. Uncommonly a fracture may result. The EP should carefully inspect the postreduction radiographs, not only for successful reduction but also for any fractures that may have resulted as a complication of the procedure or were not detected on the initial radiographs because of the distorted anatomy of the dislocated joint.

In terms of clinical assessment, much emphasis has been given to the "5 Ps" of a compartment syndrome: pain, pallor, paresthesias, pulselessness, and paralysis. Of these, however, only pain, resulting from muscular ischemia, is reliable. The pain is often of a burning character out of expected proportion to the original injury, worsens over time, and is exacerbated by passive stretch of the structures running through the involved compartment. Paresthesias, resulting from nerve ischemia, may only occur if the involved compartment contains a major nerve. In the appropriate clinical circumstances pain, with or without paresthesias, should prompt consideration of ALCS at an early enough stage to prevent significant morbidity.

Box 6
Needle-manometer technique

Equipment (Fig. 17)

Sterile skin preparation (povidone-iodine solution or chlorhexidine)

Local anesthetic with syringe and small-gauge needle for superficial infiltration

Two sets of intravenous extension tubing

One 18-gauge needle

One 3-way stopcock

One 10-mL syringe

One vial of sterile water or saline

One radial or mercury column manometer from a manual blood pressure cuff

Procedure

1. Anesthetize and sterilize puncture site

2. Connect 18-gauge needle to one end of intravenous tubing A and connect 3-way stopcock to the other end

3. Connect syringe to the 3-way stopcock

4. Turn stopcock lever to close the remaining, open stopcock port

5. Pierce vial with needle, and using syringe withdraw fluid until it reaches halfway along tubing A. Note, or mark with a marker, the position of the meniscus in tubing A

6. Turn stopcock lever to close tubing A port

7. Pull back on plunger to fill syringe with air

8. Connect one end of intravenous tubing B to the stopcock's remaining port, and fit the other to the rubber tubing of the manometer. If using a radial manometer with a connected balloon, turn the dial to close balloon

9. Insert needle at a 90° angle to the compartment and sufficiently deep to enter the selected compartment

10. Turn stopcock lever to bottom so that all ports are open

11. Slowly press the syringe plunger while observing the meniscus in tubing A

12. When the meniscus in tubing A begins to move toward the needle, stop depressing the plunger and turn the stopcock lever to close the tubing B port, which will "lock in" the measurement reading (the value on the manometer is equal to the ICP)

13. Remove needle and dress the puncture site

Data from Carter MA. Compartment syndrome evaluation. In: Roberts JR, Hedges JR, editors. Clinical procedures in emergency medicine. 5th edition. Philadelphia: Saunders; 2009. p. 986–99.

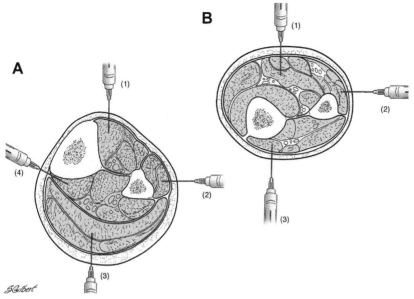

Fig. 17. Needle insertion sites to measure intracompartmental pressures. *A,* The leg compartments: anterior (1), lateral (2), superficial posterior (3), and deep posterior (4); *B,* The forearm compartments: anterior (1), mobile wad (2), and posterior (3).

Box 7
Handheld compartment pressure monitor

Equipment (Fig. 18)

Sterile skin preparation (povidone-iodine solution or chlorhexidine)

Local anesthetic with syringe and small-gauge needle for superficial infiltration

Stryker handheld ICP monitor

One 3-mL syringe

Sterile saline

One device side-port needle

Onedevice diaphragm chamber

Procedure

1. Anesthetize and sterilize puncture site

2. Attach needle to end of diaphragm chamber

3. Draw up 3-mL sterile saline in syringe and connect syringe to diaphragm chamber

4. Connect syringe to diaphragm chamber

5. Raise device cover, seat diaphragm chamber into device, and close cover

6. Aim device at a 45° upward angle and depress syringe plunger to clear air and prime needle with fluid

7. Turn on device, hold device at 90° to compartment, press button to "ZERO"

8. When monitor reads "00," puncture needle into intended compartment; pressure reading will be shown on device

9. Remove needle and dress puncture site

Data from Carter MA. Compartment syndrome evaluation. In: Roberts JR, Hedges JR, editors. Clinical procedures in emergency medicine. 5th edition. Philadelphia: Saunders; 2009. p. 986–99.

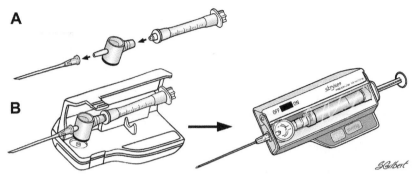

Fig. 18. Measuring intracompartmental pressure with the Stryker system. *A*, The contents of the quick pressure monitor pack are assembled; *B*, The assembled needle-diaphragm-syringe is placed onto the monitor.

Box 8
Arterial/central venous pressure transducer

Equipment (Fig. 19)

Sterile skin preparation (povidone-iodine solution or chlorhexidine)

Local anesthetic with syringe and small-gauge needle for superficial infiltration

One 18-gauge needle

High-pressure tubing

Pressure transducer with cable

Pressure monitor

Sterile saline

Transducer stand

One 3-way stopcock

One 20-mL syringe

Procedure

1. Anesthetize and sterilize puncture site

2. Connect transducer to monitor

3. Assemble system as shown in **Fig. 19**

4. Fill syringe with 15 mL saline, place one stopcock on syringe. Open stopcocks to allow filling of transducer, high-pressure tubing, and needle. Once filled, close stopcock to high-pressure tubing

5. Open top stopcock to air and place transducer at same level of compartment being measured; calibrate system to "0"

6. Open lower stopcock attached to high-pressure tubing

7. Insert needle into compartment

Data from Carter MA. Compartment syndrome evaluation. In: Roberts JR, Hedges JR, editors. Clinical procedures in emergency medicine. 5th edition. Philadelphia: Saunders; 2009. p. 986–99.

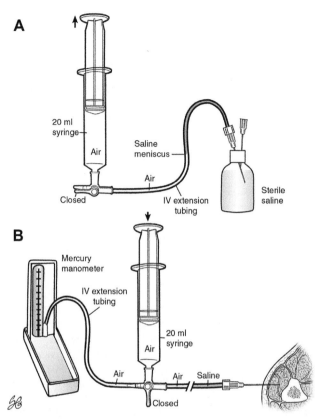

Fig. 19. The needle manometer technique. *A*, The initial system setup; *B*, The final system should form a closed system of space from the manometer through the tissue space.

If clinical signs and symptoms are clearly diagnostic of a compartment syndrome, no further testing is necessary. In less certain cases, direct measurement of compartment pressure is indicated.[52] Stated simply, "if one starts to think about tissue pressure measurements, then one should probably be making them."[50] There are no absolute contraindications to invasive measurement of compartment pressure.

The specific setup and steps for obtaining compartment pressures depends on the technique and equipment chosen for the procedure. Use of 3 of the most common and simplest methods, the needle manometer, handheld device (in this case the Stryker intracompartmental pressure monitor device), and arterial/central venous transducer, are described here. Each of these techniques (when performed properly) yields sufficiently accurate readings.[52,53]

For each of these techniques the patient should be supine, with the affected limb position that the level of the heart. The skin at the puncture site should be sterilized, and the puncture site anesthetized with local anesthesia. The patient must also receive adequate analgesia or, if necessary, procedural sedation, to tolerate the procedure (**Boxes 6–8**).[52]

Compartment Pressure Interpretation

Although various values have been proposed, there is no specific ICP that defines ALCS and mandates a fasciotomy, because tissue perfusion depends on the arteriolar pressure exceeding the ICP. When ICP equals $P_{arteriolar}$, tissue perfusion ceases. Although $P_{arteriolar}$ is lower than systemic circulatory pressures, it is supported by those pressures and thus depends on the body's hemodynamic state. As a result, a substantially lower ICP may result in ALCS in a hypotensive patient as opposed to a normotensive patient. Therefore, a more physiologic variable is appropriate for the decision to perform fasciotomy. This variable is the ΔP, the difference between diastolic pressure (some use mean arterial pressure) and the ICP.[52,53] A ΔP less than 20 mm Hg (or less than 30 mm Hg if based on mean arterial pressure) has been validated as an appropriate value for fasciotomy.

REFERENCES

1. Reichman E, Waddell R. Arthrocentesis. In: Reichman E, Simon R, editors. Emergency medicine procedures. New York: McGraw-Hill; 2004. p. 559–84.
2. Till S, Snaith M. Assessment, investigation, and management of acute monoarthritis. J Accid Emerg Med 1999;16(5):355–61.
3. Parillo S, Morrison D, Panacek E. Arthrocentesis. In: Roberts JR, Hedges JR, editors. Clinical procedures in emergency medicine. 5th edition. Philadelphia: Saunders Elsevier; 2010. p. 971–85.
4. Holdsworth BJ, Clement DA, Rothwell PN. Fractures of the radial head—the benefit of aspiration: a prospective controlled trial. Injury 1987;18(1):44–7.
5. Fye KH, Morehead K. Chapter 2. Joint Aspiration & Injection. In: Imboden JB, Hellmann DB, Stone JH, editors. Current Rheumatology Diagnosis & Treatment. 2nd edition. New York: McGraw-Hill; 2007. Available at: http://www.accessmedicine.com/content.aspx?aID=2725312. Accessed November 2, 2012.
6. Brannan SR, Jerrard DA. Synovial fluid analysis. J Emerg Med 2006;30(3): 331–9.
7. Schumacher HC. Monoarticular joint disease. In: Klippel J, Stone J, Crofford L, editors. Primer on rheumatic diseases. 13th edition. New york: Springer; 2008. p. 42–6.
8. Schumacher HR. Arthrocentesis of the knee. Hosp Med 1997;33(7):60–4.
9. Bettencourt RB, Linder MM. Arthrocentesis and therapeutic joint injection: an overview for the primary care physician. Prim Care 2010;37(4):691–702.
10. Thumboo J, O'Duffy J. A prospective study of the safety of joint and soft tissue aspirations and injections in patients taking warfarin sodium. Arthritis Rheum 1998;41(4):736–9.
11. Sibbitt WL Jr, Kettwich LG, Band PA, et al. Does ultrasound guidance improve the outcomes of arthrocentesis and corticosteroid injection of the knee? Scand J Rheumatol 2012;41(1):66–72.
12. Wiler JL, Costantino TG, Filippone L, et al. Comparison of ultrasound-guided and standard landmark techniques for knee arthrocentesis. J Emerg Med 2010;39(1): 76–82.
13. Adams B, Lowery D. Arthritis. In: Marx J, Hockberger R, Walls R, editors. Rosen's emergency medicine: concepts and clinical practice. Philadelphia: Mosby; 2010. p. 1472–87.
14. Margaretten ME, Kohlwes J, Moore D, et al. Does this adult patient have septic arthritis? JAMA 2007;297(13):1478–88.
15. Frazee BW, Fee C, Lambert L. How common is MRSA in adult septic arthritis? Ann Emerg Med 2009;54(5):695–700.
16. Li SF, Cassidy C, Chang C, et al. Diagnostic utility of laboratory tests in septic arthritis. Emerg Med J 2007;24(2):75–7.

17. Perron A, Germann C. Approach to musculoskeletal injuries. In: Wolfson A, Hendey G, Ling L, et al, editors. Harwood-Nuss' clinical practice of emergency medicine. Philadelphia: Lippincott Williams & Wilkins; 2010. p. 246–56.

18. Hutson A, Rovinsky D. Casts and splints. In: Reichman E, Simon R, editors. Emergency medicine procedures. New York: McGraw-Hill; 2004. p. 669–88.

19. Johnson M, Reichman E. Common fracture reduction. In: Reichman E, Simon R, editors. Emergency medicine procedures. New York: McGraw-Hill; 2004. p. 655–68.

20. Stanton T. Hip dislocation: is reduction timing key? American Academy of Orthopaedic Surgeons Now 2011; 2012 (May 2011). Available at: http://www.aaos.org/news/aaosnow/may11/clinical2.asp. Accessed January 3, 2012.

21. Hougaard K, Thomsen PB. Traumatic posterior dislocation of the hip—prognostic factors influencing the incidence of avascular necrosis of the femoral head. Arch Orthop Trauma Surg 1986;106(1):32–5.

22. Comes J. Ankle joint dislocation reduction. In: Reichman E, Simon R, editors. Emergency medicine procedures. New York: McGraw-Hill; 2004. p. 648–54.

23. Pappas AM, Goss TP, Kleinman PK. Symptomatic shoulder instability due to lesions of the glenoid labrum. Am J Sports Med 1983;11(5):279–88.

24. Daya M. Shoulder. In: Marx J, Hockberger R, Walls R, editors. Rosen's emergency medicine: concepts and clinical practice. Philadelphia: Mosby; 2006. p. 670–701.

25. Bond MC. Orthopedic emergencies. Emerg Med Clin North Am 2010;28(4): xv–xvi.

26. Travlos J, Goldberg I, Boome RS. Brachial plexus lesions associated with dislocated shoulders. J Bone Joint Surg Br 1990;72(1):68–71.

27. Fitch RW, Kuhn JE. Intraarticular lidocaine versus intravenous procedural sedation with narcotics and benzodiazepines for reduction of the dislocated shoulder: a systematic review. Acad Emerg Med 2008;15(8):703–8.

28. Eachempati KK, Dua A, Malhotra R, et al. The external rotation method for reduction of acute anterior dislocations and fracture-dislocations of the shoulder. J Bone Joint Surg Am 2004;86-A(11):2431–4.

29. Sineff SS, Reichman EF. Shoulder joint dislocation reduction. In: Reichman E, Simon R, editors. Emergency medicine procedures. New York: McGraw-Hill; 2004. p. 593–613.

30. Simon R, Brenner B. Orthopedic procedures. emergency procedures and techniques. Philadelphia: Lippincott Williams & Wilkins; 2002. p. 234–95.

31. Ufberg JW, Vilke GM, Chan TC, et al. Anterior shoulder dislocations: beyond traction-countertraction. J Emerg Med 2004;27(3):301–6.

32. Brady WJ, Knuth CJ, Pirrallo RG. Bilateral inferior glenohumeral dislocation: luxatio erecta, an unusual presentation of a rare disorder. J Emerg Med 1995;13(1):37–42.

33. Ebrahimzadeh MH, Amadzadeh-Chabock H, Ring D. Traumatic elbow instability. J Hand Surg Am 2010;35(7):1220–5.

34. Hildebrand KA, Patterson SD, King GJ. Acute elbow dislocations: simple and complex. Orthop Clin North Am 1999;30(1):63–79.

35. Campen A, Kelly S. Elbow joint dislocation reduction. In: Reichman E, Simon R, editors. Emergency medicine procedures. New York: McGraw-Hill; 2004. p. 614–20.

36. Hogan T. Hip joint dislocation reduction. In: Reichman E, Simon R, editors. Emergency medicine procedures. New York: McGraw-Hill; 2004. p. 632–9.

37. Ufberg J, McNamara R. Management of common dislocations. In: Roberts J, Hedges J, editors. Clinical procedures in emergency medicine. Philadelphia: Saunders Elsevier; 2010. p. 869–908.

38. Hak DJ, Goulet JA. Severity of injuries associated with traumatic hip dislocation as a result of motor vehicle collisions. J Trauma 1999;47(1):60–3.
39. Clegg TE, Roberts CS, Greene JW, et al. Hip dislocations—epidemiology, treatment, and outcomes. Injury 2010;41(4):329–34.
40. Walden PD, Hamer JR. Whistler technique used to reduce traumatic dislocation of the hip in the emergency department setting. J Emerg Med 1999;17(3):441–4.
41. Edwards GA, Sarasin SM, Davies AP. Dislocation of the knee: an epidemic in waiting? J Emerg Med 2011. Nov 4. [Epub ahead of print].
42. Pandit S, Kassutto Z. Knee joint dislocation reduction. In: Reichman E, Simon R, editors. Emergency medicine procedures. New York: McGraw-Hill; 2004. p. 644–7.
43. Peskun CJ, Levy BA, Fanelli GC, et al. Diagnosis and management of knee dislocations. Phys Sportsmed 2010;38(4):101–11.
44. Perron AD, Brady WJ, Keats TE. Orthopedic pitfalls in the ED: acute compartment syndrome. Am J Emerg Med 2001;19(5):413–6.
45. Elliott KG, Johnstone AJ. Diagnosing acute compartment syndrome. J Bone Joint Surg Br 2003;85(5):625–32.
46. Gourgiotis S, Villias C, Germanos S, et al. Acute limb compartment syndrome: a review. J Surg Educ 2007;64(3):178–86.
47. Newton EJ. Acute complications of extremity trauma. Emerg Med Clin North Am 2007;25:751–61.
48. Azar FA. Traumatic disorders. In: Canale ST, Beaty JH, editors. Campbell's operative orthopaedics. 11th edition. Philadelphia: Mosby; 2007. p. 2737–88.
49. Erdös J, Dlaska C, Szatmary P, et al. Acute compartment syndrome in children: a case series in 24 patients and review of the literature. Int Orthop 2011;35(4):569–75.
50. Twaddle BC, Amendola A. Compartment syndrome. In: Browner BD, Jupiter JB, Levine AM, et al, editors. Skeletal trauma. 4th edition. Philadelphia: W.B. Saunders; 2008. p. 341–66.
51. Tiwari A, Haq AI, Myint F, et al. Acute compartment syndromes. Br J Surg 2002;89(4):397–412.
52. Carter MA. Compartment syndrome evaluation. In: Roberts JR, Hedges JR, editors. Clinical procedures in emergency medicine. 5th edition. Philadelphia: Saunders; 2009. p. 986–99.
53. Leversedge FJ, Moore TJ, Peterson BC, et al. Compartment syndrome of the upper extremity. J Hand Surg Am 2011;36(3):544–59.

Critical Trauma Skills and Procedures in the Emergency Department

Jorge L. Falcon-Chevere, MD[a],*, Joanna Mercado, MD, MSc[a],
Dana Mathew, MD[b,c], Maria Uzcategui-Corder, MD[a],
Angelisse Almodovar, MD[a], Evan Richards, MS-IV[d]

KEYWORDS

- Chest tube thoracotomy • Resuscitative thoracotomy • Cricothyrotomy
- Venous cutdown • Diagnostic peritoneal lavage • FAST • Compartment syndrome

KEY POINTS

- Emergency physicians (EP) must be familiar with trauma emergencies.
- EP must be dexterous while performing trauma-related procedures, such as chest tube thoracotomy, emergency department thoracotomy, surgical airway, early recognition of compartment syndrome, and venous cutdown.
- It is of paramount importance for the practitioner to be dexterous while performing these procedural skills to maintain function while avoiding complications and improving trauma patient outcomes.

INITIAL EVALUATION OF TRAUMA PATIENTS

In the initial evaluation of trauma patients, it is crucial that adequate coordination between prehospital services and emergency medicine departments is established for proper management. The American College of Surgeons has designed the advanced trauma life support (ATLS) guidelines for omanagement of trauma patients. The creation of the ABCDE mnemonic facilitates the identification of life-threatening injuries and creates a systematic approach following logical and sequential treatment priorities.

[a] Department of Emergency Medicine, University of Puerto Rico School of Medicine, Hospital UPR Dr Federico Trilla, 65th Infantry Avenue Km 3.8, Carolina, PR 00985, USA; [b] WakeMed Health & Hospitals, Emergency Services Institute, 3000 New Bern Avenue, Raleigh, NC 27610, USA; [c] Emergency Medicine, University of North Carolina, 170 Manning Drive, CB #7594, Chapel Hill, NC 27599-7594, USA; [d] Uniformed Services University of the Health Sciences, 4301 Jones Bridge Road, Bethesda, MD 20814-4799, USA
* Corresponding author. PMB-209 PO Box 6022, Carolina, PR 00984.
E-mail address: jfalconc@gmail.com

Emerg Med Clin N Am 31 (2013) 291–334
http://dx.doi.org/10.1016/j.emc.2012.09.004
0733-8627/13/$ – see front matter © 2013 Elsevier Inc. All rights reserved.

PREHOSPITAL MANAGEMENT

Coordination efforts should be established between the emergency medical services (EMS) network and the emergency medicine department to alert physicians of patients' injuries, hemodynamic status, and estimated time of arrival. Efforts should be made to minimize the time on scene, facilitate preparation for arrival, and to direct patients to facilities with the required services. Prehospital management should focus on airway maintenance, bleeding control (avoidance of exsanguination), and immobilization.[1] In unstable patients, transport to the closest facility is indicated. Whenever possible, immediate transfer to a trauma center should be done. **Table 1**[2] lists the transfer criteria to a level 1 trauma center.[2]

EMERGENCY DEPARTMENT MANAGEMENT

The initial approach should be focused on immediate identification of life-threatening injuries.[3] On arrival to the emergency department (ED), it is vital to gather useful information from EMS personnel regarding the mechanism of injury, hemodynamics on route, and prehospital management (medications administered, fluids given, needle decompression, intubation). Patients are evaluated based on the types and mechanism of their injuries in addition to vital signs.

PRIMARY SURVEY

The priority of the primary survey is to identify life-threatening injuries and to correct them as soon as possible. This systematic approach was designed to assess airway, breathing, circulation, disability, and expose patients to identify occult injuries. **Box 1** describes the primary survey.

For continuous vital signs monitoring, patients should be connected to a cardiac monitor, a pulse oximeter, and a noninvasive blood pressure cuff. If not intubated, 100% oxygen delivered through a non-rebreather mask should be placed. If patients are able to communicate verbally, this may indicate airway patency.[1] If patients are unconscious, intoxicated, or have suffered distracting injuries, the cervical spine should be immobilized. In unconscious patients, a definite airway should be established by rapid sequence intubation.[3,4] The indications for intubation are listed in

Table 1
Transfer criteria to a level 1 trauma center

Physiologic Abnormalities	Type of Injury	Mechanism of Injury
Systolic blood presume <90 mm Hg	Penetrating trauma to head, neck, or torso	MVC with intrusion of >12 in into passenger compartment
Glasgow Coma Scale <14	Gunshot wound to proximal extremities	MVC with major vehicular deformity
Need for immediate intubation or inadequate airway control	Extremity with neurovascular compromise	Ejection from vehicle
	Amputation of extremity	MVC with entrapment or prolonged extrication >20 min
	Central nervous system injury of paralysis	Fall from >20 ft
	Flail chest	MVC with death of a passenger within the same compartment
	Suspected pelvic fracture	Auto-pedestrian or auto-bicycle collision >5 mph
		Vehicular rollover

Abbreviation: MVC, motor vehicle collision.

| **Box 1** |
| **Primary survey** |

Airway

    Assessment of patency

    Bleeding (oral/laryngeal)

    Obstruction (from foreign body, facial fractures, trachea deviation)

    Jaw thrust/chin lift

    Suctioning

    Intubate

    Surgical airway

Breathing

    Assessment of lung ventilation

    Visual inspection (symmetric vs asymmetric chest wall movement)

    Palpation (chest wall defects, rib fractures, subcutaneous emphysema)

    Auscultation (breath sounds)

    Oxygenate with 100% oxygen (O_2)

    Monitor O_2 saturation

    Needle decompression for suspected tension pneumothorax

Circulation

    Control bleeding (manual direct pressure)

    Assess for blood volume status, check pulses

    Establish peripheral intravenous access and start warm crystalloid infusion

    Skin color (pale, pink, ash, blue)

    Assess heart rate

    Consider central venous access if peripheral access could not be established

    Perform focused abdominal sonography for trauma examination

    Consider pericardiocentesis if suspected pericardial tamponade

Disability

    Neurologic status:

        Check pupil size and reactivity

        Motor strength and movement

        Glasgow Coma Scale

        Orientation

    Perform glucose scan by finger stick in patients with altered mental status

Exposure

    Remove all clothing and examine

    Prevent hypothermia

    Roll patients to both sides with cervical spine control

    Inspect spine, buttocks, flanks, and back

Data from Ref.[1–3]

Box 2. For intubation, the cervical collar may be removed and in-line stabilization of the neck should be performed.[1] If a tension pneumothorax is suspected, needle decompression is indicated. Intravenous (IV) access should be established, preferably in the superior extremities. Two large-bore (14–18 G) IV lines should be placed, and 2 L of crystalloid solution should be infused.[1,2] Draw blood work for typing, crossmatch, and samples for the baseline blood count. After the initial fluid bolus, vitals signs need to be reassessed. If unresponsive to isotonic infusion, blood transfusion of type O negative group may be indicated.[1] Early recognition for transfer to a level 1 trauma center is essential. Immediate efforts should be made for rapid transportation to a trauma center in the case of patients who have fulfilled the criteria for transfer.

SECONDARY SURVEY

The secondary survey should not be started until the primary survey has been completed, resuscitation has been initiated, and normalization of vital signs is observed.[1–3] This sequence of steps was designed to systematically perform a more thorough head-to-toe examination for the identification of undiagnosed injuries. A complete history should also be obtained. Periodic reassessment of vital signs should be continuous. **Box 3** mentions the different physical examination steps for the rapid identification of injuries[1,2]

Whenever there are patients with facial fractures or suspected basilar skull fracture, insert the nasogastric tube through the mouth.[2] Limited bedside focused abdominal sonography for trauma (FAST) examination should be performed to identify free intra-peritoneal or pericardial fluid. This examination may be a useful tool, particularly in hemodynamically unstable patients because it may be used to screen injuries that can be triaged directly into the operating room without the need for a computed tomography (CT) scan.[5] In patients that have sustained blunt abdominal trauma, serial abdominal examinations should be performed (preferably by the same examiner).[1] Patients with blunt abdominal trauma can be a challenge, consultation with trauma surgeon should be done in timely manner. In patients with penetrating abdominal trauma who have tenderness, distention, and/or hypotension, emergent surgery is indicated.[2] If there is a high-riding or displaced prostate on digital rectal examination, blood in the urethra in the genitalia examination, or if there is a suspected pelvic fracture, a retrograde urethrography needs to be performed before placing a Foley catheter.[1,2] In patients with multisystem trauma, a tertiary survey is recommended before the first 24 hours to decrease the likelihood of undiagnosed injuries. The most common missed injures are orthopedic.[2] In stable patients, necessary imaging studies should be ordered, including radiographs and CT scan. In the case of patients with hemodynamic instability, they should never be transported to the CT scan until the physiologic status improves. Fluid inputs and outputs should be measured and charted. It is important to remember that most of these trauma patients are

---

Box 2
Indications for endotracheal intubation

Failure to maintain airway patency

Failure to ventilate

Failure to oxygenate

Decreased level of consciousness (Glasgow Coma Scale <8)

Anticipation of deterioration of clinical course

Box 3
Physical examination steps for rapid identification of injuries

Head

    Identify and control bleeding from lacerations, abrasions (apply direct pressure, suture, place surgical clips)

Eyes, ears, nose, mouth

    Identify facial instability and anticipate potential airway deterioration

    Assess for hemotympanum

    Identify epistaxis, nasal septal hematoma, place nasal packing if bleeding is profuse

    Evaluate visual acuity

    Identify ocular injuries

    Evaluate ocular mobility

    Identify avulsed teeth

Neck

    Palpate assessing for subcutaneous emphysema

    Auscultate carotid arteries and listen for bruits

    Observe for expanding hematoma or distended neck veins

Chest

    Identify penetrating injuries

    Order a chest radiograph

    Palpate bony structures

    Auscultate

    Perform pleural ultrasound

    Place chest tube if necessary

Abdomen

    Inspect for distention, ecchymosis

    Evaluate for tenderness

    Perform focused abdominal sonography for trauma examination

    Identify penetrating injuries

Genitalia

    Inspect perineum for hematomas, lacerations

    Assess pelvic stability, place pelvic wrap if fracture is suspected

    Evaluate the urethral meatus for blood

    Inspect vagina for bleeding, perform digital and speculum examination to identify lacerations

    Perform rectal examination to assess for bleeding, high riding prostate, and evaluate sphincter tone

Extremities

    Check peripheral pulses

    Identify deformities

    Reduce limb-threatening dislocations, splint fractures

undergoing a substantial amount of pain. Management should be focused on initiating analgesia/anxiolysis judiciously and monitoring for hemodynamic compromise because some analgesics may have undesired adverse effects.[1]

DISPOSITION

Most of these patients are going to be admitted to the hospital for the management and treatment of the injuries sustained.[3] The patients who have hemodynamic instability should be transported to the operating room or should be transferred to a facility that can offer definitive treatment of their injuries.[2] In the case of transportation to a trauma center, a trained health professional capable of resuscitation should accompany the patients. When evaluating patients who have suffered major trauma without evidence of major injuries, the recommended time for observation is 4 hours. In the case of intoxicated patients, more time may be required. Serial physical examinations may be repeated for periodic assessments. Early consultation with the pertinent surgical services is essential for rapid management.

CRICOTHYROTOMY

Cricothyrotomy is an uncommon but life-saving procedure. It must be considered when other available techniques to oxygenate and ventilate have been unsuccessful. One 10-year study documented a significant decrease in cricothyrotomy rates because of possible emergency medicine residency, rapid sequence intubation techniques, and intubating trauma patients despite possible cervical spine injury. The rate was initially 1.8% and dropped to 0.2% over the decade.[6] Although decreasing in rate, it is an essential skill for emergency physicians, particularly in trauma when most cases are likely to occur. In the same article, Chang and colleagues[6] described that 32% of all cricothyrotomies involved facial fractures, 32% blood or vomitus in the airway, and 7% traumatic airway obstruction. Bair and colleagues[7] also noted similar numbers in that 76% of the cricothyrotomies over 5 years at their institution were performed on trauma patients.

CONTRAINDICATIONS

Because a cricothyrotomy is a surgical emergent airway caused by failed attempts with other oxygenating or ventilating techniques, there are no absolute contraindications in adults. However, there are relative contraindications to at least consider as well as age considerations. A surgical cricothyrotomy is not recommended in a child younger than 10 to 12 years of age because of the anatomic variations in the pediatric airway leading to an increased risk of subglottic stenosis. Other patient populations to consider are coagulopathic patients, patients with previous neck surgery or radiation therapy, a transected trachea, or a fractured larynx. In the setting of transected trachea, and fractured pharynx, direct intubation of the proximal portion of the trachea or tracheostomy should be considered as an alternative management. In all cases, if the choice is a failed airway and ultimately death versus possible complications but a secured airway, the choice becomes simple **Box 4**.

PROCEDURE

There are several options for a cricothyrotomy: open technique, rapid 4–step technique (RFST), and the Seldinger technique. A bougie-assisted technique has also been described, although essentially it is RFST with bougie confirmation of position and aid of placement. The RFST is an open technique that has been modified to

---

Box 4
Mnemonic for difficult cricothyrotomy

Surgery (history of neck surgery, presence of surgical scar)

Hematoma

Obesity

Radiation (history or evidence of radiation therapy)

Trauma (direct laryngeal trauma with disrupted landmarks)

Data from RJ Vissers, AE Bair. Surgical airway techniques. In: Walls RM, Murphy MF, Luten RC, et al, editors. Manual of emergency airway management, 2nd edition. Philadelphia: Lippincott Williams & Wilkins; 2004. p. 1–6, 15.

---

decrease the instruments and steps needed. The best choice is made based on institutionally provided instruments, physician comfort level, and type of patient. All techniques suggest neck preparation, appropriate draping, and local anesthetic if time permits.

OPEN TECHNIQUE

Box 5.

OPEN CRICOTHYROTOMY TECHNIQUE STEPS

- Identify the cricothyroid membrane (**Fig. 1**).[8]
- Make a vertical incision through the skin, approximately 4-cm horizontal incision of the cricothyroid membrane (**Fig. 2**).
- Stabilize the larynx with a tracheal hook at the inferior aspect of the thyroid cartilage (**Fig. 3** and **4**).
- Dilate the ostomy with curved hemostats.
- Place the trousseau dilator in the incision, with dilatation of the ostomy.
- Place the tracheostomy tube in the trachea.

Box 5
Equipment

No. 11 blade scalpel

Trousseau dilator

Tracheal hook

Hemostats

10-mL syringe

Tracheostomy tube (No. 4 or No. 6 cuffed) obturator

Inner cannula

Circumferential tie

Bag-valve-mask and ventilator tubing suction

Data from Bair AE, Wolfson AB. Emergent surgical cricothyrotomy (cricothyroidotomy). UpToDate 19.2:2011.

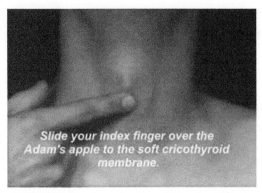

Fig. 1. Slide your index finger over the Adam's apple to the soft cricothyroid membrane. (*Courtesy of* Operational medicine: health care in military settings, CAPT Michael John Hughey, MC, USNR, bureau of medicine and surgery, department of the navy, NAVMED P-5139, January 1, 2001.)

RFST

- Identify the cricothyroid membrane.[8]
- Place horizontal incision through the skin and membrane with a scalpel.
- Stabilize the larynx with a tracheal hook at the inferior aspect of the ostomy (on the cricoid cartilage) providing caudal traction.
- Place the tracheostomy tube in the trachea.

SELDINGER TECHNIQUE

- Identify landmarks and use the nondominate hand for larynx control as with all techniques.
- Use an 18-gauge introducer needle into the cricothyroid membrane at 45° caudally. Maintain negative pressure on the syringe until aspiration of air.
- Remove the syringe and use the guidewire through the needle, then remove the needle holding the guidewire in place.

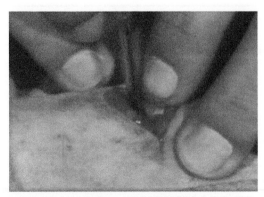

Fig. 2. Make a vertical incision through the skin, approximately 4-cm horizontal incision of the cricothyroid membrane. (*Courtesy of* Operational medicine: health care in military settings CAPT Michael John Hughey, MC, USNR bureau of medicine and surgery, department of the navy, NAVMED P-5139 January 1, 2001.)

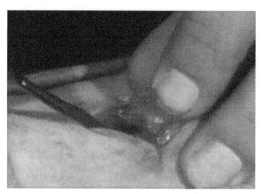

Fig. 3. Stabilize the larynx with a tracheal hook at the inferior aspect of the thyroid carti-lage. *(Courtesy of* Operational medicine: health care in military settings, CAPT Michael John Hughey, MC, USNR bureau of medicine and surgery, department of the navy NAVMED P-5139 January 1, 2001.)

- Make a small skin incision to enable the airway and dilator to pass through the tissue more easily.
- Insert the tissue dilator-airway catheter over the guidewire and advance into the trachea.
- Remove the dilator and guidewire.
- Inflate the cuff and then confirm the airway and secure.

Complications

Complications (**Box 6**) do exist; but as stated previously, the option of a complication versus lack of a necessary airway makes a physician's decision easy. The most impor-tant complication to avoid is failure to consider the cricothyrotomy early enough in a patient's failed airway. Multiple attempts with failed intubation or alternative airway techniques for ventilation and oxygenation lead to severe hypoxic injury. The inci-dence of all complications is approximately 20%.[9]

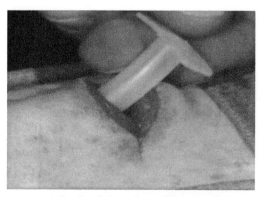

Fig. 4. Place tracheostomy tube in the trachea. (Photograph *courtesy of* Operational medicine: health care in military settings, CAPT Michael John Hughey, MC, USNR, bureau of medicine and surgery, department of the navy, NAVMED P-5139, January 1, 2001.)

Box 6
Complications of surgical airway management

Hemorrhage

Pneumomediastinum

Laryngeal/tracheal injury

Cricoid ring laceration

Barotrauma (TTJV [Trans-tracheal jet ventilation])

Infection

Voice change

Subglottic stenosis

Data from RJ Vissers, AE Bair. Surgical airway techniques. In: Walls RM, Murphy MF, Luten RC, et al, editors. Manual of emergency airway management, 2nd edition. Philadelphia: Lippincott Williams & Wilkins; 2004. p. 1–6, 15.

CHEST TUBE THORACOSTOMY

Chest trauma is a major cause of morbidity and mortality. Whether the mechanism was blunt or penetrating, many of the resultant injuries have the indication for chest tube insertion into the pleural cavity for evacuation of air, blood, or both. Once the indication for chest tube insertion (**Box 7**) is established, the necessary equipment (**Box 8, Fig. 5**) must be gathered, and the potential complications (**Box 9**) need to be anticipated for successful procedure performance.

There is only one absolute contraindication for chest tube thoracostomy, which is complete adherence of the lung to the chest wall.[1,10] Relative contraindications include coagulopathy, pulmonary adhesions from preexisting pulmonary structural disease, or skin infection over the insertion site.

Box 7
Indications for chest tube thoracostomy in trauma patients

Pneumothorax

- Open: sucking chest wound
- Closed
- Simple
- Tension: after needle decompression
- In any mechanically ventilated patient

Hemothorax

Hemopneumothorax

Hemodynamically unstable patients with a chest-wall penetrating injury

Patients with penetrating chest trauma who are or could potentially be placed on mechanical ventilation

Recommended for patients with chest trauma who are going to be air-lifted and can potentially develop a pneumothorax

---

Box 8	
Equipment for chest tube thoracostomy	
Face shield
Sterile gloves and gown
Antiseptic solution for skin cleansing (povidone-iodine or chlorhexidine)
Sterile drapes
Sterile gauze
Local anesthetic solution (lidocaine 1% or 2%)
Syringes and needles
Scalpel and blade
Suture (silk 1.0 or 2.0)
Instrument for blunt dissection (Kelly clamp or round-tip forceps)
Guidewire and dilator if Seldinger technique will be used (preferred for smaller tubes)
Chest tube
Connecting tubing
Closed drainage system
Sterile water if underwater seal system will be used
Dressing

PREPROCEDURAL EVALUATION AND RISK ASSESSMENT

A portable chest radiograph should always be ordered in the initial evaluation of stable trauma patients.[1,10–13] Another useful tool is the bedside ultrasound, which can be reliably used to identify pneumothorax and pleural effusion. It is especially beneficial in unstable patients.[10,11] In patients with a known history of coagulopathy, routine complete blood count and coagulation panel should be ordered. Preprocedure assessment of platelet count and prothrombin time should be evaluated. For elective chest tube thoracostomy, warfarin should be discontinued and time allowed for its

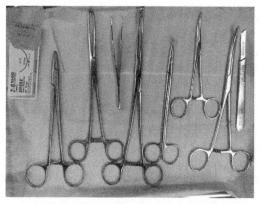

Fig. 5. Chest tube tray. From left to right: silk suture 2.0, Webster needle holder, Allis towel clamps, Adson Tissue Forceps, Standard hemostat, Metzembaum Scissors curved, Hemostats curved, Scalpe.

Box 9 **Complications of chest tube thoracostomy**			
Insertional	Positional	Infectious	Drainage
Laceration of the intercostal neurovascular bundle, which can result in conversion of pneumothorax into a hemothorax or neuritis/neuralgia	Dislodgement	Insertion site infection (cellulitis, necrotizing fasciitis)	Clotting
Perforation of lung parenchyma, intra-abdominal organs, heart, esophagus or mediastinal structures	Subcutaneous emphysema	Empyema	Kinking
Wrong side of insertion	Cardiogenic shock from compression of the right ventricle		Blocked drain
Cardiac dysrhythmias Chylothorax	Nerve injuries		
Data from Ref.[1,14,15]			

effects to resolve. There is no reported evidence that abnormal blood clotting or platelet counts could increase the incidence of bleeding complications of chest tube insertion.[10] However, if time permits, it is good practice to correct any coagulopathy or platelet defect before tube insertion.[10,13,14] Chest tube insertion is an extremely painful procedure; analgesia/sedation should be given in addition to local anesthesia. The preferred sedatives include benzodiazepines and opioids.[10,12,13] It is important to avoid the one-size-fits-all approach when preparing for chest tube selection.[12] If there is an existing stab wound or soft tissue defect surrounding or adjacent to the site of insertion, the chest tube should not be inserted through. A new surgical incision must be performed to avoid potential complications.[15]

CHEST TUBE SIZE SELECTION

The following recommendations should be followed at the moment of chest tube selection[10,13]:

- Pneumothorax: small-sized bore 10 to 18 F
- Pneumothorax in mechanical ventilated patients: medium-sized bore 20 to 24 F
- Hemothorax: large-sized bore greater than 24 F

CHEST TUBE THORACOSTOMY BLUNT DISSECTION TECHNIQUE

Patients should be placed in the supine position or at 30° to 45°. Flex the arm ipsilateral to the lesion with the hand behind the head exposing the axilla.[13,14] Identify the landmarks of the safe triangle, which is comprised of the anterior border of the latissimus dorsi, the lateral border of the pectoralis major, and a horizontal line from the nipple to the midaxillary line.[10,13] The area is prepped with cleansing solution and sterile drapes are placed.[1,10,14] Administer IV sedation/analgesia.[10] Use a 25-gauge needle to infiltrate 5 to 10 mL of lidocaine in the incision site.[14] Switch to an 18-gauge needle to infiltrate 10 to 20 mL of lidocaine into subcutaneous tissue, intercostal muscles, and periosteum.[1,14] Apply negative pressure on the syringe; advance the needle over the superior border of the rib until fluid or air enters the chamber, which indicates that the pleural space is entered. Inject lidocaine into the pleural cavity.[14] Perform a 2- to 3-cm incision parallel to the level of the fourth or fifth intercostal space midaxillary line (**Fig. 6**).[1,14] Use the round-tip forceps or Kelly clamp to do a blunt dissection of the subcutaneous tissue and muscle and create a tract projecting one intercostal space above the incision site.[14] Use the index finger to palpate the path and palpate the superior border of the rib.[14] Advance the closed forceps or Kelly clamp over the superior border of the rib until the pleura is punctured, open and spread the instrument to separate the pleura and intercostal muscle tissue (**Fig. 7**).[1] Use the index finger to palpate the pleural space to confirm proper positioning and to exclude the presence of adhesions.[12,16] Small adhesions may be disrupted with a gentle sweep of the finger.[14] Clamp the tube with the forceps or Kelly clamp in the proximal end, advance the tube into the pleural space and remove the instrument, and introduce the tube until all the holes are inside the pleural cavity.[1,14] In the case of a pneumothorax, the chest tube should be directed anterior and apically; when drainage of fluid is desired, the chest drain should be directed posterior and basally.[10,13,14] Use suture silk 1.0 or 2.0 to close the skin incision with the mattress technique and tie the loose ends around the tube to anchor it (**Fig. 8**).[10,14] Connect the tube to an underwater seal; bubbles should be seen in the chamber in the case of a pneumothorax, and blood accumulation should be noted in the case of a hemothorax.[1,14] A chest radiograph must be ordered to confirm the position of the chest tube.[1,14] Once the chest tube position is confirmed, wrap sterile petroleum gauze around the incision site and secure the tube to the chest wall with adhesive material.

CHEST TUBE THORACOSTOMY GUIDEWIRE (SELDINGER) TECHNIQUE

The procedure is prepped as mentioned earlier. Inject local anesthesia intrapleurally. Use a large-bore needle, create negative pressure in the chamber of the syringe, and advance the needle over the superior border of the rib of the fourth or fifth intercostal space in the midaxillary line. Once air or fluid enters the chamber, the pleural cavity has been reached. Disconnect the syringe from the needle maintaining proximal control. A guidewire is advanced though the hub.[13] Remove the needle with the guidewire in place. Perform a small superficial incision with a blade on the point of entry of the guidewire. Introduce a dilator over the wire to enlarge the incision site. Insert the chest

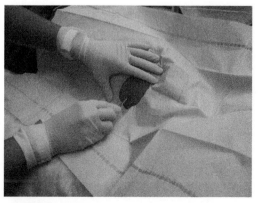

Fig. 6. A 2- to 3-cm incision parallel to the level of the fourth or fifth intercostal space midaxillary line is performed.

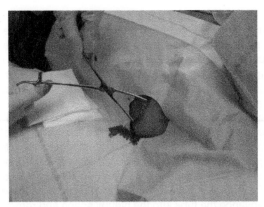

Fig. 7. Advance the closed forceps or Kelly clamp over the superior border of the rib until the pleura is punctured; open and spread the instrument to separate pleura and intercostal muscle tissue.

tube over the wire until all the holes are within the pleural cavity. Remove the guide-wire.[13] Connect the tube to an underwater seal system. Suture the chest tube to the chest wall. Obtain a chest radiograph to confirm the position of the chest drain.[10] Once confirmed, secure the tube, place sterile petroleum gauze around the point insertion site, and place adhesive material to secure the tube to the chest wall.[10]

CHEST TUBE MANAGEMENT

All chest tubes should be connected to a single flow drainage system (eg, underwater seal or flutter valve).[10] In the case of pneumothorax, condensation through the tube may confirm proper positioning.[13] When hemothorax is drained, the respiratory swing of the blood in the chest tube may be used to evaluate tube patency and confirm the intrapleural position of the tube.[10] A bubbling chest tube should never be clamped.[10,16]

As a rule, surgical intervention is indicated if 1500 mL of blood are evacuated immediately through the chest tube, if drainage is more than 200 mL in 2 to 4 hours, or if

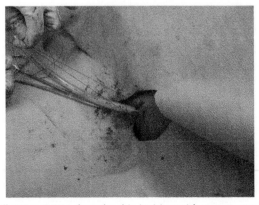

Fig. 8. Use suture silk 1.0 or 2.0 to close the skin incision with mattress technique, and tie the loose ends around the tube to anchor it.

a blood transfusion is required.[1] Controversies exist regarding the use of antibiotics in this setting. The recommendation is to treat with first-generation cephalosporins for the first 24 hours. Some studies showed a decrease in the risk for empyema, pneumonia, and pneumonitis. However, evidence is limited.[12,14,17,18]

COMPLICATIONS

Multiple complications have been reported, which can generally be divided into insertional, positional, infectious, and technical involving the drainage system.[15] The most common complications are recurrent pneumothorax and chest tube misplacement. **Box 9**[14] mentions common reported complications of chest tube thoracostomy.

Other complications described are large primary leak, leak at the skin around the chest tube (suction on the tube is too strong), failure of lung expansion caused by a plugged bronchus, and allergic reaction to anesthesia or surgical preparation material.[1] Uncommonly, nerve injuries have been reported as a result of chest tube malpositioning[17]:

- Horner syndrome
- Phrenic nerve injury that has resulted in diaphragmatic paralysis
- Long thoracic nerve injury
- Ulnar neuropathy

Most of the mentioned nervous injuries improve after repositioning of the tube. Another rare but potentially fatal complication is re-expansion pulmonary edema.[11] The cause is unknown. Risk factors include age less than 40 years, lung collapse for more than 3 days, large pneumothorax (>30%), rapid lung expansion, and application of negative pleural pressure suction. Treatment is supportive.[13,17]

ED THORACOTOMY
Introduction

ED thoracotomy (EDT) can be lifesaving. Rehn[19] first described emergency department thoracotomy (EDT) in 1894 while managing a right ventricle stab wound with associated pericardial tamponade.[19,20] Ever since its first description, it has been a controversial procedure, complicated, and potentially harmful to the provider. Penetrating chest trauma is a major cause of morbidity and mortality. EDT has been described as the last resource to save the life of patients in extremis.[21] Once the indications for EDT (**Box 10**) are established and contraindications (**Box 11**) considered, the necessary equipment (**Box 12**) must be gathered, and the potential complications (**Box 13**) need to be anticipated for successful procedure performance.

Technique

Place patients in the supine position. Once the left fifth intercostal space is detected, the area is prepped with cleansing solution and sterile drapes are placed.[22,23] Perform

Box 10
Indications
Penetrating chest trauma with loss of vitals signs during transport or in the ED
Penetrating chest trauma with rapid clinical deterioration without response to fluid resuscitation
Blunt trauma with loss of vital signs in the hospital

> **Box 11**
> **Contraindications**
>
> *Thoracotomy contraindications*
>
> Signs of death
>
> Hemodynamically stable patients
>
> Chest blunt trauma with associated cardiorespiratory arrest in the scene

an incision laterally, extending from the left side of the sternum along the intercostal space to the midaxillary line. The incision must be done in the superior border of the sixth rib to avoid neurovascular injury. The incision should go through all layers in a single attempt. Use the Mayo scissors to cut the remaining intercostal muscles. Insert a rib retractor with the handle proximal to the bed; it will extend the laceration if needed. Once the pleura is visible, perform an incision with the scalpel and complete it with scissors. Open the retractor to expose the hemithorax and inspect the visible area for injury and act according to need. Remove blood and check for bleeding. If hemorrhage is present, apply pressure (use a staple or sutures). Inspect the pericardium and open it, grasp it with a nick in a cephalocaudad direction using scissors. It is important to identify the phrenic nerve to avoid damage. Once the pericardium is open, check the myocardium for wounds and clots. If a wound is found, the physician can occlude the wound using a finger. Another alternative is to use a Foley catheter to occlude the wound, inflate the balloon, and apply traction followed by a purse-string suture, then remove the catheter. Finally, any cardiac laceration can be sutured using the horizontal mattress technique with Teflon (DuPont, Wilmington, Delaware) pledgets.

If no injury is found in the left hemithorax, the chest incision may be extended across the sternum using a sternotomy knife or a Gigli saw to have a better evaluation of right atrium and ventricle. If intra-abdominal hemorrhage is suspected, aorta cross clamping is imperative.

> **Box 12**
> **Equipment**
>
> Prep materials: iodine–povidone solution, towels
>
> No. 10 scalpel
>
> Rib spreader
>
> Mayo scissors
>
> Metzembaum scissors
>
> Tissue forceps
>
> Hemostats
>
> Vascular clamps
>
> Lebsche knife with mallet
>
> Sponges
>
> 3–0 cardiovascular suture
>
> Jumbo applicators

Box 13
Thoracotomy complications
Infection
Dysrhythmias
Pericarditis
Postpericardectomy syndrome
Heart, coronary arteries, lung, esophageal, and phrenic injuries

Internal cardiac massage is indicated in the absence of cardiac activity while performing an open thoracotomy.

Disposition

Once vital signs are obtained after EDT, patients must be transferred to the operating room for definitive treatment. EDT will remain an indispensable tool in the treatment of severely injured trauma patients.[24]

DIAGNOSTIC PERITONEAL LAVAGE VERSUS FAST

Diagnostic peritoneal lavage (DPL) has been a mainstay in the evaluation of blunt abdominal trauma (BAT) for decades; it was first described in 1965.[25] However, in recent years, DPL has fallen out of favor as the more noninvasive modalities of FAST (see **Box 14** for comparison) and CT scanning have gained popularity and comfort. In fact, Rhodes and colleagues,[26] in a 2011 12-year retrospective study at a level 1 trauma center recommended that with the substantial decrease in DPL occurrence, proposed that the American College of Surgeons consider changing DPL instruction to an optional component of ATLS. Therefore, DPL is no longer taught as a mandatory in ATLS course.[27] However, DPL continues to have a place in trauma evaluation when FAST and CT scan are not an option because of facilities or patient hemodynamic instability. In that light, it is still a necessary skill to discuss, although as less surgeons and emergency physicians become comfortable with the procedure during training, it will continue to fall from favor.

Box 14	
Comparison of DPL versus extended FAST	
Ultrasound	*DPL*
Rapid	Relative speed
Noninvasive	Invasive
No complications	Approximately 1% complication rate
Portable	Ability to detect early viscous injury
High specificity of intraperitoneal fluid	No contrast or radiation
Can evaluate for pericardial fluid	Rapid triage of multisystem unstable trauma
No radiation or contrast exposure	patients
Affordable	
Repeatable	
Easy to learn	
Poor evaluation of retroperitoneal injury	
Cannot distinguish blood from ascites	
Can detect pneumothorax	

Indications

Abdominal evaluation is essential in any trauma patient, both blunt trauma and penetrating trauma. Both modalities have increased significance in patients with altered mental status or spinal cord injury. DPL is also indicated in anterior abdominal penetrating wounds when local wound exploration is positive, although there is no standard accepted red blood cell count in penetrating trauma and it does not detect retroperitoneal injuries. FAST evaluation in blunt trauma is accepted with little downside to evaluation. Ultrasound benefits use, in penetrating trauma is still controversial, but Udobi and colleagues[28] found that there may be a role as an adjunct modality.

Contraindications

The FAST has no contraindications because it is noninvasive, rapid, and can be performed in concert with the trauma survey. Its utility will be decreased in obese patients and patients with subcutaneous air or ascites. The only absolute contraindication to DPL is obvious need for laparotomy.[29] Relative contraindications include previous abdominal surgery, coagulopathy, advanced cirrhosis, morbid obesity, second- or third-trimester pregnancy, and pelvic fractures. The concern for previous abdominal surgery is that adhesions will increase the risk of iatrogenic injury. It could also compartmentalize the intraperitoneal fluid, resulting in a false-negative result. In pregnancy and patients with pelvic fractures, a supraumbilical open approach is the only possible option to avoid trauma to the uterus or destabilization of a pelvic hematoma.

DPL PROCEDURE

DPL has the option of a closed, semiopen, or open technique. Each is described later. The closed technique will be familiar to most physicians because it has the same basic principles already practiced with central lines.[27,30]

- Place the patient in a supine position and decompress the bladder and stomach.
- Prep and drape the periumbilical area (**Figs. 9** and **10**).
- Use local anesthetic of 1% lidocaine with epinephrine to decrease cutaneous bleeding and consider conscious sedation if necessary.

Semiopen

- A vertical midline incision is made 2 cm below (or above in a supraumbilical DPL) the umbilicus.
- Identify the linea alba.
- Retract the skin and subcutaneous tissue bilaterally.
- Grasp the fascia bilaterally with hemostats.
- Insert an 18-gauge needle filled with saline at a 45° angle caudally
- Once the needle has transversed the peritoneum, the saline will flow freely into the peritoneal cavity.
- Pass a guidewire through the needle; if there is any resistance, remove the needle and wire.
- Remove the needle but maintain control of the wire.
- Pass a dilator over the wire.
- Remove the dilator and pass the DPL catheter into the peritoneal cavity.
- Remove the wire.
- Then aspirate, if 10 mL of blood are obtained the result is positive for intra-abdominal injury (**Fig. 11**).

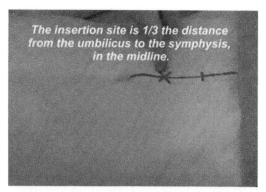

Fig. 9. The insertion site is 1/3 the distance from the umbilicus to the symphysis, in the midline. (*Courtesy of* Operational medicine: health care in military settings CAPT Michael John Hughey, MC, USNR bureau of medicine and surgery, department of the navy NAVMED P-5139 January 1, 2001.)

- If there is less than 10 mL, connect to warm lactic Ringer's solution (LR) via IV tubing and allow it to flow in freely (**Fig. 12**).
- Rock the patient back and forth, and then use gravity to allow at least 30% of the original amount to return (in a child infuse 10–15 mL/kg) (**Fig. 13**).
- Once the effluent has been obtained, remove the catheter.
- Place 4-0 nylon interrupted sutures or staples to the skin and dress the wound appropriately.

OPEN TECHNIQUE

- Make a vertical midline incision 2 cm below (or above) the umbilicus extending 5 to 6 cm; the vertical extension should be inferiorly if infraumbilical and superiorly extended if supraumbilical.
- Retract the skin and subcutaneous tissue.
- Incise the fascia (**Fig. 14**).
- Grasp and elevate the peritoneum with Allis clamps.
- Insert the lavage catheter into a small peritoneal incision (<5 mm) angled caudally (**Fig. 15**).

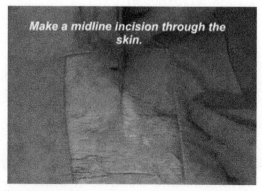

Fig. 10. Make a midline incision through the skin. (*Courtesy of* Operational medicine: health care in military settings CAPT Michael John Hughey, MC, USNR Bureau of Medicine and Surgery, Department of the Navy NAVMED P-5139.)

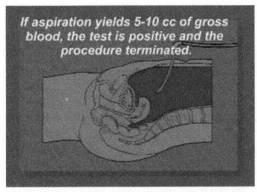

Fig. 11. If aspiration yields 5-10 cc of gross blood, the test is positive and the procedure terminated. (*Courtesy of* Operational medicine: health care in military settings. CAPT Michael John Hughey, MC, USNR bureau of medicine and surgery, department of the navy NAVMED P-5139.)

- Continue as described earlier for evaluation of the effluent.
- Once the effluent has been obtained, remove the catheter.
- Close the fascia with a No. 0 monofilament polyglyconate synthetic absorbable sutur, monofilament, nonabsorbable polypropylene, polyglactin 910 absorbable, or braided, monofilament synthetic absorbable suture in a running fashion; you do not need to close the peritoneum.
- Close the skin with 4-0 nylon interrupted sutures or staples and dress the wound appropriately (**Fig. 16**).

CLOSED TECHNIQUE

- In the middle line of abdomen, 1 or 2 cm below the umbilicus, advance the introducer needle at a 45–angle caudally and use continuous negative pressure on the syringe.

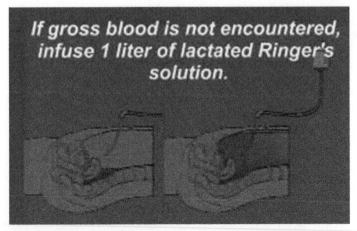

Fig. 12. If gross blood is not encountered, infuse 1 liter of lactated Ringer's solution. (*Courtesy of* Operational medicine: health care in military settings CAPT Michael John Hughey, MC, USNR bureau of medicine and surgery, department of the navy NAVMED P-5139 January 1, 2001.)

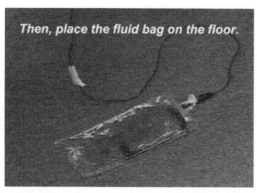

Fig. 13. Place the fluid bag on the floor. (*Courtesy of* Operational medicine: health care in military settings CAPT Michael John Hughey, MC, USNR bureau of medicine and surgery, department of the navy NAVMED P-5139 January 1, 2001.)

- Feel for the penetration (pops) of the skin, fascia, and peritoneum, and then advance another 2 mm.
- If you get a blood return, this is a positive aspirate and you can stop.
- If no blood returns, remove the syringe and advance the guidewire. You should not have resistance with this process.
- Withdraw the needle and make a small incision adjacent to the guidewire.
- Advance the lavage catheter over the guidewire until it is against the abdominal wall.
- Hold the lavage catheter securely and remove the guidewire.
- Attach the warmed LR or normal saline solution via IV tubing and proceed as described earlier.
- After effluent is obtained, remove the lavage catheter and dress the wound appropriately.

FLUID EVALUATION

- Blunt abdominal trauma (BAT) red blood cell count (RBC) more than 100 000/mm^3

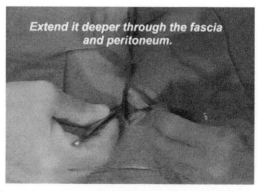

Fig. 14. Incise the fascia. (*Courtesy of* Operational medicine: health care in military settings CAPT Michael John Hughey, MC, USNR bureau of medicine and surgery, department of the navy NAVMED P-5139.)

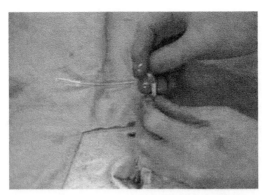

Fig. 15. Insert the lavage catheter into a small peritoneal incision (<5 mm) angled caudally. (*Courtesy of* Operational medicine: health care in military settings CAPT Michael John Hughey, MC, USNR bureau of medicine and surgery, department of the navy NAVMED P-5139.)

- For penetrating trauma, there is no consensus and depends on the area of trauma; in the anterior abdomen, more than 100 000/mm^3 RBC is accepted
- More than 500/mm^3 white blood cell count
- Presence of enteric or vegetable matter

FAST Examination

- Place the patient in a supine position and evaluate using a 3.0- to 5.0-MHz transducer.
- Orient the ultrasound probe indicator toward the patient's right side or head at all times to maintain proper orientation.
- Morrison pouch evaluation: Place the transducer at the costal margin in the anterior axillary line with the indicator pointed toward the patient's head for the sagittal plane.
- Morrison pouch evaluation in the coronal plane: Place the transducer at the costal margin with the indicator toward the patient's head, placed in the midaxillary line.

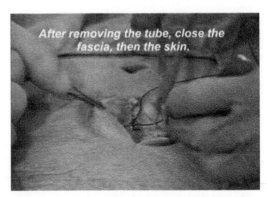

Fig. 16. After removing the tube, close the fascia, then the skin. (*Courtesy of* Operational medicine: health care in military settings CAPT Michael John Hughey, MC, USNR bureau of medicine and surgery, department of the navy NAVMED P-5139. January 1, 2001.)

- Splenorenal recess evaluation: The probe is placed at the posterior axillary line at the inferior costal margin with the indicator pointed toward the patient's head.
- Subxiphoid anterior transverse plane: Place the transducer with the indicator toward the patient's right side, placed in the midline abdomen and angled toward the right scapula using the liver as a window.
- Suprapubic evaluation (pouch of Douglas): The transducer probe should be pointed to the head and rotated to the patient's right to obtain the transverse and sagittal views. The transducer is placed 2 cm superior to the pubic symphysis and angled inferiorly.
- (EFAST) extended FAST evaluation for pneumothorax: Place the transducer in the midclavicular line of the anterior chest wall. Look for the bat sign (rib shadowing) and look for the normal respiratory motion and artifact.
- EFAST: In M mode, orient the transducer parallel to the ribs in the intercostal spaces. The granular artifacts below the pleural line, also, called seashore, are indicating of normal respiratory movement.

COMPLICATIONS

Because ultrasound is rapid and quick, there are no direct complications from the procedure. However, with a sensitivity range of 65% to 95% depending on the study, false negatives are a definite possibility and could delay treatment. Ultrasound detection of fluid is also variable based on the amount of intraperitoneal fluid.[31–34]

Because DPL is an invasive procedure, certain complications are noted, although rare, and include infection; injury to the bowel, mesentery, or iliac vessels; bladder punctures; or abdominal wall infusions. Overall rate of complications ranges from 0.8% to 1.7%.[27]

COMMON PITFALLS AND SUGGESTIONS
DPL

- If the fluid does not flow freely into the peritoneal cavity but seems to drip slowly, consider placement erroneously in the abdominal wall and assess for repositioning.
- If the effluent does not readily return, consider blockage by the omentum. Use firm pressure on the abdomen or slight repositioning of the catheter for improved flow.
- If there is any difficulty advancing the wire through the peritoneal cavity or pain is reported remove the wire then the needle to avoid wire shearing into the peritoneal cavity.
- Stabilize the needle securely to avoid intra-abdominal organ lacerations.
- In pelvic fractures, there may be a false positive FAST (**Figs. 17–25**).
- Infuse fluid in the bladder catheter or place the catheter after evaluation of the pouch of Douglas to avoid a false negative from a poor sonographic window.
- The left kidney is more difficult to visualize because of its superior position. Directing the patient to take a deep breath in may help visualize the splenorenal angle better.
- A distended stomach can prevent visualization of the pericardium in the subxiphoid view; decompression with an nasogastric tube may be necessary.
- Move the probe around to visualize the entire area; rib shadows can hide a positive finding.
- Perirenal fat may appear hypoechoic.
- Use the Trendelenburg position to evaluate the paracolic gutters for free fluid and the reverse Trendelenburg position for pelvic evaluation.

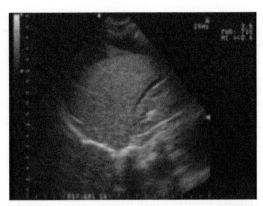

Fig. 17. FAST, fluid in Morison's pouch. (*Courtesy of* Robert Park, MD.)

ACUTE LIMB COMPARTMENT SYNDROME

Acute limb compartment syndrome (ALCS) is a surgical emergency and is caused by raised pressure within a closed fascial space (**Box 15**). An increase of the intra-compartmental pressure (ICP) reduces the capillary perfusion lower than a level necessary for tissue viability.[35,36] The limbs are comprised of superficial and deep fascia that cover and divides the limbs into skeletal muscle groups, neurovascular bundles that accompany them into different compartments.[35,36]

An increase in the ICP may reduce the capillary blood inflow if decompression is not performed promptly, leading to arteriolar compression, muscle and nerve ischemia, muscle infarction, and nerve damage.[35,36]

The most important determinant of a poor outcome from ALCS after injury is delay in diagnosis. The complications are usually disabling and include infection, contractures, deformity, and amputation.[35–37]

The normal pressure of the skeletal muscle compartment at rest is less than 10 mm Hg. One study demonstrated that when tissue pressure within a closed compartment increases to within 10 to 30 mm Hg of the patient's diastolic blood pressure, inadequate perfusion ensues, resulting in relative ischemia of the involved limb.[35–37]

Blood flow to tissues depends on the A-V gradient in capillary beds. If reduced less than a critical level, oxygen delivery is impaired and metabolism becomes anaerobic.

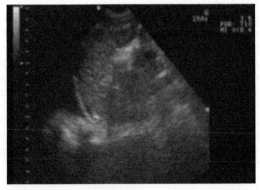

Fig. 18. FAST, left hemothorax and splenodiaphragmatic interface. (*Courtesy of* Robert Park, MD.)

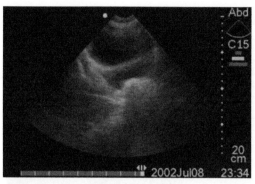

Fig. 19. FAST, pelvis fluid. (*Courtesy of* Robert Park, MD.)

A drop in blood pressure, an increase in compartment pressure, or a combination of the two can reduce A-V gradients and lead to insufficient blood flow to tissues causing ischemia, leading to compartment syndrome.

Sensory changes, like paresthesia and hypesthesia, develop after 30 minutes of ischemia. The irreversibility of damage is directly related to the time of compartment syndrome onset. After 4 to 8 hours of compartment syndrome onset, irreversible functional changes in the muscle occur. Then, between 12 to 24 hours of onset, irreversible damage takes place.[35,36]

INDICATIONS AND CONTRAINDICATIONS

The diagnosis of compartment syndrome is primarily clinical, supplemented by direct measurement of compartment pressures. The history of substantial trauma and the presence of severe injuries should raise clinical suspicion. But, in patients in which clinical findings are inconclusive or subtle, such as: children, unresponsive, uncooperative patients or patients with distracting injury, or when it is particularly difficult to assess the history and physical examination, then high index of suspicion will grant a compartment pressure measure.

Severe and spontaneous pain is the earliest and most frequent sign of compartment syndrome among others (**Box 16**).[38] Serial examinations are necessary to prevent complications and manage in a timely manner.[38]

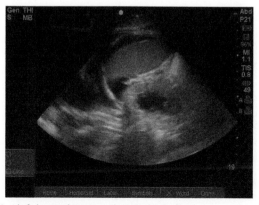

Fig. 20. FAST, positive left hemothorax and perisplenic fluid. (*Courtesy of* Robert Park, MD.)

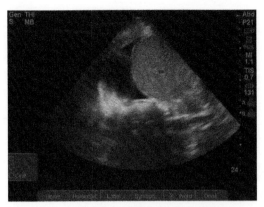

Fig. 21. FAST, right hemothorax. (*Courtesy of* Robert Park, MD).

There are not absolute contraindications for compartment pressure measure but if there is cellulitis or severe trauma to site of needle placement counts for contraindications.[37]

PREPARATION FOR THE TECHNIQUE

There are some ways for measure the compartment pressure depends on the devices available. Depends on the devices to be used the equipment will vary as technique needs. Therefore, the emergency physician should familiarize with the device that is available in the institution for which is work. For the purpose of this paper, three of the methods will be discussed: mercury manometer measure, Stryker and arterial line methods. Although, all of them are used there is agree that the mercury method is the less accurate in comparison with the other two.[37]

Obtain informed consent and explain procedure to patient. Local anesthesia as well as conscious sedation will be needed for most patients. The extremity being studied should be at the level of the heart and in a position that permits insertion of the needle perpendicular to the compartment being measured. This may require an assistant to hold an extremity above the stretcher. Any obstruction to needle entry and all structures that may put pressure on the compartment should be removed because them can raise falsely the compartment pressure. Use sterile technique at all times.[37]

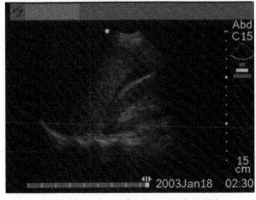

Fig. 22. FAST, hepatorenal fluid. (*Courtesy of* Robert Park, MD.)

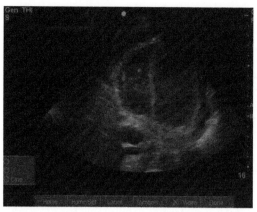

Fig. 23. Pericardial effusion: apical view. (*Courtesy of* Robert Park, MD.)

PRESSURE MEASUREMENT SYSTEMS

Box 17.

PROCEDURE TECHNIQUE

Anesthetize and sterilize the puncture site. Connect an 18-gauge needle to one end of the plastic IV tubing (as shown in **Fig. 26**) and connect the 3-way stopcock to the other end. Connect a 20-mL syringe to the 3-way stopcock. Turn the stopcock lever to close to the remaining IV tube, and open the stopcock port. Pierce the vial with a needle and, using an 18-gauge syringe, withdraw fluid until it reaches halfway along the IV tubing. Annotate, or mark with a marker, the position of the meniscus in the IV tubing (**Fig. 27**). Turn the stopcock lever to close the IV tubing proximal to the skin, pull back on the plunger to fill the syringe with air, and connect one end of the IV tubing to the stop-cock's remaining port and fit the other to the rubber tubing of the manometer (see **Fig. 26** B). If using a radial manometer with a connected balloon, turn the dial to close the balloon. Insert a needle at a 90° angle to the compartment and sufficiently deep to enter the selected compartment. Turn the stopcock lever to the bottom so that all ports are open. Slowly press the syringe plunger while observing the meniscus in the IV tube. When the meniscus in the IV tube begins to move toward the needle,

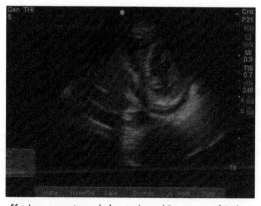

Fig. 24. Pericardial effusion parasternal short view. (*Courtesy of* Robert Park, MD.)

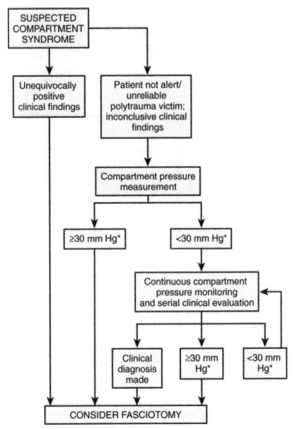

Fig. 25. Clinical decision-making algorithm when evaluating patients with suspected compartment syndrome. * pressure threshold.

stop depressing the plunger and turn the stopcock lever to close the IV tube port, which will lock in the measurement reading (the value on the manometer is equal to the intracompartmental pressure). In some instances, 3 readings are recommended to achieve an agreement. Remove the needle and dress the puncture site.[37]

STRYKER HANDHELD PRESSURE METHOD

Box 18

TECHNIQUE

Anesthetize and sterilize the puncture site and attach the needle to the end of the diaphragm chamber. Draw up a 3-mL sterile saline in the syringe and connect the syringe to the diaphragm chamber. Raise the device cover, place the diaphragm chamber into the device, and close the cover. Aim the device at a 45° upward angle and depress the syringe plunger to clear the air and prime the needle with fluid. Turn on the device, hold the device at 90° to the compartment, press the button to ZERO. When the monitor reads 00, puncture the needle into the intended compartment; the pressure reading will be shown on the device. Later, remove the needle and dress the site as shown in **Fig. 27**.

Box 15
Common causes of ALCS

Orthopedic (fracture related)

    Tibial fracture

    Distal radial and ulna fractures: supracondylar fracture; femoral and calcaneal fractures

Vascular

    Arterial and/or venous injuries

    Revascularization procedures

    Phlegmasia caerulea dolens

    Intra-aortic balloon pumping

    Isolated limb perfusion

Iatrogenic

    IV/intra-arterial drug injection

    Tourniquet

    Pneumatic anti-shock garment

    Patients with hemophilia

    Anticoagulation

    Extravasation of fluid after an arthroscopic procedure

    Prolonged surgery

Soft tissue

    Crush injury without fractures

    Burn

    Edema or intramuscular hematoma

    Drug or alcohol overuse induced stupor snakebite

Data from Gourgiotis S, Villias C, Germanos S, et al. Acute limb compartment syndrome: a review. J Surg Edu 2007;64(3):178–86; and Köstler W, Strohm PC, Südkamp NP. Acute compartment syndrome of the limb. Injury 2004;35(12):1221–7.

Box 16
Symptoms and signs of ALCS

Pain (spontaneous and disproportionate)

Pain on passive stretching of the involved muscles

Swollen and tense compartment

Rapid progression of signs over a short time

Paresthesia (initially affecting 2-point discrimination)

Pulselessness (usually in vascular injury)

Paralysis (latest symptom)

Box 17
Mercury manometer system

Equipment

Two 18-gauge simple or spinal needles

Two plastic extension tubes

One 20-mL syringe

One 3-way stopcock

One vial of sterile normal saline

One mercury manometer

ARTERIAL LINE SYSTEM

Box 19

TECHNIQUE

Anesthetize and sterilize the puncture site. Connect the transducer to the monitor and assemble the system as shown in **Fig. 28**. Fill the syringe with 15 mL of saline. Place one stopcock on the syringe. Open the stopcocks to allow filling of the transducer, high-pressure tubing, and needle. Once filled, close the stopcock to the high-pressure tubing. Open the top stopcock to air and place the transducer at the same level of the compartment being measured; calibrate the system to 0, and then close the top stopcock. Open the lower stopcock attached to the high-pressure tubing. Insert the needle into the compartment. Squeeze slightly the intended compartment or passive movement to the muscle in the compartment to provoke a spike on the monitoring. After a few seconds, measure the mean compartment pressure.

TECHNIQUE FOR NEEDLE PLACEMENT

The needle placement is an essential part of the compartment pressure measure technique. Accurate placement allows reliable measures. This section reviews the anatomy and placement of the needle.

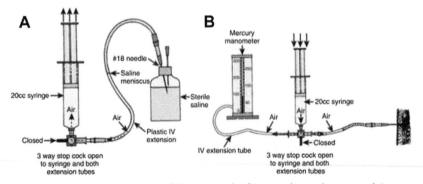

Fig. 26. Mercury monitor technique. (*A*) Connect the first IV tube to the stopcock in one end and 18-gauge needle to another, followed by connection of 20-mL syringe. (*B*) Connect the second IV tube to a manometer and open this remaining port to start with the measures.

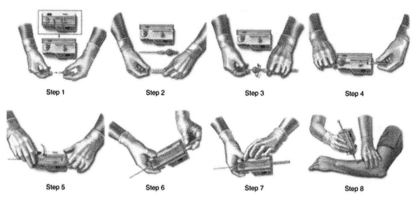

Step 1   Step 2   Step 3   Step 4

Step 5   Step 6   Step 7   Step 8

Fig. 27. Handheld compartment pressure monitor. Set up the Stryker 295 (Srtyker Instruments, Kalamazoo, MI, USA).

The lower leg is the most common place for compartment syndrome to occur; the anterior compartment is the most common involved.[37] The lower leg consists of 4 compartments: anterior tibial, deep posterior, posterior, and lateral. The anterior tibia compartment can reach 1 cm lateral to the anterior border of the tibia, and the needle should be placed 1 to 3 cm in depth (**Fig. 29**). The lateral compartment is in the lateral aspect of the fibula. Place the needle anterior to the posterior border of the fibula, about 1 cm in depth (**Fig. 30**B). The deep posterior compartment can be reached when the needle is placed posterior to the medial border of the tibia and directed to the posterior border of the fibula as shown in **Fig. 30**A. Then the posterior compartment is reached in the posterior aspect of the leg at the level of the calf. Insert the needle 2 to 4 cm in depth as shown in **Fig. 30**C.

Gluteal compartment syndrome is very uncommon. But in some instances, compartment syndrome may occur: prolonged immobilization and significant contusions to this area. Since the body habitus may vary, the compartment sites vary from patient to patient, then, insert 18-gauge spinal needle about 4 to 8 cm in depth, where the maximal point tenderness exists,[37] as shown in the **Fig. 31**.

The foot compartment syndrome results from crush injuries. The number of compartments in the foot is still controversial, but for the purpose of the measure 3 different sites are identified as shown in the **Fig. 32**.

| **Box 18** |
| **Stryker method equipment** |
| Sterile skin prep (povidone-iodine solution or chlorhexidine) |
| Local anesthetic with syringe and small-gauge needle for superficial infiltration |
| Stryker (Stryker Instruments, Kalamazoo, MI, USA) handheld intracompartmental pressure monitor |
| (1) 3-mL syringe |
| Sterile saline |
| (1) Device side-port needle |
| (1) Device diaphragm chamber |

> **Box 19**
> **Equipment for arterial line system**
>
> Sterile skin prep (povidone-iodine solution or chlorhexidine)
>
> Local anesthetic with syringe and small-gauge needle
>
> (1) 18-gauge needle
>
> High-pressure tubing
>
> Pressure transducer with cable
>
> Pressure monitor
>
> Sterile saline
>
> Transducer stand
>
> (2) 3-way stopcocks
>
> (1) 20-mL syringe

COMPLICATIONS

The late diagnosis of compartment syndrome results in muscle ischemia and loss of function and ultimate contractures (Volkmann contracture). Then the emergency physician should be able to perform the compartment pressure measure with proficiency and accuracy. Even though the procedure will be performed with proficiency, some complications may occur. Local and systemic infection is considered one of the complications of the measures methods.[39,40] Using aseptic conditions and universal precautions should diminish this possibility. Pain associated with needle insertion and patient movement during measurement (proper analgesia should be given) can also complicate the procedure.[39,40]

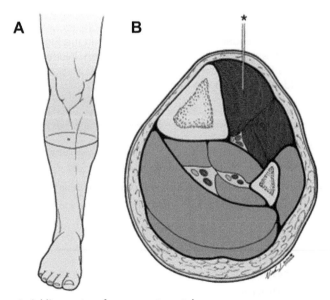

Fig. 28. The arterial line system for compartmental pressure measure.

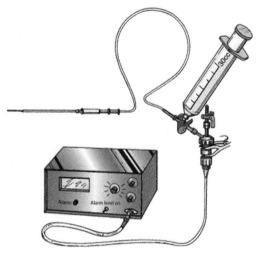

Fig. 29. Anterior compartment of the lower leg.

TREATMENT OF ALCS

Patients should be immediately referred to a surgeon for urgent consideration of fasciotomy in the presence of ALCS (**Box 20**). A fasciotomy should be performed as soon as possible, preferably within 6 hours and definitely within 12 hours (if at all possible),

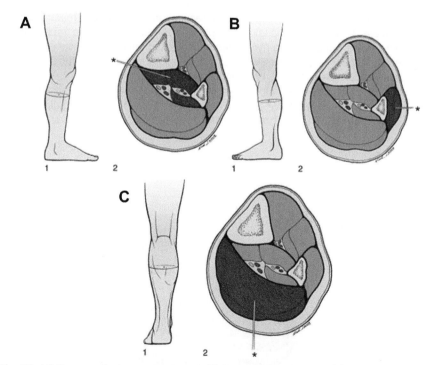

Fig. 30. (*A*) Deep posterior compartment. (*B*) Lateral compartment. (*C*) Posterior compartment. Note the asterisk suggest the needle entrance place.

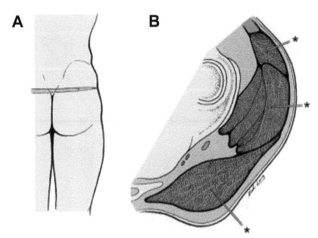

Fig. 31. Gluteal compartment. Note the asterisk suggests the needle entrance place. (*A*) A, transverse cut of gluteal compartments. (*B*) Gluteal compartments.

once the diagnosis of ALCS has been done.[41] There are specific techniques depending on the compartment that is involved. **Table 2** describes the different compartments and the proper approach to achieve successful decompression.[39]

VENOUS CUTDOWN

One of the first steps during a trauma patient resuscitation is circulation achieved by vascular access. Vascular access takes first place in seriously ill patients, moderate to severe dehydrated patients, and hypovolemic shock patients. The challenge begins when vascular access is not achieved by conventional peripheral modality; then alternatives route should be explored, like venous cutdown.

Although venous cutdown is no longer taught in the ATLS course as mandatory skill, still as an alternative for vascular access when other less invasive modalities have failed.[42] The venous cutdown modality have been displaced for the over-the-wire

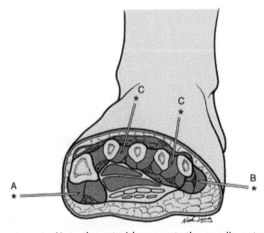

Fig. 32. Foot compartments. Note the asterisk suggests the needle entrance place.

> **Box 20**
> **Indications for fasciotomy**
>
> Absolute pressure greater than 30 mm Hg
>
> Perfusion pressure (diastolic blood pressure compartment pressure) less than 30 mm Hg
>
> *Data from* Mubarak SJ, Owen CA, Hargens AR, et al. Acute compartment syndromes: diagnosis and treatment with the aid of the wick catheter. J Bone Joint Surg Am 1978;60(8):1091–5; and Hargens AR, Schmidt DA, Evans KL, et al. Quantitation of skeletal-muscle necrosis in a model compartment syndrome. J Bone Joint Surg Am 1981;63(4):631–6.

percutaneous catheters (known commonly as central lines), however, for infants and children, among others, still as an alternative vascular access route as shown in **Box 21**.[43] In hypovolemic shock, the venous cutdown has advantages because of the rapid flow rate. When the large-bore catheter is inserted directly into the vein, the blood flow increases 15% to 30%.[44] Thus, one blood unit can be transfused in 3 minutes; therefore, large-bore lines placed by venous cutdown are excellent mechanism to treat severe hypovolemia.[44]

The saphenous vein is the most common vein used for venous cutdown. Its superficial location and usually predictable anatomy permit more rapid dissection. In addition, it is preferable in the setting of cardiac arrest because it is distant from chest compressions and resuscitative efforts.[45] Other veins that are chosen for venous cutdown are the basilic and cephalic veins. Even though these sites are not commonly used, it is useful to know their anatomy in such cases as bilateral leg amputation or burned legs.[43]

Venous cutdown is contraindicated when less invasive vascular access has been achieved. In addition, if the technique execution is prolonged, it is also contraindicated.[1,5–23,46,24–45,47–50] Detailed knowledge of anatomy and the equipment to be used can reduce the time to perform the procedure as discussed in **Table 3** and **Box 22**, respectively (**Fig. 33**).

TECHNIQUE
Isolation of the Veins

The venous cutdown technique is quite the same no matter what vein is to be cannulated. However, as expected, the isolation depends on the location and the vein to be catheterized. For the purpose of this section, the isolation is discussed as a different section but the technique per se is discussed as a whole.

The saphenous vein is the longest vein of the body and begins on the ankle and ends at level of the thigh when it joins the femoral vein. At ankle level, it is named the

Table 2
Fasciotomy procedures and extremities involved

Extremity	Fasciotomy Procedures
Forearm	Volar/dorsal fasciotomy: requires decompression of nerve and muscle.
Hand	Volar fasciotomy should be extended to the palm and carpal tunnel released
Thigh	All 3 compartments can be decompressed with lateral incision
Lower leg	Single lateral incision with or without fibulectomy or double incision with medial and lateral incisions Skin incision long to ensure decompression of all muscles

---

Box 21
Clinical examples for venous cutdown

Venous cutdown indications

Infants and children

Shock

IV drug abusers

Severely burned or scarred patients

Skin or anatomy distorted

Cardiac arrest without palpable femoral pulse

---

saphenous vein. It arises from the dorsal venous arch of the foot and then ascends cephalad 2 cm anterior to the malleolus.[51] The leg should be extended and externally rotated to expose the medial malleolus. Then, apply counter-traction on the skin, and the 3-cm incision will be performed across the anterior tibial surface (not too deep). Separate the overlying tissue with a hemostat or mosquito. At the knee, the incision for isolation should be performed 1 to 4 cm below the knee and posterior to the tibia; beware of the proximity to saphenous branch of the genicular artery and the saphenous vein.[43,51] This approach could fail when the knee is bent or flexed because the line could kink. The greater saphenous vein at the level of proximal thigh is another portion of the vein that can be used for cannulation. Actually, this site is the most recommended when treating hypovolemia because of the large caliber and easy access. This portion raises anteromedial in the proximal thigh. It could be found 4 cm inferior

---

Table 3
Anatomy of great saphenous and saphenous, basilica, and cephalic veins

Vein	Anatomy	Incision Site
Saphenous	Begins at the ankle, crosses 1 cm anterior to medial malleolus and then up to the anteromedial aspect of the leg (preferable site for venous cutdown); in the knee, lies superficial on the medial aspect (less used because of the risk of injury of saphenous nerve and genicular artery)	Ankle: 1 cm anterior to medial malleolus (preferable site for children) Knee: 1–4 cm below the knee and immediately posterior to the tibia
Great saphenous	Begins on medial aspect of the knee, then crosses anterolaterally, ascends until it joins the femoral vein	Anterior thigh: 3–4 cm below inguinal ligament and 3 cm lateral to pubic tubercle (preferable site for hypovolemia because of the large caliber)
Basilic	At level of midforearm, crosses anterolaterally; it is found at 1–2 cm lateral to the medial epincondyle	Antecubital fossa 2 cm above and 2–3 cm lateral to the medial epicondyle
Cephalic	Begins on radial aspect of the wrist and crosses anteromedially toward antecubital fossa	Most common site: antecubital fossa at the distal flexor crease

> **Box 22**
> **Equipment for venous cutdown**
>
> *Equipment*
>
> Plastic dilator-lifter
>
> Scalpel
>
> Blade No. 10 or No. 11
>
> Curved hemostat
>
> 0–0 silk sutures
>
> Iris scissors
>
> Plastic venous dilator
>
> Large-bore IV catheter
>
> IV tubing
>
> Tape

and 3 cm lateral to the pubic tubercle or approximately 2 cm inferior to the site of percutaneous femoral line placement. Another cited landmark is 4 cm below the inguinal ligament.[51] A transverse 5- to 6-cm incision should be done distal to where labial/scrotal fold meets the thigh. With a hemostat blunt dissection should be done but if muscle or investing fascia is found the dissection is too deep. Then reassessment of the landmarks should be done.

The basilic vein can be cannulated, as an alternative, in the setting of leg amputation, leg trauma, or deformity. To find the basilic vein, the arm should be abducted 90°, flexed at 90°, and externally rotated. The incision should be done on the medial aspect of the arm 2 cm proximal and 2 to 3 cm lateral to the medial epicondyle. Superficial incision may be done until subcutaneous tissue is revealed.[43,51] Blunt dissection is recommended to avoid injury to the brachial artery and median nerve.

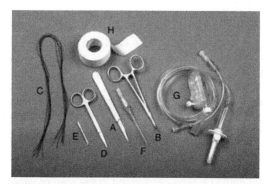

Fig. 33. Equipment for venous cutdown. Venous cutdown tray. Note the small plastic vein dilator-lifter (E), which is especially useful in children. Equipment: (*A*) scalpel No. 11 blade, (*B*) curved hemostat, (*C*) No. 0–0 silk suture, (*D*) iris scissors, (*E*) plastic venous dilator, (*F*) large-bore IV catheter, (*G*) IV tubing, and (*H*) tape for securing catheter. (*From* Custalow CB. Color atlas of emergency department procedures. Philadelphia: Elsevier Saunders; 2005. p. 163.)

The cephalic vein is subcutaneous in the antecubital fossa, overlying the lateral aspect of the biceps muscle. Careful incision should be done in the antecubital fossa in the lateral aspect.[51] Although the cephalic vein ascends until deltoid muscle area, this site is very difficult to access and interferes with the resuscitative efforts.[51]

TECHNIQUE

Once the vein is selected for the procedure, prepare and clean the chosen area with povidone-iodine or other antiseptic solution. Place a tourniquet proximal to the chosen site for venous cutdown.[43] Anesthetize the place of venous cutdown if the patient is awake. With a No. 10 or No. 11 scalpel, incision in the site should be done perpendicular following the landmarks for vein isolation as described in the previous section ("Isolation of the Veins") (see **Fig. 33**). Use the hemostat for blunt dissection of the vein, spreading the subcutaneous tissue until the vein is exposed. Use the hemostat to place distal and proximal silk ties. Then, tie the distal silk, but the proximal one should remain untied (the proximal tie will be used for maneuvering the vein, bleeding control, and/or tubing placing). Nick the vein with a No. 10 or 11 scalpel blade in 45° to transect one-third to one-half the diameter of the vein, not too large because the vein will be transected completely and not too small because false lumen may occur.[43,51] To avoid false lumen insertion, a vein dilator can be used, especially in children. If a vein dilator is not available, a 20-gauge needle is bent at a 90° angle (to use it as a vein dilator or elevator).[43]

In case the catheter does not have a tapered tip, make a bevel in the catheter at a 45° angle before introducing it. Introduce the catheter, but do not force it. If the catheter is large, grasp the proximal edge of the vessel with small forceps or a mosquito hemostat. After introducing the catheter, flush air from the cannula and then connect it to the IV tubing. The proximal ligature should be tied around the vein and the cannula. Then remove the tourniquet; once the catheter is tied, the IV infusion can begin. Fix the catheter to the skin and proceed to repair the incision wound. Topical antibiotic may be beneficial at the wound site. Do not delay the fluid infusion despite wound closure.[43]

Mini-venous cutdown is an alternative modality of venous cutdown. With this method, the time-consuming part of the venous cutdown of placing the catheter is avoided.[1–26,28,29,46,27,30–45,47–52] Identify the vein and isolate it as described previously. Instead of placing the tourniquet and tying the vein, the vein will be canalized under direct vision but with a percutaneous infusions catheter (**Fig. 34** and **35**). After identifying the vein, make an incision over it and with blunt dissection expose it. Then stab the skin with the percutaneous catheter below the incision for visualization.[1–23,46,24–43,47–49] Remove the needle and a cannula will stay inside the vein. Then close the wound and fix it to the skin. This method is designed for chronically ill patients, obese patients, and children. Flow rates and infusions are the same as classic venous cutdown, as discussed previously.

COMPLICATIONS

The venous cutdown could be time-consuming in the step of venous catheterization that may result in patient deterioration. This complication can be overcome with a vein dilator or elevator. Detailed knowledge of anatomy is required to avoid secondary damage to surrounding structures, such as arteries or nerves. Other complications are local hematoma, infection, sepsis, phlebitis, embolization, and wound dehiscence. Using topical antibiotics can diminish the incidence of infection.

Step 1

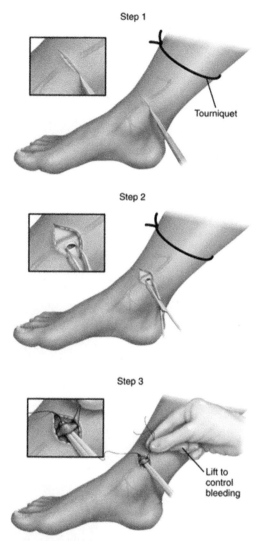

Tourniquet

Step 2

Step 3

Lift to
control
bleeding

Fig. 34. Venous cutdown technique: procedural steps for venous cutdown. Step 1: Saphenous vein approach. The saphenous vein at the ankle can be found approximately 1 cm anterior to the medial malleolus. Place a tourniquet and use a topical antiseptic. Make a skin incision perpendicular to the course of the vein. Step 2: Bluntly dissect, isolate, and mobilize the vein. Step 3: Use a hemostat to isolate the vein and to pass the silk ties under the vein proximal and distal to the proposed cannulation site. Step 4: Tie the distal suture only. Step 5: Incise the vein while retracting the proximal ligature. Lift the proximal untied suture to control back bleeding. Step 6: Using the plastic venous dilator to lift the flap, advance the catheter into the vein. Attach IV tubing to the catheter. Step 7: Tie the proximal silk suture around the vein and catheter. Remove proximal suture and suture skin. (*From* Custalow CB. Color atlas of emergency department procedures. Philadelphia: Elsevier Saunders; 2005. p. 164.)

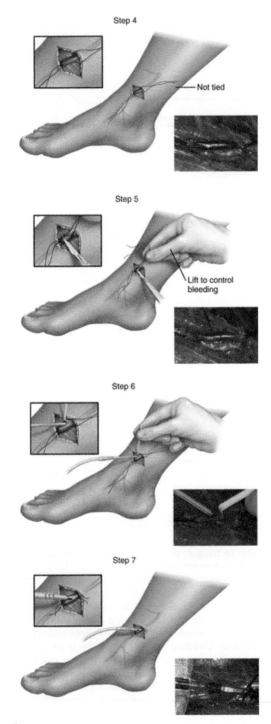

Fig. 34. (continued)

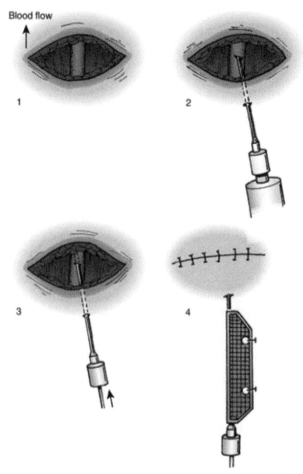

Fig. 35. Mini-venous cutdown technique. Mini-cutdown technique is an alternative to the venous cutdown method. The vein is cannulated under direct vision using standard percutaneous catheters. A separate entry site (shown) may be used or the vein can be cannulated through the skin incision. Note that the vein is not tied off with this technique. A standard Angiocath IV (BD Angiocath™ Franklin Lakes, NJ USA) set may also be used instead of the through-the-needle catheter shown here.

This procedure is not permanent and should be removed as soon as possible to avoid complications.

SUMMARY

Emergency physicians must be proficient in the acute management of trauma patients. Most injuries related to trauma are initially evaluated in the ED; this evaluation may be complex depending on the age of the patient, associated mechanism of injury, and comorbidities at the moment of trauma. Conditions, such as hemopneumothorax, hemorrhages, and surgical airway, require prompt intervention and proficiency in the execution of procedures to avoid complications and functional impairment while improving outcomes. It is of paramount importance for the practitioner to be dexterous while performing these procedural skills.

REFERENCES

1. Advanced Trauma Life Support, 8th edition, The evidence for change. J Trauma 2008;64:1638–50.
2. Tintinalli J. Tintinalli's emergency medicine: a comprehensive study guide. New York: McGraw Hill Companies Inc.; 2011. p. 1671–76E.
3. Trauma L. A comprehensive emergency medicine approach. New York: Cambridge University Press; 2011. p. 11–23.
4. Bruner D. Rapid sequence intubation in trauma. Trauma Rep 2011;12(1):1–11.
5. Lee B. The utility of sonography for the triage of blunt abdominal trauma patients to exploratory laparotomy. Am J Roentgenol 2007;188(2):415–21.
6. Chang RS, Hamilton RJ, Carter WA. Declining rate of cricothyrotomy in trauma patients with an emergency medicine residency: implications for skills training. Acad Emerg Med 1998;5:247.
7. Bair AE, Panacek EA, Wisner DH, et al. Cricothyrotomy: a 5-year experience at one institution. J Emerg Med 2003;24(2):151–6.
8. Holmes JF, Panacek EA, Sakles JC, et al. Comparison of 2 cricothyrotomy techniques: standard method versus rapid 4-step technique. Ann Emerg Med 1998; 32:442–7.
9. Vissers RJ, Bair AE. Surgical airway techniques. In: Walls RM, Murphy MF, Luten RC, et al, editors. Manual of emergency airway management. 2nd edition. Philadelphia: Lippincott Williams & Wilkins; 2004. p. 1–6,15.
10. Laws D. BTS guidelines for the insertion of a chest tube. Thorax 2003;58:53–9.
11. Mowery N. Practice management guidelines for management of hemothorax and occult pneumothorax. J Trauma 2011;70(2):510–8.
12. Sharma A. Principles of diagnosis and management of traumatic pneumothorax. J Emerg Trauma Shock 2008;1(1):34–41.
13. Gareeboo S. Tube thoracostomy: how to insert a chest drain. Br J Hosp Med 2006;67(1):16–8.
14. Legome E. Trauma: a comprehensive emergency medicine approach. New York: Cambridge University Press; 2011. p. 601–3.
15. Maritz D. Complications of tube thoracostomy for chest trauma. S Afr Med J 2009; 99:114–7.
16. Funk G. Clamping thoracostomy tubes: a heretical notion? Proc (Bayl Univ Med Cent) 2009;22(3):215–7.
17. E Kesieme. Tube thoracostomy: complications and its management. Vol. 2012, article ID 256878 (2011), doi:10.1155/2012256878.
18. Olgac G. Antibiotics are not needed during tube thoracostomy for spontaneous pneumothorax: an observational case study. J Cardiothorac Surg 2006. http://dx.doi.org/10.1186/1749-8090-1-43.
19. Rehn L. Ueber penetrirende herzwunden und herznaht. Archiv für Klinische Chirurgie 1897;55:315–29.
20. Seamon MJ, Chovanes J, Fox N, et al. The use of emergency department thoracotomy for traumatic cardiopulmonary arrest. Injury 2012;43(9):1355–61.
21. Siram S, Oyetunji T, Johnson SM, et al. Predictors for survival of penetrating trauma using emergency department thoracotomy in an urban trauma center: the Cardiac Instability Score. J Natl Med Assoc 2010;102(2):126–30.
22. Rosen P, Chan TC, editors. Atlas of emergency procedures. St. Louis (MS): Mosby; 2001. p. 46–55.
23. Tintinalli J, editor. Tintinalli's emergency medicine: a comprehensive study guide. 7th edition. New York: McGraw Hill; 2011. p. 1761.

24. Passos EM, Engels PT, Doyle JD, et al. Societal costs of inappropriate emergency department thoracotomy. J Am Coll Surg 2012;214:18–25.
25. Root HD, Hauser CW, McKinley CR. Diagnostic peritoneal lavage. Surgery 1965; 57:633.
26. Rhodes CM, Hayden LS, Sidwell RA. Utility and relevance of diagnostic peritoneal lavage in trauma education. J Surg Educ 2011;68(4):313–7.
27. Whitehouse JS, Weigelt JA. Diagnostic peritoneal lavage: a review of indications, technique, and interpretation. Scand J Trauma Resusc Emerg Med 2009;17:13.
28. Udobi KF, Rodriguez A, Chiu WC, et al. Role of ultrasonography in penetrating abdominal trauma: a prospective clinical study. J Trauma 2001;50:475–9.
29. Isenhour J, JA Marx. General approach to blunt abdominal trauma in adults. UpToDate; 19.2: 2011.
30. Nagy K. Chapter 55. Diagnostic peritoneal lavage. In: Reichman EF, Simon RR, editors. Emergency medicine procedures. New York: McGraw-Hill; 2004. Available at: http://www.accessemergencymedicine.com/content.aspx?aID=51517. Accessed December 15, 2011.
31. Holmes JF, Harris D, Battistella FD. Performance of abdominal ultrasonography in blunt trauma patients with out-of-hospital or emergency department hypotension. Ann Emerg Med 2004;43:354.
32. Dolich MO, McKenney MG, Varela JE, et al. 2,576 ultrasounds for blunt abdominal trauma. J Trauma 2001;50:108.
33. Griffin XL, Pullinger R. Are diagnostic peritoneal lavages or focused abdominal sonography for trauma safe screening investigations for hemodynamically stable patients after blunt abdominal trauma? A review of the literature. J Trauma 2007; 62:779–84.
34. American College of Emergency Physicians. Use of ultrasound imaging by emergency physicians. Ann Emerg Med 2001;38:469–70.
35. Gourgiotis S, Villias C, Germanos S, et al. Acute limb compartment syndrome: a review. J Surg Educ 2007;64(3):178–86.
36. Köstler W, Strohm PC, Südkamp NP. Acute compartment syndrome of the limb. Injury 2004;35(12):1221–7.
37. Roberts J, Hedges JR, editors. Clinical procedures n emergency medicine. 5th edition. Philadelphia: WB Saunders; 2010. p. 986–99.
38. Frink M, Hildebrand F, Krettek C. Compartment syndrome of the lower leg and foot. Clin Orthop Relat Res 2010;468(4):940–50.
39. Wall CJ, Lynch J, Harris IA, et al. Clinical practice guidelines for the management of acute limb compartment syndrome following trauma. ANZ J Surg 2010;80(3): 151–6.
40. Shadgan B, Menon M, O'Brien PJ, et al. Diagnostic techniques in acute compartment syndrome of the leg. J Orthop Trauma 2008;22(8):581–7.
41. Finkelstein JA, Hunter GA, Hu RW. Lower limb compartment syndrome: course after delayed fasciotomy. J Trauma 1996;40(3):342–4.
42. Committee on Trauma. American College of Surgeons: advanced trauma life support instructor manual. Chicago: American College of Surgeons; 2008.
43. Roberts J, Hedges, editors. Clinical procedures n emergency medicine. 5th edition. Philadelphia: WB Saunders; 2010. p. 411–7.
44. Dronen SC, Yee AS, Tomlanovich MC. Proximal saphenous cutdown. Ann Emerg Med 1981;10:328.
45. Taghizadeh R, Gilbert PM. Long saphenous venous cutdown revisited. Burns 2006;32(2):267–8.

46. Bair AE, Wolfson AB. Emergent surgical cricothyrotomy (cricothyroidotomy). UpToDate 19.2: 2011.

47. Soderstrom CA, DuPriest RW, Cowley RA. Pitfalls of peritoneal lavage in blunt abdominal trauma. Surg Gynecol Obstet 1980;151:513–8.

48. Mubarak SJ, Owen CA, Hargens AR, et al. Acute compartment syndromes: diagnosis and treatment with the aid of the wick catheter. J Bone Joint Surg Am 1978; 60(8):1091–5.

49. Hargens AR, Schmidt DA, Evans KL, et al. Quantitation of skeletal-muscle necrosis in a model compartment syndrome. J Bone Joint Surg Am 1981;63(4): 631–6.

50. Knopp R. Venous cutdowns in the emergency department. JACEP 1978;7:429.

51. Chappell S, Vilke GM, Chan TC, et al. Peripheral venous cutdown. J Emerg Med 2006;31(4):411–6.

52. Shiu MH. A method for conservation of veins in the surgical cutdown. Surg Gynecol Obstet 1972;134:315.

Critical Procedures in Pediatric Emergency Medicine

Fernando Soto, MD[a],*, Alison Murphy, MD[b], Heather Heaton, MD[c]

KEYWORDS

- Pediatric emergency medicine • Pediatric respiratory arrest
- Pediatric oral lacerations • Pediatric thoracostomy • ENT foreign bodies

KEY POINTS

- Pediatric respiratory arrest offers different challenges than in the adult population: limited ventilatory reserve, the trachea is more anterior and superior, intraoral and supraglottic structures are relatively large and floppy, and neck extension might decrease airway size considerably.
- Bag-valve mask ventilation is an invaluable skill when dealing with pediatric respiratory arrests. It may be performed for a prolonged period in difficult airway situations. Consider inserting a nasogastric tube.
- Intraosseous vascular access can be used in all ages. When peripheral access cannot easily be obtained, the other preferred vascular approaches in the pediatric population include the external jugular, scalp veins, or femoral veins.
- When dealing with ear and nose foreign bodies, the size, shape, consistency, and depth of the object will determine the ideal extraction equipment. Avoid repeated attempts. Order radiographs when looking for button batteries and magnets.
- Small spontaneous pneumothoraces could be observed or aspirated through a needle; consider inserting a pigtail catheter in selected patients.
- Oral lacerations are seldom sutured. Antibiotic coverage remains controversial.
- When considering an infected ventricular shunt, consider performing a lumbar puncture in selected patients instead of directly tapping the shunt.
- To improve success rates in performing lumbar punctures, increase hip flexion; neck flexion rarely helps and may increase the risk of apnea in infants.
- An equally sized Foley catheter may be used to replace gastrostomy tubes.

[a] Pediatric Emergency Medicine Section, University of Puerto Rico School of Medicine, PO Box 29207, San Juan, PR 00929, USA; [b] Department of Pediatric Emergency Medicine, Wolfson Children's Hospital, 820 Prudential Drive, Suite 713, Jacksonville, FL 32207, USA; [c] Department of Emergency Medicine, University of North Carolina Hospitals, 1st Floor Physicians Office Building, 170 Manning Dr, CB#7594, Chapel Hill, NC 27599-7594, USA
* Corresponding author.
E-mail address: sotomd13@yahoo.com

Emerg Med Clin N Am 31 (2013) 335–376
http://dx.doi.org/10.1016/j.emc.2012.09.003
0733-8627/13/$ – see front matter © 2013 Elsevier Inc. All rights reserved.

AIRWAY

Effective management of the pediatric airway is an essential skill for emergency medicine physicians. Pediatric airways provide unique challenges given the differences in anatomy between pediatric and adult populations, and the airways of infants and children are more susceptible to obstruction. **Box 1** details key principles that must be remembered when dealing with pediatric airways.

Noninvasive Airway Management

Noninvasive management of the airway in pediatrics is similar to adults, with 2 main maneuvers available for health care providers: chin-lift and jaw-thrust. Both allow the airway to remain in a neutral position, and therefore allow for better oxygenation and ventilation. In the chin lift, one hand is placed under the mandible, which gently lifts the chin anteriorly, while the other hand is placed on the forehead to tilt the head into a neutral position. The jaw thrust should be used when trauma is suspected given the ability to maintain cervical spine immobilization. To perform, a hand should be placed at the angle of the lower jaw on each side and the mandible should be moved forward.

Airway adjuncts, like oral and nasopharyngeal airways, are also useful in pediatric airway management. Oral airways lift the tongue and soft tissues off the posterior pharynx and should be used only in unconscious children. To choose an appropriate-sized oral airway, measure along the side of the child's face (the tip of the airway should reach the angle of the mandible). They are easily placed with the assistance of a tongue depressor. Nasopharyngeal airways are useful in conscious patients with obstructions caused by tongue and pharyngeal airway obstructions. The correctly sized nasopharyngeal airway should extend from the nostril to the tragus of the patient's ear. After lubricating the airway, it should easily slide into the nostril.

Rapid Sequence Intubation

When the emergency medicine physician is unable to maintain an adequate airway with noninvasive measures, rapid sequence intubation can be safely performed in children.[1,2] Although there is often little time to obtain consent before the intubation, if possible, parents should be counseled on the medications, procedure, and alternatives if intubation is unsuccessful (**Table 1**).

Indications/contraindications

There are no contraindications to performing an endotracheal intubation in patients unable to ventilate or oxygenate, or are presenting with altered mental status with unsecured airway; however, lack of equipment or expertise should be considered when encountered with this situation. Studies have shown that bag-valve mask ventilation can prove just as efficient in providing oxygenation and ventilation as

---

Box 1
Anatomic principles of pediatric airways

The airway is more anterior; hyperextension of the neck can obstruct the airway.

Airways are smaller and more susceptible to obstruction and edema.

Neonates and infants have large occiputs causing neck flexion.

Children have larger tongues that fall into the hypopharynx and cause obstruction.

The narrowest portion of the pediatric airway is the subglottic space.

Table 1
Medications used in pediatric airway management

	Dose	Indications	Contraindications
Atropine	0.02 mg/kg IV, minimum single dose 0.1 mg, maximum single dose 0.5 mg	Can be considered in pretreatment approximately 2 min before intubation in all children less than 5 y old to help prevent bradycardia.[9]	
Lidocaine	1.5 mg/kg IV	Pretreatment in patients with suspected increased intracranial pressure and asthma.[9]	
Etomidate	0.3 mg/kg IV	Sedation in patients with hemodynamic instability	Transient adrenal corticosuppression is a potential complication.[10]
Ketamine	1–2 mg IV	Safe for use in patients with hemodynamic instability as well as bronchospams	Avoid in patients with increased intracranial pressure.[11]
Succinylcholine	Infants and young children: 2 mg/kg IV, older children: 1–1.5 mg/kg IV	Depolarizing agent with rapid onset (45–60 seconds) and short duration (6–10 minutes)	Avoid in patients with chronic myopathies, denervating neuromuscular disease, within 48–72 hours after burn, crush or denervating injury, malignant hyperthermia or in patients with pre-existing hyperkalemia.[12,13]
Rocuronium	0.6–1.2 mg/kg IV	Nondepolarizing neuromuscular blocking agent; rapid onset and short duration	

endotracheal intubations, especially in the prehospital field.[3,4] There are alternatives to orotracheal intubation such as supraglottic airway devices (i.e. LMA's, King LT's, Combitubes, etc), among other supraglottic airway rescue devices that may aid in intubation before securing an airway through endotracheal intubation (see the following).

Procedure

Before intubation, the patient should be placed on a continuous cardiac monitor that follows the heart rhythm, respiratory rate, and oxygen saturation along with a noninvasive blood pressure monitor. Supplemental oxygen must be available as well. In preparation for the procedure, the patient should be preoxygenated with 100% inspired oxygen. Place the patient in the "sniffing position" to align the pharyngeal, tracheal, and oral axes and maintain airway patency. Further equipment required includes suction, bag valve mask (BVM), airway adjuncts (oropharyngeal airways, nasopharyngeal airways), rescue devices, such as laryngeal mask airways, Combitube, King airway, or a gum elastic bougie in case the endotracheal tube cannot be placed. An end-tidal CO_2 detector is also required at the bedside to confirm successful placement.

When choosing the appropriate endotracheal tube, the literature supports the use of cuffed tubes in all pediatric patients outside of the newborn age as long as cuff pressures remain less than 20 cm H_2O.[5,6] For uncuffed endotracheal tube sizing, the age-based formula 4+ (age in years/4) can be used, whereas cuffed tubes should be one-half size smaller than the age-based calculation recommendation.[7,8] Additionally, the clinician should have a tube one size smaller and one size larger easily accessible during the procedure. Place a stylet in the endotracheal tube to improve the firmness of the tube, but the tip of the stylet should not extend farther than the tip of the endotracheal tube.

Laryngoscope blades can be either curved or straight. The curved blade tip is placed in the vallecula, whereas the straight blade tip extends into the glottic opening for lifting of the epiglottis. Frequently, straight blades are preferred in infants and young children because they have a large floppy epiglottis. Blade sizes range from 00 for premature infants to 4 for large adults. Generally, size 0 to 1 can be used in most infants and size 2 can be used for most 2-year-olds. The blade should adequately move the tongue and soft tissues to allow for direct visualization of the vocal cords.

Rapid sequence intubation consists in applying interventions and medications in a continuous fashion in order to decrease the risk for aspiration. **Table 1** includes the indications and dosing of the most common medications. Once the medications are administered, apply cricoid pressure to help prevent gastric insufflation and regurgitation. Open the mouth using the scissor technique or with extension of the head. The provider should insert the laryngoscope into the patient's mouth to the appropriate position based on the blade type and sweep the tongue to the left. Lift the handle up to move the soft tissue structures out of the way and to improve visualization. Avoid "rocking" the blade backward onto teeth. Once the epiglottis is visualized, continue lifting up to expose the vocal cords. With the endotracheal tube in the right hand, slide the tube through the vocal cords and pull the stylet out. The endotracheal tube tip should be midpoint between the thoracic inlet and the carina. Intubation should be confirmed immediately. After visualizing the tube pass through the cords, watch for visible chest rise and mist in the endotracheal tube. Further, breath sounds should be audible in both axillae, but not over the stomach. Continuous pulse oximetry and end-tidal CO_2 should also confirm placement. Secure the tube and minimize head movement to decrease the chances of tube dislodgement.

Approach to the Difficult Airway

When definite airway management is necessary and intubation is either not possible or has failed, different methods of emergency airway access must be considered. Needle cricothyroidotomy can be performed in patients of any age, but is considered preferable to a surgical cricothyroidotomy in infants and children up to age 10 to 12 years because it is easier to perform and less likely to cause permanent damage.[14–17] The main indication to undergo this procedure is inability to maintain an airway with standard airway procedures. Contraindications include any injury to the larynx, cricoid cartilage, or trachea (ie, laryngeal fracture or tracheal rupture). Relative contraindications include situations in which a potential anatomic distortion is present.

Setup for a needle cricothyroidotomy includes universal precautions (gown, cap, mask, eye protection, sterile gloves), iodine for site cleansing, sterile drapes, 1%

lidocaine without epinephrine for local anesthesia, 10 mL syringe filled with sterile saline, and a large-bore catheter (infants and young children: 16 to 18 gauge; adolescents and adults: 12 to 18 gauge). Connectors should also be available to connect to a BVM or oxygen tubing. The patient is placed on a continuous cardiac monitor. The insertion site is identified by localizing the cricothyroid membrane region and is prepared with basic sterile technique procedures. The site is cleansed with iodine and local anesthestic should be injected if needed. The trachea is held in place with skin tension using the provider's nondominant hand. The needle is attached to the half-filled saline syringe and inserted at the inferior margin of the cricothyroid membrane, directed toward the patient's feet. Advance the needle while applying continuous negative pressure on the syringe until air bubbles are seen, then slide the catheter off the needle into the trachea and remove the syringe and needle. Hold the catheter in place at all times, even after it has been secured.

Special Considerations: Permanent Tracheotomies

Pediatric patients with permanent tracheotomies present a unique set of challenges for emergency medicine providers. On presentation, these patients should be placed in a room with advanced airway equipment, including multiple endotracheal tubes and tracheostomy tubes.

If a patient with a tracheostomy presents with respiratory distress, check for obstruction with a foreign body, blood, or mucus. If an obstruction is not obvious during examination, suction through the cannula. If the patient continues to have distress, the tracheostomy should be removed, inspected, and cleaned. Insert a catheter through the tracheostomy tube before removing the tube to ensure proper replacement, especially if the tracheostomy site is less than 4 weeks old. When replacing the tracheostomy, lubricate the cannula and advance with a semicircular motion as it curves into the trachea. If tracheostomy tubes are not immediately available, one can also place an endotracheal tube through a tracheostomy opening. Do not force the tube, as this may create false passages within the soft tissue of the neck.

VASCULAR ACCESS

Obtaining vascular access is of vital importance in providing care for children. Intravenous fluid administration, antibiotics, and other therapies are commonly provided parenterally. Although commonly needed, venous access can still prove to be a challenge for even experienced health care providers. Access is usually obtained in the dorsum of the hand or foot, or in the antecubital fossa; however, these can be difficult in well-nourished or chronically ill patients, or in certain critical situations. Approaches are different in the pediatric population, including a predilection for the femoral vein if central access is to be considered, the potential for cannulation of scalp veins, and the widespread use of intraosseous access. For all of these procedures, it is important to address parental issues and discuss options.

To perform the procedure, the child should be kept in a stable and fixed position, minimizing movement. The procedure site is draped and cleansed in the usual manner before performing the procedure. After venous access is obtained, the catheter is fixed in place and covered with a clear protective adhesive shield. See **Table 2** for a description of each of the procedures.

PROCEDURAL SEDATION

Certain procedures in the emergency department (ED) require cooperation by the patient. Others are deemed too traumatic or painful to be performed in awake

Table 2
Venous access procedures

Site/Procedure	Population	Materials	Procedure	Complications
Scalp cannulation	Neonates and infants	22- to 25-gauge catheters or butterfly needles	Place rubber band cephalad to eyebrows and cannulate veins	Arterial cannulation is identified by blanching of scalp after saline infusion[18]
External jugular	All ages	22-gauge to 24-gauge catheters in younger children; 16-gauge to 18-gauge in adolescents	Place in Trendelenburg to increase venous return	Arterial cannulation is possible; if noted by pulsations visualized on the catheter, remove and apply pressure
Central line: femoral, subclavian, internal jugular. Femoral is preferred site initially	All ages	Use Seldinger technique kits and consider ultrasound-guided approach	As per available kit use over the wire approach after localizing the vein.	Air embolus, bleeding, arterial cannulation, site infection, thrombus formation
Umbilical vessels	Vein – up to 2 wk after birth. Artery – 24 h to 1 wk of age[18,19]	A feeding tube or catheter (5F FT/ 3.5F PT) is attached to a 5 mL syringe filled with NS and the system is flushed. Tie or sutures to tie purse string at base of umbilical cord	Tie cord or purse string stitch at the base of umbilical cord, cut the stump with a scalpel approx 2 cm from the abdominal wall and inserted into the large, thin walled vein normally at the 12 o'clock position on the cord. Introduce 4–5 cm until blood returns. Tie with sutures	Thrombosis, embolism, vessel perforation, infection, tissue ischemia and damage, hepatic necrosis, hydrothorax, and multiple cardiac complications[20]
Intraosseous access (IO)	All Ages Preferred sites in Peds–2 cm below tibial tuberosity or distal tibia superior to medial malleolus	18 gauge needle, Bone marrow needles, or any commercially available IO kit	Firm, steady pressure is used during placement. Bone cortex is evidenced when sudden decrease in resistance is noted. Confirmation is made when able to aspirate marrow or blood with a 5–10 mL syringe	Avoid placement along areas of infection Common complications include discomfort with infusion, infection and extravasation of fluids (localized swelling). Less common complications include fat and air emboli, growth plate injuries, as well as tibial fractures[21–24]

Abbreviations: FT, full term; IO, intraosseous; NS, normal saline; PT, Preterm.

Box 2
Basic definitions used in analgesia and sedation

Analgesia: Pain relief without purposely producing a sedated state.

Minimal sedation: Patient is able to respond normally to verbal commands but cognitive function and coordination may be impaired. Patient is able to maintain his or her own airway and cardiovascular function.

Moderate sedation: Patient responds purposefully to verbal commands with or without light touch and maintains his or her own airway and cardiovascular function.

Deep sedation: Patient cannot be easily aroused but does respond purposefully to painful stimuli. Occasionally requires assistance to maintain airway but cardiovascular function is normally maintained.

Dissociative sedation: Trancelike cataleptic state associated with profound analgesia and amnesia, but able to protect airway and maintain hemodynamic stability.

---

patients. Pediatric patients pose significant challenges in that they have limited understanding and coping mechanisms and in these cases sedation is useful. For basic definitions frequently used in sedation, please refer to **Box 2**.[25–27]

Before sedation, patients are assessed thoroughly with an in-depth history, including last oral intake, and physical examination. Prior reactions to anesthesia as well as family reactions to sedation and general anesthesia should be ascertained. To limit the risk of aspiration, fasting recommendations include a minimum of 2 hours for clear liquids, 4 hours for breast milk, and 6 hours for formula, nonhuman milk, and solids.[28] Further, American Society of Anesthesiologists (ASA) physical status classification should be assigned (see **Box 3**).[26]

The decision to place a patient under sedation should not be undertaken lightly, and the care provider must be able to deal with emergency airway management, adverse medication effects, and unintended deep sedation.[28,29] Children with ASA class I and II are suitable candidates for procedural sedation; however, those who qualify for class III or IV have special needs, or anatomically abnormal airways should only be sedated with the assistance of anesthesiology and possibly in the controlled setting of an operating room.[26]

In addition to the physician managing the sedation, a nurse should be present to monitor the patient. All patients should be placed on a continuous cardiac monitor so as to monitor heart rate, respiratory rate, pulse oximetry, and noninvasive blood pressure.

The American College of Emergency Physicians developed a clinical policy describing use of medications for sedation and analgesia in the ED, focusing on the following medications in **Box 4**.[30]

Box 3
American Society of Anesthesiologists physical status classifications

Class I: healthy patient

Class II: mild systemic disease (eg, mild asthma)

Class III: severe systemic disease (eg, moderate to severe asthma, pneumonia)

Class IV: severe systemic disease that is a constant threat to life (eg, advanced cardiac disease)

Class V: moribund patient not expected to survive without the operation/procedure (eg, septic shock, severe trauma)

> **Box 4**
> **Medications used in sedation and analgesia in the ED**
>
> Etomidate
>
> Fentanyl/midazolam
>
> Ketamine
>
> Methohexital
>
> Pentobarbital
>
> Propofol

Dosing, side effects, and contraindications are discussed in **Table 3**.

In addition to sedative and analgesic medications, nitrous oxide can be used in light sedation cases. Nitrous oxide is usually mixed with 50% oxygen and provides mild analgesia, sedation, amnesia, and anxiolysis.[34–36] While using nitrous oxide, patients are able to maintain their airway without assistance and remain hemodynamically stable. Minimal side effects include nausea, vomiting, and dysphoria. Contraindications include nausea and vomiting, pregnancy, and any situation in which gas is trapped, such as bowel obstructions.[25]

Before discharge, the patient should be easily arousable and talking if age appropriate, able to sit up without assistance if appropriate, have a patent airway and stable cardiovascular status, and be able to maintain oral hydration.

THORACOSTOMY PROCEDURES

Thoracostomy is the surgical formation of an opening into the chest cavity. It is an uncommon emergency procedure in pediatric patients.[37,38] Certain characteristics that make pediatric chest trauma unique include limited pulmonary reserve, compact vital structures, and small lung volumes.[37] In neonates and young children, emergent thoracostomies are performed either during the neonatal period as part of treatment for conditions such as meconium aspiration or a simple pneumothorax,[39] whereas in older children, it is usually observed following blunt or penetrating trauma.[40,41] Other indications (eg, empyema, effusion) are usually treated by pediatric surgeons or in the intensive care unit. Because trauma is the leading cause of death and disability in patients ages 1 through 40 years,[42] most of the thoracostomies that an emergency physician will perform will be either spontaneous or secondary to trauma. Being that pediatric chest trauma remains an uncommon occurrence, most studies are small and descriptive with no randomized control trials available.[38,42] These focus mainly on epidemiology, descriptive findings, pathophysiology, and offer no recommendations to the preferred method of pleural fluid drainage.[38]

Various types of thoracostomy procedures have been described: needle thoracostomy, catheter thoracostomy (Seldinger method), and tube thoracostomy are the most common.[43] These techniques and equipment have different success rates depending on the fluid to be removed and few have studies performed in the ED. There is a lack of evidence for treatment in traumatic pneumothoraces, especially in pediatric patients; however, there is a growing body of evidence about the expected treatment of primary spontaneous pneumothorax.[44–49]

Chest radiography has been established as the standard for the initial approach to diagnosing and assessing pneumothorax size[50]; however, ultrasound is emerging as a useful tool in the treatment of pleural fluid collections.[51,52] More and more pneumothoraces (traumatic, spontaneous, or iatrogenic) are being diagnosed by bedside ultrasound in the ED.[53,54] Even after diagnosis takes place, bedside US can be used to treat the pneumothorax by guiding placement and monitoring complications. Some studies have shown ultrasound to improve placement of pigtail catheters for successful drainage of pleural effusions.[55,56]

Whatever the approach, this procedure follows a similar process with the goal of accessing the pleural cavity, removing the offending agent, and eventually reexpanding the lung while decreasing the potential for reaccumulation and further complications. The next sections provide recommendations for the drainage of fluid in the pleural space.

Needle Thoracostomy

Indications

Needle thoracostomy is the immediate insertion of a small catheter or needle into the pleural space for the temporary relief of pressure. Concern has been raised recently that this procedure may not be as effective as once thought. Investigators claim that, at least in adults, the recommended length for catheters (5 cm) may not drain the air in as many as 30% of patients.[57–59] Regardless, this procedure is necessary for the immediate removal of air causing a tension pneumothorax and the stabilization of the patient. Even if uncertain as to which side is affected, the procedure should be performed empirically in those clinically presenting the symptoms. If no improvement is noted after procedure, decompression of the contralateral side is indicated.

Contraindications

There are no absolute contraindications for the procedure but diagnosis of pneumothorax in the youngest patients, especially neonates, may prove challenging. In stable patients, relative contraindications include clotting disorders (which should be addressed before placement, if possible) (**Box 5**).

Procedure

The preferred site for needle thoracostomy is the second or third intercostal spaces at the midclavicular line, but these can be modified depending on the patient's position. Cleanse the area with chlorhexidine or povidone-iodine solution. Administer anesthetic to the area. Attach the angiocath to a syringe with 3 mL of normal saline. Introduce the needle in the aforementioned space just until there is a change in resistance. The presence of bubbles as the pleural space is entered confirms the presence of a pneumothorax. The needle is removed while the catheter is left in place to continue draining the pneumothorax. The catheter can be attached to a cutoff surgical glove or a Heimlich valve to avoid air entering the pleural space.

In neonates, the procedure is similar, but a butterfly needle is used, placed in the same space as a syringe aspirates the air and bubbles are seen. The butterfly needle is left in place and the tubing is submerged in 4 mL water in a cup or baby bottle so that air continues to come out while creating a seal. More than one needle may be necessary to resolve the condition and, ultimately, a chest tube is placed.[39]

Tube Thoracostomy

Indications

Tube thoracostomy should be considered in all but the simplest pneumothoraces encountered (see earlier in this article). Spontaneous pneumothoraces may be observed in as many as 2% of neonates (particularly in the neonatal intensive care setting). In older children and adolescents, the most common indications for this

Table 3
Medications for sedation and analgesia in the ED

	Description	Dose	Side Effects	Contraindications
Etomidate	Nonbarbiturate hypnotic agent with 5–30 sec until onset and duration of 5–15 min. Does not affect hemodynamic stability or intracranial pressure.	0.1–0.3 mg/kg IV	Has been associated with transient adrenal suppression.	Not recommended for use in children under age 10.
Fentanyl	Synthetic opioid providing analgesia. Rapid onset (2–3 min) and short duration (30–60 min).	1–4 μg/kg IV	Hypoxia, respiratory depression. Chest wall and glottic rigidity have been reported in neonates.	
Midazolam	Short acting benzodiazepine with rapid onset; provides sedation but no analgesia, often combined with opioids like fentanyl	6 mo to 5 y: 0.05–0.1 mg/kg IV, may repeat every 2–3 min as needed with max 0.6 mg/kg total 6–12 y: 0.025–0.05 mg/kg IV x1, repeat every 2–3 min as needed, max 0.4 mg/kg total >12 y: 0.5–2 mg IV x1, repeat every 2–3 min	Can result in respiratory depression when combined with fentanyl	

Drug	Description	Dose	Adverse effects	Contraindications
Ketamine	Phencyclidine derivative that acts as a dissociative sedative. Rapid onset and short duration of action.	>3 mo: 1.5 mg/kg IV over 1 min >3 mo; 4–5 mg/kg IM	Can be associated with laryngospasm, more commonly when given IM. Vomiting, increased salivation can also be seen. Older children (>15 y/o) can experience unpleasant hallucinations.	Younger than 3 mo, airway instability, hypertension, angina/heart failure, increased intracranial pressure, increased intraocular pressure, porphyria, thyroid disease, psychosis all are contraindications for use.
Methohexital	Very short acting barbiturate with onset within 30–60 seconds when given IV and duration of 5–10 min	>1 mo: 6.6–10 mg/kg IM	Hypotension, respiratory depression potentiated when used with other sedatives or opiates[31]	Do not use in children with temporal lobe epilepsy[32] or porphyria.
Pentobarbital	Barbiturate with 3–5 minutes until onset when given IV and duration of 30–45 min	2–6 mg/kg IM 1–3 mg/kg IV	Hypotension, respiratory depression potentiated when used with other sedatives or opiates[31]	Do not use in patients with porphyria.
Propofol	Nonopioid, nonbarbiturate sedative hypnotic with immediate clinical effect. Also has some antiemetic properties.	1–18 years old: 1 mg/kg IV × 1 (max 40 mg), then 0.5 mg/kg IV (max 20 mg) as needed	Hypotension, oxygen desaturation, apnea. Because of the quick onset, it is difficult to tatrate[33]	Children with allergies to egg and/ or soybeans should not receive propofol.

Box 5
Materials required for needle thoracostomy

Skin-cleansing materials, such as chlorhexidine or povidone-iodine solution

Gauze

Angiocath (16–20 gauge) or butterfly-type needle (23–25 gauge; 19 or 25 mm in length) for neonates[a]

Syringe filled with 2–3 mL of sterile normal saline (optional)

Flutter valve, underwater seal, such as a cup of water, or a commercially available 1-way valve (Heimlich)

[a] Depending on the age and weight of the infant, variable catheter sizes should be available ranging from 25 gauge in premature infants to 16 gauge in adolescents.

---

procedure are hemothorax or pneumothorax secondary to penetrating or blunt trauma.

Contraindications

There are no absolute contraindications for this procedure, especially if the patient is symptomatic.

Materials

As this should be a sterile procedure, the area should be cleansed and draped with sterile solution, such as chlorhexidine or povidone-iodine solution. The provider should wear sterile gloves and mask, and work on a sterile field (**Box 6**).

Procedure

If the patient is unstable and a tension pneumothorax is considered, release of air from the pleural space by needle thoracostomy is of vital importance.

In the intubated unstable patient, consider opening the chest cavity to release air in selected patients. Perform an incision in the upper ribs at the midaxillary line and bluntly dissect the tissues until reaching the pleural space. A "popping sound" followed by a gush of air may indicate arrival into the pleural space. After initial

---

Box 6
Materials required for chest tube placement (materials will vary depending on technique used)

Sedation and analgesia as needed	Dressing gauzes (may apply antibiotic for protection and further aid in seal)
Oxygen by nasal cannula or mask if required	Needle holder
Cleansing solution (povidone-iodine or chlorhexidine)	2–0 silk sutures
No. 10 scalpel	Seldinger kit or percutaneous drainage catheterization kit or other minimally invasive approach as indicated and available
Lidocaine 1% with epinephrine	Gauze (4 × 4 inches)
Large straight scissors	Chest tubes: size depending on patient's weight and anatomy (see **Fig. 1**)
Curved Mayo scissors	Suction tubing and adaptors
Large clamps	Suction or water seal device or Heimlich valve

stabilization, that wound may be closed as a chest tube is inserted to drain that space or a tube may be placed inside that same wound for drainage.

In stable patients, the procedure should be discussed and consent (or assent if the patient understands), should be obtained. Sedation of the patient is invaluable, especially in younger, uncooperative patients, who may not understand or follow commands. Even with sedation and local anesthesia, some degree of restraint may be required. To select the adequate chest tube size, a length-based tape can be consulted or see **Fig. 1** for the recommended size based on weight.[42] Consider the reason for tube placement, as larger tubes will be required for draining fluid (eg, blood) whereas smaller tubes might be used to drain air.

Select the appropriate area for placement and make sure the equipment is ready. Although most needle thoracostomies are performed at the midclavicular line, most tube thoracostomies are performed laterally, at the anterior axillary line at the fourth through sixth level; however, they may be placed anteriorly as well. Drape the area and cleanse. Anesthetize the intercostal space to be incised. Perform a small incision at the site. The incision should be approximately 3 times longer than the tube diameter.

Perform a blunt dissection with a finger or hemostat to create a subcutaneous tract, superiorly to a rib above the initial level so that the subcutaneous tissue further helps in covering and affixing the tube. Introduce the hemostat into the pleural space just above the rib by performing a blunt dissection into the intercostal muscles or by carefully cutting or pushing through the intercostal muscle. Make sure that the point of entry is immediately on the superior surface of the rib, as the neurovascular bundle for each rib is directly underneath it.

There are different modifications to this procedure. For example, in the Seldinger technique, the needle is introduced into the pleural space followed by a wire, which is used to guide the placement of either a catheter or dilators of increasing size (**Fig. 2**). Once the desired gauge is acquired, the smallest tube possible to get the specific fluid out optimally is introduced. A systematic review by Argall and Desmond[60] published in 2003 searched for any studies comparing these methods and found only

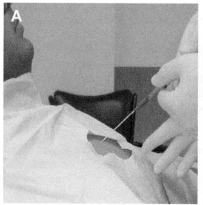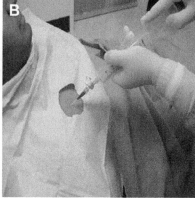

Fig. 1. Needle aspiration of a primary spontaneous pneumothorax. Midclavicular line second or third space is prepped and draped while the patient is placed at 45°. The area is anesthetized and the catheter (attached to a 3-way valve) and a syringe is introduced. Pneumothorax is suctioned on multiple occasions until no more air returns. (*From* Zehtabchi S, Rios CL. Management of emergency department patients with primary spontaneous pneumothorax: needle aspiration or tube thoracostomy? Ann Emerg Med 2008;51:91–100; with permission.)

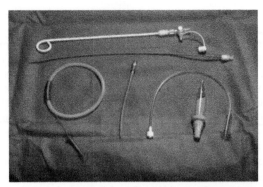

Fig. 2. Pigtail catheter equipment. Pigtail equipment (Cook system). (*From* Kulvatunyou N, Vijayasekaran A, Hansen A, et al. Two-year experience of using pigtail catheters to treat traumatic pneumothorax: a changing trend. J Trauma 2011;71(5):1104–7; with permission.)

3 relevant studies. There was no evidence to support that the Seldinger technique was superior to traditional methods.[60,61]

There is some evidence to suggest that use of small catheters, such as the pigtail catheter, which is usually placed following the Seldinger (over the wire) technique, may be successful in removing the offending agent and reexpanding the lungs. Roberts and colleagues[62] studied the treatment of pneumothoraces and pleural effusions in a Pediatric intensive care unit. The investigators showed this procedure might be effective in draining both air and fluid from the pleural space. They concluded that this procedure was successful in draining chylous effusions and "somewhat less efficacious" in draining hemothorax or pneumothorax.

On a different study, Dull and colleagues[43] published a small retrospective study, in which it was shown that pigtail catheters were comparably as effective as the classic pneumothorax technique in draining both traumatic and spontaneous pneumothoraces. Patients were less likely to require analgesics than their chest tube counterparts. In this study, it was also demonstrated that pediatric emergency physicians are capable of performing this procedure and successfully placing pigtail catheters in the ED.

Finally, after the catheter or chest tube is placed, it should be affixed to the skin with sutures and attached to a suction source to continue the lung expansion and drainage of the fluid (**Fig. 3**). Commercially designed units are available that allow for tubing from the chest tube or catheter to be connected to a reservoir. This, in place is connected to wall suction, which can be modified depending on the level of suction required.

Monitoring and complications

Complications and monitoring recommendations are similar for tube as well as needle thoracostomies, yet they present different incidence of complications depending on the selected approach. During the procedure, any number of injuries may occur, including surrounding organs, lungs, ribs, blood vessels, and nerves. Specific injuries will require specific treatments, which reach beyond the scope of this article.

Many pneumothoraces, hemothoraces, or other collections may recur, requiring suction for a longer period. Subcutaneous placement is more common with closed (classic) chest tube placement than with pigtail placement.[43,63–65] Incidences of tube kinking or dislodgement are similar.[63] These complications require that the tube be repositioned.

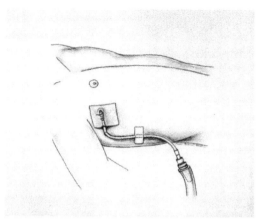

Fig. 3. Pigtail catheter secured at the skin. Pigtail is affixed at the skin with sutures, taped to the chest and connected to a suction device. (*From* Roberts JS, Bratton SL, Brogan TV. Efficacy and complications of percutaneous pigtail catheters for thoracostomy in pediatric patients. Chest 1998;114(4):1116–21; with permission.)

For hemothorax, the presence of more than 15 mL/kg of blood initially or more than 3 to 4 mL/h of blood are indications for surgical thoracostomy in the operating room. Close monitoring for any signs of clinical deterioration is crucial. Pediatric patients have a higher rate of complications and require early surgical intervention more often than adults.[38]

EAR, NOSE, AND THROAT FOREIGN BODY REMOVAL

Evolving from their curious nature, pediatric patients are prone to place foreign bodies (FBs) into their ears and noses. Close to 90% of nasal FBs occur in patients younger than 4 years of age.[66] And although most cases can be found in the pediatric population, certain psychiatric, mentally delayed, or other types of patients may present with this condition. Despite their uncommon presentation, they are a challenge to the practitioner and may be potentially life threatening.[66–71]

Common FBs in children include toys, beads, pieces of foam, earrings, paper, or food, such as popcorn and peanuts.[66–70] Notorious for damaging tissues if ingested or placed in certain orifices are button batteries, which may cause tissue necrosis in a matter of hours and should be promptly removed.[72–77] On the other hand, the most common ear FBs in adults are insects (ie, cockroaches) that crawl into the ear.[68] As part of the initial evaluation, the emergency physician should include inspection of the both ears and nostrils, in search for potential FBs. Many patients may be asymptomatic on presentation, especially if early in the course.[78] Signs of ear FBs include ear pain, decreased hearing, dizziness, or vertigo or bleeding. In one study, 30% of pediatric patients presented with decreased hearing.[66] In nasal FBs, the most common symptoms are pain and discomfort and classic findings include foul-smelling nasal discharge and halitosis.

As time progresses, the FBs will accumulate bacteria, fester, swell, and/or mineralize and eventually will become symptomatic, such as purulent rhinitis with unilateral vestibulitis on examination, seen in **Fig. 4**.[79] Atypical presentations of common conditions, such as chronic sinusitis and otitis media, may prompt the examiner to consider FBs as likely etiology for the persistent symptoms. Rare occurrences of a calcified FBs

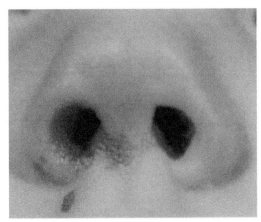

Fig. 4. Unilateral vestibulitis as evidence of nasal foreign body in a child with purulent rhinitis. (*From* Kalan A, Tariq M. Foreign bodies in the nasal cavities: a comprehensive review of the etiology, diagnostic pointers, and therapeutic measures. Postgrad Med J 2000;76(898):484–7; with permission.)

have been noted in the literature. Chronic sinusitis or persistent epistaxis should prompt the physician to consider calcified nasal FBs as a possible cause.[80–83]

Ear Canal Foreign Body Removal

Indications/contraindications

Most FBs found in the EAC do not require immediate removal. It is crucial that the patient be cooperative and that the object is easily visible. Some experts claim that because most EAC FBs are removed easily, more than one attempt or using more than one technique should prompt an ear, nose, and throat (ENT) referral.[66,69] Blind attempts can cause harm and should be avoided. Consider ENT consultation for any challenging removal.

Irrigation, in particular, has special considerations. Avoid this procedure if the suspected agent might be vegetable matter (popcorn, peas, beans, and so forth), as these tend to swell up during the process and further decrease the chance of removal. Other contraindications for irrigation include symptoms of otitis externa, uncooperative patient, myringotomy tubes, inner ear disturbances, suspicion of tympanic membrane perforation, or history of inner or middle ear disease (**Box 7**).[84]

Procedure

Explain the procedure to the patient and caretaker. Consider instilling a few drops of topical anesthetic into the canal before attempting removal. In the case of insects,

Box 7	
Materials for ear FB removal	
Adequate lighting from head light, surgical light or held by assistance	Sterile water
Alligator forceps	12-French Foley catheter or No. 4 or 5 vascular Fogarty catheter
Cyanoacrylate (glue) with 20-mL syringe with 16-gauge catheter tip	Suction equipment (Frazier or soft tip)
	Forceps
	Right hook or paper clip-shaped at an angle

instilling microscopic immersion oil, "baby oil," or viscous lidocaine will paralyze the vermin in less than 2 minutes.[85] Consider sedation with sedatives or dissociative agents like ketamine.[86]

Depending on the type of FB, different approaches for a successful removal can be made. The site, consistency, origin, and depth of the FB also play a role in its successful removal (**Fig. 5**).

Irrigation

First, gather history of any suspicion of tympanic membrane rupture. If this is a concern, irrigation should not be used (see previous section). Change the patient into a gown and cover the area of the head with towels. Place the patient on his or her side with the affected ear up. Warming the water closer to body temperature will decrease the chance of vestibular response and secondary nausea or vomiting through caloric stimulation. Ask an assistant to gently pull on the pinna to straighten the canal.

Using a 20-mL syringe and a 16-gauge or 18-gauge catheter, flush the saline forcefully.[84] An alternative to this procedure includes using the tubing from a butterfly needle after cutting the wings and needle off and placing it in the canal. Guide the irrigation toward the superior-posterior portion of the canal. Certain commercially available systems are available for this procedure. If the offending agent is cerumen, consider applying hydrogen peroxide or other cerumenolytics before performing the procedure. If the patient complains of sudden pain or tinnitus during the procedure, stop the procedure, as this may signal a tympanic membrane (TM) perforation.[84]

Suction-tip catheters

This technique is effective in removing round and rubber objects, which may otherwise be difficult to grasp. The noise could startle small patients, so appropriate restraining

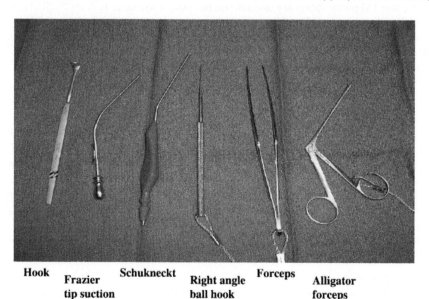

Hook   Frazier   Schukneckt   Right angle   Forceps   Alligator
        tip suction   ball hook   forceps

Fig. 5. Equipment for ear foreign body removal. Different equipment and techniques should be available to the practitioner. The position and consistency of the FB will determine the ideal technique used. (*From* Kalan A, Tariq M. Foreign bodies in the nasal cavities: a comprehensive review of the etiology, diagnostic pointers, and therapeutic measures. Postgrad Med J 2000;76(898):484–7; with permission.)

should be anticipated and be in place before performing the procedure. To prevent iatrogenic injury, inform the patient of the impending noise to prevent sudden movements from a startle reflex. Place either the blunt or the soft plastic tip against the object and slowly withdraw. If using a suction instrument with a thumb-controlled release valve (as with the Frazier suction), remember to cover the port to activate the suction.

Place the patient on his or her side and make sure there is adequate visualization of the FB before removal attempt by having an assistant gently pull on the pinna to straighten the EAC. Press the suction to the FB before activating the suction. Avoid the skin or sealing tightly around the canal since the creation of a vacuum may cause TM rupture.

Manual instrumentation

For manual removal, the patient is placed in a position similar to the prior techniques and the operating otoscope is used to visualize the FB. An assistant should handle the pinna to line up the canal to gain optimal visibility. The nondominant hand is used to grasp the otoscope while the dominant hand stabilizes against the head of the patient while the instrument is introduced. There are multiple different types of instruments to remove specific objects. If the object is a round and smooth, like a bead or plastic pellet, a right angle hook is advanced past the object, rotated 90° and placed posterior to the object before pulling it out slowly. Small alligator forceps may be used to remove soft materials like paper, foam, or other organic materials.

Complications and monitoring

Examine both ears after performing the procedure to assess for any other FBs, remaining particles, bleeding, or TM rupture. Damage to ossicles, external ear lacerations, and TM perforations are uncommon but potentially serious complications, and should be documented. A small amount of bleeding from small abrasions and lacerations can be expected from the procedure and should be documented. These generally heal spontaneously with no complications.[66–69] If the FB cannot be successfully removed, the patient should be referred to ENT for removal. Otherwise, no further follow-up is usually required.

Nasal FB Removal

Indications

Indications for nasal FB removal include any FB presenting after initial evaluation. A complete examination of ears and nose is warranted. In some instances in which there is evidence of chronic infection or recurrent epistaxis (even in the absence of a history of FB insertion) a full examination is indicated. Some FBs require prompt removal, such as magnets and button batteries, because, according to some reports, batteries may cause necrosis in just a few hours after insertion.[72,81,87–89] Magnets, such as those used to imitate piercing, may cause septal necrosis if they remain place long enough.

Contraindications

Some authorities believe that superiorly located FBs (close to the cribriform plate) should be referred to ENTs for removal, fearing possibility of trauma to this area, which may increase the risk of perforating into the meninges. Also, if the FB cannot be removed or if the patient cannot be sedated, consider referral for removal. Keep in mind that some require immediate consultation, such as for button batteries, magnets, or those presenting respiratory complaints (**Box 8**).

Box 8	
Materials for nasal foreign body removal[a]	
Adequate lighting form head light, surgical light, or held by assistance	Right hook[a]
Nasal speculum(optional)	12-French Foley catheter or No. 4 or 5 vascular Fogarty catheter[a]
1% Lidocaine without epinephrine (max 0.3 mL/kg)	Alligator forceps[a]
Nasal decongestant: oxymethozaline, epinephrine (1:1000), or neosynephrine	Suction equipment[a]

[a] Depending on the level of comfort, the location, and the consistency of the FB, different types of materials may be used.

Procedure

Engage the caretakers as well as the child (especially if verbal) and explain the procedure. If there is a concern or doubt about the nature of the FB, consider skull radiographs (anteroposterior and lateral) to exclude rhinolithiasis, magnets, or button batteries (**Fig. 6**).[80–83,90] Attempts to reduce parental or child anxiety may prove useful, because successful removal is directly linked to patient cooperation. Have more than tool for removal easily accessible at to anticipate every possibility. If, at any point, the patient is too distressed to tolerate the procedure, consider conscious sedation. Ketamine is ideal for manual removal; especially if there have been other failed attempts.[88] If sedation is to be used, cardiovascular monitoring and advanced airway equipment should be readily available at the bedside (see previous section).

Generally speaking, the shape and consistency of the FB will determine the optimal removal technique. For example, rugged, irregular foreign bodies may be removed with alligator forceps, whereas round and smooth FBs may be removed with positive-pressure, curettes, or a Fogarty apparatus, such as the Katz method.[91,92] Age and level of anxiety by the caretakers, as well as the patient, should also be gauged to determine the ideal approach to removal. Position and lighting are of paramount importance. A headlight or surgical light that allows the physician to work with both hands are invaluable for this procedure.

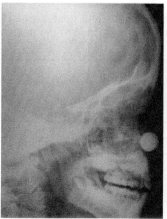 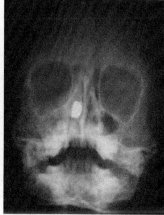

Fig. 6. Lateral and anteroposterior views of a 9-year-old male with a button battery in the nose. (*From* Dane S, Smally AJ, Peredy TR. A truly emergent problem: button battery in the nose. Acad Emerg Med 2000;7:204–6; with permission.)

Positive-pressure method

For some FBs, especially those that occlude most or all of the nasal passage, an ideal method is to perform positive pressure while occluding the contralateral nostril. Older children may be able to attempt this on their own. The patient is asked to close the unaffected nostril and blow. Another way of replicating this process is to ask the parent to blow into the patient's mouth hard and fast while occluding the contralateral nostril. This "parent's kiss" has been shown to be effective in some studies and has the advantage that it can be performed without restraints or sedation, by someone known to the patient. It can significantly reduce anxiety.[93–95] This may also be performed by placing the patient in the semi-sitting or prone position and holding the patient down gently. The unaffected side is occluded and a bag valve mask is placed covering only the mouth and creating a seal. A short, quick blow from a bag valve mask is done. More than one attempt may be required for successful removal.[96,97]

Modifications to the positive pressure method as discussed include blowing through a straw instead of direct contact of the parent's mouth but this is not indicated in children who cannot create an adequate seal around the straw. Another option is to perform this procedure by closing the mouth and placing rubber tubing in the unaffected nostril before blowing hard. A small study claims success in removing close to 40 FBs with no complications.[98]

A few drops of epinephrine (1:1000) or phenylephrine may be used as decongestants to decrease the nasal swelling and aid in passage of the FB while using this method. The practitioner must make sure the FB is large enough as to diminish the chance of aspiration. It is believed that the reduction in swelling from these vasoconstrictors may reduce edema and loosen the FB before extraction by positive pressure.[91]

Mechanical extraction

Success in removing FBs by mechanical extraction depends on the position of the FB as well as the shape. For direct visualization, a nasal speculum is placed in the anterior-posterior position as to avoid pressure on the septum. Visualization can also be obtained by using the thumb to gently elevate the nose to visualize the nares. Blind attempts at removal are discouraged, as they may cause undue harm without any success. For recommendations about removal approach based on the type of FB, see **Table 4**.[91]

Anterior FBs may be removed by placing a curette or hook posterior and superior to it and performing gentle traction. Foreign bodies positioned in the posterior aspect

Table 4
Recommended approaches of nasal foreign body removal based on FB type, location, and degree of obstruction

Procedure	FB Type	Location	Degree of Obstruction
Positive pressure	Any	Ant/post[a]	Complete
Washout	Friable	Ant/post	Complete
Hooks	Hard	Ant	Incomplete
Forceps	Soft	Ant	Incomplete
Catheter	Any	Ant/post	Incomplete
Magnet	Metallic	Anterior	Complete/incomplete

[a] Ant, anterior; FB, foreign body; post, posterior.

Data from Kiger JR, Brenkert TE, Losek J. Nasal foreign body removal in children. Pediatr Emerg Care 2008;24(11):785–92.

undergo a similar process in which a Fogarty or Foley catheter is placed, passing the object superior and posterior to it. The catheter is filled with saline: 1 mL for a Fogarty catheter or 2 to 3 mL for a Foley catheter and the object is gently retracted. Commercially available versions of this catheter are available (**Fig. 7**).

Complications and further monitoring

Bleeding and localized swelling are the most common complications but are usually self-limited and resolve with a few minutes of pressure. In some instances, the patient may aspirate the FB during removal. If there is any airway compromise, the patient should be stabilized. If the patient develops respiratory symptoms during or after the procedure, the patient should consult an otolaryngologist for a rigid bronchoscopy.

If the procedure is a success, no specific follow-up will be required. If symptoms of chronic sinusitis or otitis media were noticed, a course of antibiotics may be considered.[91]

ORAL LACERATIONS
Introduction

Trauma to the oral cavity is common in pediatric emergency practice.[99,100] Evaluation of the oral cavity includes attention to the face, head, and neck, as well as to the mouth and any other trauma observed. Isolated tooth trauma is promptly referred to a dentist for evaluation depending on the severity of dental trauma. As a general rule, dental repair is undergone before gingival suturing to avoid displacing the sutures. Consider radiographs if there are severe injuries associated with dental fractures to exclude teeth fragments in the soft tissue.[100]

There are certain areas of controversy in the treatment of oral trauma. For example, treating tongue lacerations by primary closure with sutures is controversial, with some studies showing no benefit.[101,102] Furthermore, prescription of antibiotics has also shown to be controversial.[103] Despite these controversies, both therapies remain common accepted practice.

Indications

Most lacerations to the oral mucosa require no treatment at all. Oral lacerations to the tongue or gingival that present with a flap or measure more than 1 cm should be

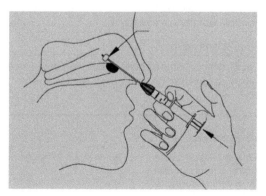

Fig. 7. Nasal foreign body removal. Example of a Katz extractor procedure. Foley and Fogarty catheters are used in the same manner for FB removal. (*From* Kiger JR, Brenkert TE, Losek J. Nasal foreign body removal in children. Pediatr Emerg Care 2008;24(11):785–92; with permission.)

approximated. Although evidence is lacking, the rationale behind closure to these wounds is to decrease the chance of food presence and therefore minimize infection.[102]

Contraindications

If the patient is unable to sit still, trauma is severe, or there are any contraindications to sedation, consider performing these repairs in the operating room. Severe lacerations include those with damage to the salivary glands or ducts, or that expose the facial nerve, as well as those too complex for the ED (which require more than 1 hour in repairing). Consult the oral surgery service for these types of injuries (**Box 9**).

Procedure

Place the patient in a comfortable position with airway equipment and cardiac monitor available at the bedside. Adequate lighting and suction equipment are crucial for adequate performance of the procedure. Administer anesthesia to the affected area. Consider blocks, such as the inferior alveolar blocks, depending on the area involved. Wash the area with saline solution. Inspect the area for any foreign bodies or damage to deep structures. The oral mucosa is generally sutured with absorbable sutures. Lacerations to the mucosa, gingiva, and tongue that do not gape or measure less than 1 cm are generally left alone. Through-and-through lacerations require approximation on both ends to decrease rate of infection and decrease healing time. Evaluate wounds for foreign bodies (ie, teeth fragments) while using radiography in selected cases to look for said fragments. External skin lacerations are approximated using nonabsorbable sutures, such as 6-0 nylon.

Special attention is given to tongue lacerations; most lacerations heal well with no interventions. For example, the small avulsions, like those encountered in a seizing patient, will heal normally without intervention. Suture those that gape, have exposed muscle, or measure more than 2 cm. The tongue must be fixed to decrease movement through the procedure. Have an assistant secure the tongue by holding it with gauze. An alternative to this is to place a suture at the tip of the anesthetized tongue to keep the tongue still. Uncooperative patients should undergo sedation with a dissociative or sedative agent. Ketamine is a good choice because it does not cause respiratory depression. Consider the concomitant administration of atropine to decrease salivation during the procedure. Administer lidocaine with epinephrine locally or by lingual block. Begin the repair with either a local infiltration of anesthetic or a lingual block. To close the wound, use absorbable 4-0 sutures. Sutures should be deep, anchoring levels of muscle and knots should be buried if possible to decrease the likelihood of loosening up with normal biting and movement.

Disposition and Further Monitoring

Inform caretakers that the patient should have a soft diet for the next 7 days. Through-and-through lacerations should be rechecked in 48 hours and the patient should

Box 9 Materials for oral laceration repair	
Suture equipment: 3-0 and 4-0 absorbable sutures, such as chromic gut for mucosal surfaces; for skin use 6-0 nonabsorbable sutures	Syringe with 25-gauge or 27-gauge needles
Suction equipment	Sterile gloves and mask
1% Lidocaine with epinephrine	Saline solution

follow-up with dental service or oral surgery for further evaluation. Wounds that are more likely to get infected (eg, through-and-through) lacerations should likely receive a short course of antibiotics. However, there is inconclusive evidence to suggest the use of prophylactic antibiotics for any oral laceration repaired in the ED.[103] Infections are rare but if present, consider admission to oral or dental service to avoid abscess formation that may spread in the face and neck fascial planes.

Finally, oral trauma may bring about concerns for abuse. Almost half of abused infants present with facial and intraoral lesions and it has been thought that a torn frenulum is pathognomonic for abuse. However, a recent review of the literature shows there is no evidence to support that a torn frenulum, in isolation of other injuries, means that there has been nonaccidental trauma.[104]

ORTHOPEDIC PROCEDURES
Nursemaid's Elbow Reduction

Introduction
Radial head subluxation (ie, nursemaid's elbow) usually occurs in children younger than 6 years of age, but has been reported in 6-month-old babies, as well as preteen patients, with an average age of 2.5 years. It is the most common presenting complaint in the painful upper extremity in children younger than 6 years of age.[105] The mechanism is considered to be secondary to traction of the arm with the forearm and wrist pronated.[106] This leads to a detachment (sliding or tear) of the annular ligament to the radial head.[107] When the arm is released, the ligament becomes trapped between the radial head and the capitellum.

History may be inconsistent with the classic "pulling" mechanism.[106] In one study, approximately half of the presenting patients had a history of pulling as a possible mechanism, whereas the second most common mechanism was falling from bed.[105] Patients will present with the arm adducted, mildly pronated, and minimally flexed. Pain might be referred to the wrist region, but further examination will show no point tenderness at the level of the wrist. On examination, the patient will refuse to use the arm and there might be some pain on palpation of the radial head area. Although this procedure can be undertaken without any radiographs, findings such as ecchymosis, swelling, or deformity should raise concern for other possible diagnoses and will require further studies.

Although usually unnecessary, the physician should assess if the patient will be willing to undergo the reduction without any sedation. Analgesia in the form of oral ibuprofen would most likely suffice. Care must be taken to discuss the plan and procedure with the caretakers to diminish anxiety. They should understand that there is nothing broken and that only a ligament will be fixed into position. It should also be made clear that the patient will feel pain or discomfort briefly but that the symptoms will improve shortly after the procedure.

Contraindications
If there is any evidence of pain or deformity to palpation around the shoulder, humerus, forearm, or wrist, radiographs should be evaluated to exclude fracture or dislocations, such as a Monteggia, radial head, or supracondylar fracture. Otherwise, the procedure may be attempted before radiographic testing.[108]

Procedure
The patient should be sitting comfortably in the lap of the caretaker or assistant and held. The affected arm is held in extension. The examiner is positioned in front of the child. There are 3 approaches to this reduction: supination/flexion, hyperpronation,

and forced pronation/flexion (not shown) (**Fig. 8**). Supination/flexion is the classic technique. Hyperpronation or forced pronation/flexion is perceived by caretakers and physicians to be less painful.[108–114]

Supination technique Using the hand in front of the injured arm, the practitioner should grasp the elbow with the thumb palpating the radial head. With the other hand, the wrist is grasped and guided to supination and elbow flexion. A clicking sound may be heard while the radial head is being reduced. If a click is heard or felt, it is very likely that the reduction has been a success; however, absence of a clicking sound does not suggest that the procedure has been a failure.

Hyperpronation After preparing the child in the same manner, the hand is grasped in a similar fashion as described previously. Instead of flexing the elbow, the wrist is forcefully hyperpronated. A click is sought in the same manner as previously.

Forced pronation/flexion The patient is prepared in the same manner and the grip is similar to the prior procedures. The practitioner pronates the wrist and immediately flexed the elbow. A click may be felt, indicating reduction.

Complications and disposition
After the procedure, the child should be observed and reevaluated after 10 to 15 minutes. In most cases, the child will show full use of the extremity after this observation time. Based in previous study protocols, if the child is not using the extremity after 15 to 30 minutes, the procedure may be repeated up to 3 times before ordering films.[108,112] Usually there are no complications during or after the procedure aside from the pain; brief, if successful, but more pronounced if an undiagnosed fracture is being manipulated. Sometimes movement of the arm may not be observed until after a period longer than 30 minutes. Follow-up instructions should include reevaluation with a pediatric orthopedist 24 hours after the evaluation if symptoms persist. Immobilization is not recommended unless there are recurrent symptoms.[114] Although rare, there have been reports of nonreducible nursemaid's elbows requiring visualization and repair in the operating room after radiographs and examination were found to be consistent with this pathology but the patient remained unable to move the extremity.[115]

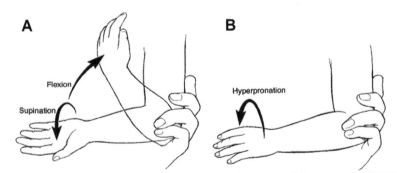

Fig. 8. Nursemaid's elbow reduction. (*A*) Supination at the wrist followed by flexion at the elbow; (*B*) Hyperpronation at the wrist. (*From* Macias CG, Bothner J, Wiebe R. A comparison of supination/flexion to hyperpronation in the reduction of radial head subluxations. Pediatrics 1998;102(1):e10; with permission.)

CENTRAL NERVOUS SYSTEM PROCEDURES
Evaluation a Ventricular Shunt

Intracranial shunts are used whenever patients require a continuous drainage of cerebrospinal fluid for conditions such as hydrocephalus.[116] Shunt failure rates approximate 14% during the first month,[117–120] and nearly half will fail within the first year.[121] Infection risks are lower but considerable, approaching 11% during the first 24 months in one series. Risk factors for shunt infections include procedure performed at a younger age, previous shunt infection, multiple prior shunt revisions, and prolonged procedure.[122,123]

Shunts may vary in shape, distal insertion site, and components, but most have a similar functionality. There are many different types of valves, which provide for access to the cerebrospinal fluid (CSF) (**Figs. 9** and **10**). There is generally proximal tubing, a valve, and a distal portion. The most common site for distal placement is the peritoneal cavity, known as the VP shunt (**Fig. 11**). Other sites include the atrium (VA shunt), venous vessels (VV shunt), or less commonly lumboperitoneal shunts (LP) may be used.[120]

The usual presentation of shunt failure or infection may be nonspecific and could include headache, vomiting, blurred vision, generalized malaise, fever, lethargy, and seizures. In children, the symptoms are usually noticed by the caretaker.[120,124] Evaluation and concurrent diagnosis of shunt failure is a challenge to the practicing emergency medicine physician, as signs and symptoms may be subtle while physical findings remain obscure. This is why the possibility of shunt failure should be entertained with any complaint presented by children with shunts as the etiology for their symptoms.

To evaluate a shunt, the clinician should carefully observe and palpate the head and neck for any signs of erythema, swelling, or tenderness, as well as any evidence of exposed hardware. Initial assessment includes a "shunt series" of radiographic studies that includes skull radiographs in the anteroposterior and lateral views, as well as chest and abdomen views, looking for shunt displacement, breakage, or kinking. Computed tomography of the head is useful, especially when comparing it with previous studies for any indication of increased or decreased ventricle size. If these studies are inconclusive, further studies are recommended and include magnetic resonance imaging, lumbar puncture, and shunt tapping.

Part of the evaluation of a shunt includes the potential for tapping the shunt to assess the pressure while excluding infection. According to a protocol published by

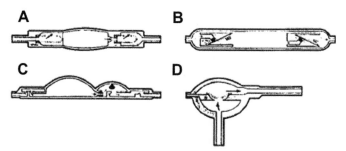

Fig. 9. Cerebrospinal fluid shunt valves. (*A*) Holter valve (*slit valve*); (*B*) Hakim valve (*ball valve*); (*C*) miter valve (on-off device to right of pumping chamber); (*D*) diaphragm valve (proximal end sits in the burr hole). (*From* Key CB, Rothrock SG, Falk JL. Cerebrospinal fluid shunt complications: an emergency medicine perspective. Pediatr Emerg Care 1995;11(5): 265–73; with permission.)

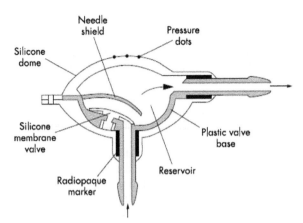

Fig. 10. Structure of a typical CSF shunt valve. (*From* Pople IK. Hydrocephalus and shunts: what the neurologist should know. J Neurol Neurosurg Psychiatr 2002;73(Suppl 1): i17–22; with permission.)

Miller and associates, most shunts may be evaluated without the use of a tap.[124] Based on this study, it was recommended that radiographic studies be performed initially. They also recommended performing a lumbar puncture in patients with a communicating hydrocephalus, stating that the information gathered from tapping the shunt would not be worth the potential risk for infection.[124]

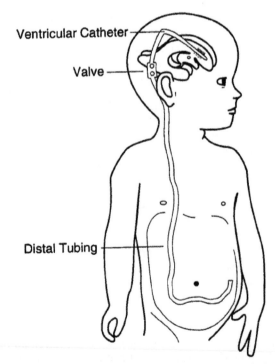

Fig. 11. Ventriculoperitoneal shunt system. (*From* Pople IK. Hydrocephalus and shunts: what the neurologist should know. J Neurol Neurosurg Psychiatr 2002;73(Suppl 1): i17–22; with permission.)

Diagnostic Tap of a Ventricular Shunt

Indications
Ventricular shunt tapping is performed whenever there is a concern for possible ventricular shunt blockage or infection and as part of a full evaluation of shunt function. Consider shunt tapping only in selected cases (see previously).

Contraindications
Evidence of cellulitis or any sign of infection around the valve site should raise concern about introducing infection into the system. Some investigators advocate that tapping the shunt is of limited value in most patients.[124] If only infection is being sought, and the patient has a communicating hydrocephalus, consider performing a lumbar puncture instead of a shunt tap. However, if patients have distorted anatomies or lower back conditions (eg, myelomeningocele), a lumbar puncture may prove close to impossible to perform, and other alternatives should be considered (**Box 10**).

Procedure
Discuss the advantages and risks of performing this procedure in the ED with the neurosurgery service at your institution. Whenever possible, consult the neurosurgeon who initially performed the shunt. Most patients with suspicion of a VP shunt malfunction or infection will require neurosurgery evaluation. So consider transferring to a tertiary institution. After gathering consent from the patient or surrogate decision maker, the area should be examined for any evidence of infection or discharge. Although there are different types of valves, most of them possess a reservoir for potential tapping.[125] Localize the valve and clear the area of any hair or particulates. Sterile lubricant can be used as a gel to part the hair and further removal of hair should be performed using scissors. Avoid shaving the area, as it may further irritate the skin. The scalp is then prepared and cleansed with povidone-iodine solution and draped in the usual sterile fashion.

The butterfly needle tubing is attached to a 3-mL syringe and it is inserted at a 30° angle. The CSF may drain spontaneously or with less than 1 mL of pressure, signifying good flow has been established. More pressure may be required on the syringe (2–3 mL) for filling but this may signify decreased flow.

Opening pressures can be determined by using a column or manometer and placing it next to the patient's ear. Document well where the column was placed so as to aid in the interpretation of this pressure. Some studies use a cutoff value of 25 cm H_2O as a diagnosis of increased pressure; yet pressures above 15 cm H_2O may be considered abnormal.

Finally, place the CSF samples into specimen tubes and send for analysis. Laboratory examination should include glucose and protein levels, cell count, Gram stain, and culture. Definitions of infection vary depending on the source. Based on a study by McGirt and colleagues,[118] shunt infection was considered if CSF culture yielded

---

Box 10
Materials for ventricular shunt tapping

Sterile gloves	Cerebrospinal fluid (CSF) manometer (optional)
Cleansing solution (povidone-iodine or chlorhexidine)	Scissors or razor for hair removal
Sterile fenestrated drape	Gauzes
Syringe	Numbered CSF tubes
Three-way stopcock	
Butterfly needles, 23 or 25 gauge	

a pathogenic organism or indicated CSF pleocytosis (white blood cell count higher than 150 per mm^3) with associated fever (38.5°C), shunt malfunction, or presence of suggestive neurologic symptoms. On the other hand, Lan and colleagues[126] defined infection when leukocytosis was greater than 100 leukocytes per mm^3 and also observed the presence of eosinophilia.

Complications and further monitoring

The patient should be monitored further for any other symptoms, such as worsening neurologic status. There is a low risk for shunt infection after a tap, but damage to the shunt secondary to the procedure could occur, requiring a revision.[127] Rare complications have been described, such as intracranial bleeding, after this procedure.[128] Most patients will require admission for observation and further workup. Although usually a safely performed procedure for both the hardware and the patient, the valve may be damaged during the tap. This will require neurosurgery evaluation. Consider early referral or transfer based on your resource capabilities. Monitor for any neurologic deterioration during and after the procedure.

Lumbar Puncture

Introduction

A lumbar puncture (LP), or "spinal tap," is performed in patients requiring evaluation and treatment of neurologic emergencies. The use of magnetic resonance imaging and the computed tomography scans (CT) have limited the use of this technique to the diagnosis of infections, inflammatory disorders, and intracranial bleeding (subarachnoid hemorrhage). The lumbar puncture remains the only way in which we can access fluid for assessment of its contents as well as to perform bacteriologic or immunologic testing of the cerebrospinal fluid.

Although useful in the diagnosis and treatment of many conditions, it is important to observe that treatment, referral, and further testing should not be delayed pending an LP. In many instances, such as meningitis, therapy should be started immediately on suspicion (eg, antibiotics) and not withheld pending completion or results to this test.[129]

Indications

The most common indication for this procedure is to evaluate for the possibility of CNS infection (meningitis or meningoencephalitis), subarachnoid hemorrhage, and inflammatory neurologic syndromes (eg, Guillan-Barré). Other rare indications include conditions such as idiopathic intracranial hypertension (pseudotumor cerebri).

Contraindications

Allergy to any of the components of the equipment or to local anesthetic is a contraindication to the procedure. Suspicion of increased intracranial pressure is a well-known, albeit controversial, contraindication for an LP. Fortunately a rare entity, it is estimated to occur in fewer than 5% of patients with bacterial meningitis.[130,131] Some investigators state that increased intracranial pressure is invariably present in all cases of meningitis and that many of those who herniate would do so with or without the procedure.[131] CT may not be enough to exclude cerebral edema or anticipate a herniation syndrome, while at the same time the physical examination may not correlate with abnormal CT findings in all patients. In those patients with focal neurologic deficits, rapidly decreasing mental status, papillary abnormalities, or recent seizures, LP should be reconsidered and perhaps delayed.[130] In many cases, it may be safer to begin treatment while further evaluation, history, or even radiographic studies are made available. In patients with a distorted anatomy, as in myelomeningocele, alternatives to the procedure should be sought. Evidence or suspicion of infection at the puncture site is another contraindication to the procedure. On the other hand, patients with bleeding diatheses (platelets <50,000 or international normalized ratio ≥1.4) or prolonged coagulation parameters should undergo correction before the procedure, so as to avoid epidural hematomas or persistent bleeding (**Box 11**).[132]

Technique

Positioning of the child presents the physician with 2 main options: lateral decubitus and sitting position. Studies have shown that interspinous processes are maximally separated in the latter one when there is maximal hip flexion.[133,134] Either position is appropriate. The assistant can hold the infant's hands between the flexed legs with one hand and then hold the head or shoulders with the other hand. The spinal cord ends at the level of L1-L2 and ideal sites for lumbar puncture are the interspaces between L3-L4 and L4-L5. Landmarks can be determined using the iliac crest, which is at the level of the L4-L5 interspace. Using a sterile technique, prepare a large area using povidone iodine. Infants and children feel pain with lumbar punctures and should have topical or local anesthesia before puncture.[135] Evidence has shown that local anesthesia does not add difficulty or increase the failure rate.[136] If topical anesthesia was not used (eg, EMLA), inject local anesthesia (1% lidocaine plain) by first injecting a small intradermal wheal and then deeper into the desired interspace. It is important to aspirate to ensure you do not inject into a vessel or into the spinal canal. After the area is anesthetized, insert the spinal needle with the bevel facing up (toward the ceiling) in the midline. A "pop" and decreased resistance can be felt once through the ligamentum flavum and then once through the dura. Remove the stylet and check for CSF, if not present replace stylet and advance slowly and check again for CSF. Once CSF is flowing, collect 1 mL in each of the tubes. Replace the stylet before removing the needle. Cleanse area and place a gauze or cover.

Complications

The most common complication of an LP is headache, usually associated with nausea and vomiting. Postdural postspinal headache (PDPH) was thought to be uncommon in younger children, yet recent data suggest a similar incidence across all age groups.[132,137,138] The incidence of postspinal headache has been shown to decrease with smaller-gauge needles and with the use of round (atraumatic) needles, instead of the classic cutting ones.[137]

Other complications include local pain at site of puncture, spinal cord bleeding, infection, and rarely a subarachnoid epidermal cyst (owing to foreign body reaction). Finally, apnea is another complication, especially in neonates. This can be prevented

Box 11 Equipment for lumbar puncture		
Povidone-Iodine Solution Assistant to help position patient	Commercial LP Tray 22-gauge spinal needles with variable lengths: 1.5 in. for <1 y old 2.5 in. for 1 y to middle childhood, 3.5 in. for older children (Consider using noncutting needles to reduce incidence of postspinal headache)	Sterile Gloves Topical anesthetic or lidocaine for local injection Cerebrospinal fluid manometer (optional)

by avoiding extreme neck flexion. In fact, a study by Abo and colleagues[133] suggests that neck flexion does not increase interspinous spaces, and should be avoided.

Perhaps the most feared complication regarding LPs is the brainstem herniation syndrome (see previously). If this should occur, the patient should be immediately stabilized, including endotracheal intubation and admitted to the intensive care unit.[130]

Monitoring
Young patients should be offered fluids to keep hydrated. They should be observed for movement of all extremities.

Older patients should be followed for any evidence of worsening back pain or decreased sensation. Lying in bed for 2 hours after the procedure has been advocated as a method to decrease the rate of PDPH, but this has not been shown to decrease this complication. The patient should be monitored closely for any worsening neurologic symptoms, weakness, sphincter tone loss, or incontinence. Disposition of the patient depends on the initial indication and results of the CSF testing. If discharged, the caretakers should be given instructions regarding proper monitoring at home.

GASTROINTESTINAL PROCEDURES
Gastrostomy Tube Replacement

Introduction
Gastrostomy tube (G-tube) placement is becoming increasingly common within the pediatric population. The most common indications for a G-tube placement include failure to thrive and swallowing disorders (ie, debilitating neuromuscular disease). Complications may occur and may be minor, such as blockage, leakage, or dislodgement, which occurs in approximately 70% of patients. Major complications, such as gastric outlet obstruction, peritonitis, septicemia, and death, may be seen in approximately 5% of cases.[139] Many of these will present to an ED for diagnosis and treatment.[140,141]

Indications
Once a gastrostomy tube inadvertently is removed, it is important to try to replace it as quickly as possible. After placement of a simple gastrostomy tube, it takes about 1 to 2 weeks to form a tract. Once the tube is out, the tract can narrow or close completely within hours. If the tube is only partially dislodged, it will need to be fully removed before replacing. It should slide out easily with minimal resistance.

Contraindications
If the tract is younger than 3 weeks old or if it is unclear how long ago it was originally placed, the patient may need operative replacement or replacement under fluoroscopy.[142] A gastrostomy tube should not be replaced in the ED if there is any evidence of infection or peritonitis, including extensive erythema, pus drainage, or warmth around the site. If active bleeding is a concern, emergent consultation should take place.

Equipment
A new tube should be used for replacement, as there may be a mechanical problem with the original device (ie, faulty balloon or balloon rupture) or if the tube is clogged. An alternative is to use a Foley catheter of similar size.[143] For a complete list of materials needed for this procedure, see **Box 12**.

Procedure
The child should be restrained in the supine position (or older, cooperative children may be most comfortable in recumbent/supine position). The tract should be gently

Box 12	
Equipment for gastrostomy tube replacement	
Gloves	New tube or Foley
Stethoscope	"External bolster"
Lubricant	Syringe (to insufflate air to check placement)
Saline	Syringe for saline (to inflate balloon)

probed with a lubricated cotton tipped swab or a blunt stylet (be careful not to form a false tract). Hold the tube between your thumb and forefinger and use the heel of your hand to stabilize the abdominal wall. Hold tube perpendicular to the abdominal wall and after lubricating tube, slide it into the tract with gentle pressure.[144] This may take 30 to 45 seconds of gentle steady pressure to allow the tube to pass. Be careful not to force it, as it can form a false tract. If the same size tube does not fit, use the next size smaller or a Foley catheter of similar size.[143] Insert the tube until the entire balloon or mushroom tip is advanced past the abdominal wall.

If the tube is inserted correctly into the stomach, it should move freely and you should be able to aspirate gastric contents. If no gastric contents are aspirated, place 30 mL of normal saline through the tube and aspirate again. If no gastric contents are aspirated or there is any doubt about placement, then tube placement can be radiographically verified by placing 20 to 30 mL of water-soluble contrast (gastrograffin, do not use barium) and then take supine abdominal x-ray within 1 to 2 minutes.[145]

Complications and monitoring

Complications with tube changes have an incidence of less than 5%.[140] These include intraperitoneal placement, minor bleeding, infection, and internal migration (if using Foley catheter may migrate causing a gastric outlet obstruction).[146] There is at least one case in the literature of esophageal rupture secondary to placement of a Foley catheter into the esophagus.[147] If no gastric contents can be aspirated or if there is any doubt about placement, then radiographic verification is recommended. Verify intragastric placement as described previously. If placement has been verified, no further workup is necessary.[148]

Incarcerated Inguinal Hernia Reduction

Inguinal hernias occur when an intra-abdominal structure protrudes through a defect in the abdominal wall. Studies describe an overall incidence of hernias in childhood of approximately 5% rising to 30% in premature infants. These can become incarcerated and commonly occur in the first year of life.[149,150] Most inguinal hernias in infants and children are indirect inguinal hernias, which occur when the processus vaginalis fails to close and intra-abdominal contents protrude through this space. According to recent studies, the risk of incarceration more than doubles if the patient has to wait more than 14 days for elective surgery.[151] Current recommendation is that they be repaired promptly after diagnosis owing to risk of incarcerations while waiting for elective repair; especially during the first 12 months of life.[150,152]

Diagnosis of a hernia is suggested by bulging present in the inguinal region. A hernia may be seen after an infant or child is crying or straining and may resolve when the child is sleeping. Therefore, spontaneously reducing hernias may be absent on examination. Techniques must be used in the very young to assess for hernias during the examination. In the very young, the child should be examined while crying. Older children can blow into a glove or straw to cause Valsalva maneuvers. If the hernia persists and is found to be tender to palpation, firm, erythematous, and edematous, it is likely incarcerated. In these cases, the child will be fussy, not wanting to feed, crying, or inconsolable. An incarcerated hernia can be organ-threatening or life-threatening if not managed quickly. Bowel, ovary, testes, or other organs can become strangulated and ischemia, necrosis, and perforation can occur. Reduction is important to allow for the edema to resolve and permit an elective repair, which has less risk to the patient.[150] Ultrasound is rapidly emerging as an invaluable tool in the evaluation and diagnosis of inguinal masses, including hernias. Differentiation between hydroceles and bowel can be easily performed at the bedside.[153,154]

Indications/contraindications
Manual reduction is required after the diagnosis of incarcerated hernia is made. It should not be attempted if the patient has any signs of systemic toxicity (including peritoneal signs, abdominal distention, bilious vomiting, or discoloration of the entrapped viscera). If any signs of toxicity are present, the patient should be resuscitated and an emergent surgical consultation obtained. Early consultation with the surgery service is recommended, because depending on their availability, they may request to be present during the attempts at manual reduction.

Procedure
The patient is placed in mild Trendelenberg position with the ipsilateral leg externally rotated and flexed. Apply uniform pressure along the incarcerated bowel by placing one hand at the hernia bulge at the upper edge of the external inguinal ring while the other hand applies steady firm pressure for up to 5 minutes. The contents of the bowel will be reduced first and then the bowel itself reduced back into the abdomen. If the hernia is not reduced after 5 minutes of steady pressure, consider sedation. If again reduction is not successful after 5 to 10 minutes with the patient sedated and comfortable, an emergent surgical consult should be obtained. When reduction is not successful it is usually secondary to an ovary or incarcerated bowel outside the inguinal ring.[144]

Complications and disposition
Common complications include pain and edema. Other complications are rare, such as damage to bowel (perforation), ovaries, and testes. There have been reported cases of associated testicular or ovarian torsion.[155] Incarcerated hernias can be successfully reduced in 80% of cases.[148] If manual reduction is unsuccessful, the bowel may progress to necrosis and gangrene. In these cases, a surgeon should be consulted for immediate reduction in the operating room. Following the reduction, patients should be admitted following herniorrhaphy once edema has subsided in 24 to 48 hours.[148] They should be monitored closely for any deterioration, signs of recurrence, or toxicity.

Rectal Prolapse

Rectal prolapsed is defined as a herniation of the rectum through the anus. It may involve the mucosa or all the layers of the rectum. Age of presentation is usually in the preschool years. Caretakers usually observe a painless episode in which a red mass protrudes from the rectum before reducing spontaneously.[156,157] Several predisposing factors include increased intra-abdominal pressure, diarrhea, neoplastic diseases, malnutrition, and conditions associated with pelvic floor weakness, as well as straining and constipation.[157,158] It is important to ask about history of cystic fibrosis, history of neonatal stooling problems, excessive straining, and prolonged sitting on the toilet. If the patient has recurrent rectal prolapse, he or she should have follow-up for cystic fibrosis testing, as close to 10% of patients with rectal prolapse may have the condition. The patient should be examined while sitting or squatting if possible. The differential diagnosis includes intussusception; this can be distinguished by inserting a finger between the mucosa of the mass and the anal wall.[159]

Indications
Many instances of rectal prolapse will reduce by itself. Rectal prolapse should be manually reduced if it fails to reduce spontaneously or is associated with passive congestion and swelling or hemorrhage.[157,158]

Contraindications
Evidence of necrosis of the bowel, strangulation, infection, or bleeding should prompt a surgical consultation (**Box 13**).[158]

Procedure
Consider sedation and position the child prone on the knees. Lubricate gloves and use gauze to hold edges of prolapsed rectum. Apply pressure with both hands on both sides alternating to reduce the prolapse. Afterward, have the child lie on his or her side. A digital rectal exam should be performed to ensure reduction complete. If the prolapse occurs immediately again after reduction the buttocks may be taped together for several hours after subsequent reduction.[157] If the reduction is difficult owing to edema or large size, up to one-half cup of topical table sugar can be applied to the mucosa, which acts as a dessicating agent to help decrease the edema and allow reduction. This may take up to 30 to 90 minutes and can reduce the edema by as much as 50%. Sugar will not irritate the tissue as salt does.[160]

Complications and disposition
Most will reduce without further complications. Patients should be discharged with instructions to avoid straining and constipation by keeping a high-fiber diet, stool softeners, and plenty of hydration.

In some cases there will be some minor bleeding and pain, which is self limited. Follow-up should be arranged with a pediatric gastroenterologist for further workup so as to seek an etiology for the prolapsed rectum.

UROLOGIC PROCEDURES
Suprapubic Bladder Aspiration

Indications
Suprapubic bladder aspiration has been considered the gold standard technique to obtain urine for diagnosis of urinary tract infection in infants and young children up to 2 years old.[161] The bladder in infants extends above the symphysis pubis into the lower abdomen when it is distended and can easily be percussed or palpated. The procedure is most likely to be successful if the bladder is palpable or able to be percussed, or if you see a full bladder on bedside ultrasound. It is more painful than transurethral catheterization; however, there is less contamination. The procedure is faster than transurethral catheterization but less efficient, as a physician needs to do the procedure instead of a nurse.[161]

Box 13	
Equipment for rectal prolapse reduction	
Gloves	Gauze
Lubricant	Sugar

Box 14
Equipment for suprapubic bladder catheterization

Sterile gloves	1.5 cm 22-gauge needle
3-mL syringe	Povidone iodine prep

Contraindications

Organomegaly, congenital abnormalities of the genitourinary or gastrointestinal tract, and volume depletion (and likely empty bladder) are all contraindications.

Procedure

Restrain patient supine in the frog leg position. Prep area to be punctured (approximately 1–2 cm superior to the pubic symphysis) with povidone iodine. Occlude the urethral opening (as the procedure may cause the infant to urinate) by applying pressure to the urethral meatus in girls or gently squeezing the penile urethra in boys. Insert the needle into the abdominal wall at an angle approximately 10 to 20° cephalad. Aspirate and slowly withdraw needle. If no urine is obtained before completely removing the needle from abdominal wall, re-angle more perpendicular to abdomen and attempt again. After the third attempt it is unlikely to be successful. At this point, waiting an hour or 2 for the bladder to fill or performing transurethral catheterization are options to consider.[145] Ultrasound can be used to determine if the bladder is full (**Box 14**).

Complications

Complications can include infection, bowel perforation, and microscopic hematuria (gross hematuria is rare).[145,161]

SUMMARY

When a child needs to undergo a procedure in the ED it can be a high-stress situation, especially in community EDs that see few children. The initial approach to critical procedures in infants and children is the same as with adults, beginning with airway, breathing, and circulation assessments. Differences in anatomy (eg, airway) and physiology (eg, limited ventilator reserve) must be taken into account when performing procedures on infants and children. Restraints should be used when applicable for the safety of the child, and may reduce pain and distress by making the procedure faster and easier for the physician. Alternatives such as distraction can also be considered when age appropriate. Keep in mind the developmental age of the child and involve the parents whenever possible, including explaining emergent procedures, such as intubation if time allows.

REFERENCES

1. Sagarin MJ, Chiang V, Sakles JC, et al. Rapid sequence intubation for pediatric emergency airway management. Pediatr Emerg Care 2002;18:417–23.
2. Brownstein D, Shugerman R, Cummings P, et al. Prehospital endotracheal intubation of children by paramedics. Ann Emerg Med 1996;28:34–9.
3. Gerritse BM, Draaisma JM, Schalkwijk A, et al. Should EMS-paramedics perform paediatric tracheal intubation in the field? Resuscitation 2008;79(2):225–9.
4. Gausche M, Lewis RJ, Stratton SJ, et al. Effect of out-of-hospital pediatric endotracheal intubation on survival and neurological outcome: a controlled clinical trial. JAMA 2000;283:783–90.

5. Fine GF, Borland LM. The future of the cuffed endotracheal tube. Paediatr Anaesth 2004;14:38–42.
6. Kleinman ME, Chameides L, Schexnayder SM, et al. Part 14: pediatric advanced life support: 2010 American Heart Association Guidelines for cardiopulmonary resuscitation and emergency cardiovascular care. Circulation 2010; 122:S876.
7. King BR, Baker MD, Braitman LE, et al. Endotracheal tube selection in children: a comparison of four methods. Ann Emerg Med 1993;22:530–4.
8. Wheeler M, Coté CJ, Todres ID. The pediatric airway. In: Coté C, Lerman J, Todres ID, editors. A practice of anesthesia for infants and children. 4th edition. Philadelphia: Saunders-Elsevier; 2009. p. 237.
9. Schneider RE, Caro DA. Pretreatment agents. In: Walls RM, Murphy MF, editors. Manual of emergency airway management. 2nd edition. Philadelphia: Lippincott, Williams & Wilkins; 2004. p. 183–8.
10. Schenarts CL, Burton JH, Riker RR. Adrenocortical dysfunction following etomidate induction in emergency department patients. Acad Emerg Med 2001;8(1):1–7.
11. Mace SE. Ketamine. In: Mace SE, Ducharme J, Murphy M, editors. Pain management and sedation. New York: McGraw Hill; 2006. p. 132–8.
12. Schneider RE, Caro DA. Neuromuscular blocking agents. In: Walls RW, Murphy MF, editors. Manual of airway management. 2nd edition. Philadelphia: Lippincott, Williams & Wilkins; 2004. p. 200–11.
13. Mace SE. Challenges and advances in intubation: Rapid sequence intubation. Emerg Med Clin North Am 2008;26:1043–68.
14. Mutzbauer TS, Munz R, Helm M, et al. Emergency cricothyrotomy—puncture or anatomical preparation? Peculiarities of two methods for emergency airway access demonstrated in a cadaver model. Anaesthesist 2003;52:304–10 [in German].
15. Sise MJ, Shackford SR, Cruickshank JC, et al. Cricothyroidotomy for long-term tracheal access. A prospective analysis of morbidity and mortality in 76 patients. Ann Surg 1984;200:13–7.
16. Craven RM, Vanner RG. Ventilation of a model lung using various cricothyrotomy devices. Anaesthesia 2004;59:595–9.
17. Chan TC, Vilke GM, Bramwell KJ, et al. Comparison of wire-guided cricothyrotomy versus standard surgical cricothyrotomy technique. J Emerg Med 1999;17:957–62.
18. Christopher NC, Cantor RM. Venous and arterial access. In: Barkin RM, editor. Pediatric medicine: concepts and clinical practice. 2nd edition. St. Louis (MO): Mosby; 1997. p. 153–4.
19. Lipton JD, Schafermeyer RW. Umbilical vessel catheterization. In: Henretig FM, King C, editors. Textbook of pediatric emergency procedures. Baltimore (MD): Williams & Wilkins; 1997. p. 515–23.
20. Green C, Yohannan MD. Umbilical arterial and venous catheters: placement, use, and complications. Neonatal Netw 1998;17(6):23–8.
21. Ribeiro JA, Price CT, Knapp DR Jr. Compartment syndrome of the lower extremity after intraosseous infusion of fluid. A report of two cases. J Bone Joint Surg Am 1993;75(3):430–3.
22. Blumberg S, Gorn M, Crain E. Intraosseous infusion: a review of methods and novel devices. Pediatr Emerg Care 2008;24(1):50–6.
23. Hasan MY, Kissoon N, Khan TM, et al. Intraosseous infusion and pulmonary fat embolism. Pediatr Crit Care Med 2001;2(2):133–8.
24. van Rijn RR, Knoester H, Maes A, et al. Cerebral arterial air embolism in a child after intraosseous infusion. Emerg Radiol 2008;15(4):259–62.

25. Krauss B, Green SM. Procedural sedation and analgesia in children. Lancet 2006;367(9512):766–80.
26. American Academy of Pediatrics, American Academy of Pediatric Dentistry, Coté CJ, et al. Guidelines for monitoring and management of pediatric patients during and after sedation for diagnostic and therapeutic procedures: an update. Pediatrics 2006;118(6):2587–602.
27. Sacchetti A, Schafermeyer R, Geradi M, et al. Pediatric analgesia and sedation. Ann Emerg Med 1994;23(2):237–50.
28. Practice guidelines for preoperative fasting and the use of pharmacologic agents to reduce the risk of pulmonary aspiration: application to healthy patients undergoing elective procedures: a report by the American Society of Anesthesiologist Task Force on Preoperative Fasting. Anesthesiology 1999;90(3):896–905.
29. Sury M, Bullock I, Rabar S, et al. Sedation for diagnostic and therapeutic procedures in children and young people: summary of NICE guidance. BMJ 2010; 341:c6819.
30. Mace SE, Barata IA, Cravero JP, et al. Clinical policy: evidence-based approach to pharmacologic agents used in pediatric sedation and analgesia in the emergency department. Ann Emerg Med 2004;44(4):342–77.
31. Coté CJ. Sedation for the pediatric patient. A review. Pediatr Clin North Am 1994;41(1):31–58.
32. Rockoff MA, Goudsouzian NG. Seizures induced by methohexital. Anesthesiology 1981;54(4):333–5.
33. Green SM, Krauss B. Propofol in emergency medicine: pushing the sedation frontier. Ann Emerg Med 2003;42(6):792–7.
34. Gamis AS, Knapp JF, Glenski JA. Nitrous oxide analgesia in a pediatric emergency department. Ann Emerg Med 1989;18(2):177–81.
35. Hennrikus WL, Simpson RB, Klingelberger CE, et al. Self-administered nitrous oxide analgesia for pediatric fracture reductions. J Pediatr Orthop 1994;14(4): 538–42.
36. Kanagasundaram SA, Lane LJ, Cavalletto BP, et al. Efficacy and safety of nitrous oxide in alleviating pain and anxiety during painful procedures. Arch Dis Child 2001;84(6):492–5.
37. Nakayama DK, Ramenofsky ML, Rowe MI. Chest injuries in children. Ann Surg 1989;210:770–5.
38. Peterson RJ, Tiwary AD, Kissoon N, et al. Pediatric penetrating thoracic trauma: a five-year experience. Pediatr Emerg Care 1994;10(3):129–31.
39. Margau R, Amaral JG, Chait PG, et al. Percutaneous thoracic drainage in neonates: catheter drainage versus treatment with aspiration alone. Radiology 2006;241(1):223–7.
40. Reinhorn M, Kaufman HL, Hirsch EF, et al. Penetrating thoracic injury in a pediatric population. Ann Thorac Surg 1996;61:1501–5.
41. Roux P, Fisher RM. Chest injuries in children: an analysis of 100 cases of blunt chest trauma from motor vehicle accidents. J Pediatr Surg 1992;27:551–5.
42. Bliss D, Silen M. Pediatric thoracic trauma. Crit Care Med 2002;30(Suppl 11): S409–15.
43. Dull KE, Fleisher GR. Pigtail catheters versus large-bore chest tubes for pneumothoraces in children treated in the emergency department. Pediatr Emerg Care 2002;18(4):265–7.
44. MacDuff A, Arnold A, Harvey J. On behalf of the BTS Pleural Disease Guideline Group Management of spontaneous pneumothorax: British Thoracic Society pleural disease guideline 2010. Thorax 2010;65(Suppl 2):ii18–31.

45. Brandler ES, Fontenette D, Stone MB. Needle aspiration of spontaneous pneumothorax. Acad Emerg Med 2010;17:e25–6.
46. Choi SH, Lee SW, Hong YS, et al. Can spontaneous pneumothorax patients be treated by ambulatory care management? Eur J Cardiothorac Surg 2007;32(1): 183.
47. Hassani B, Foote J, Borgundvaag B. Outpatient management of primary spontaneous pneumothorax in the emergency department of a community hospital using a small-bore catheter and a Heimlich valve. Acad Emerg Med 2009;16(6):513–8.
48. Cho S, Lee EB. Management of primary and secondary pneumothorax using a small-bore thoracic catheter. Interact Cardiovasc Thorac Surg 2010;11(2):146–9.
49. Liu CM, Hang LW. Pigtail tube drainage in the treatment of spontaneous pneumothorax. Am J Emerg Med 2003;21(3):241–4.
50. Sistrom CL, Reiheld CT, Gay SB, et al. Detection and estimation of the volume of pneumothorax using real-time sonography: efficacy determined by receiver operating characteristic analysis. AJR Am J Roentgenol 1996;166:317–21.
51. Elia F, Ferrari G, Molino P, et al. Lung ultrasound in postprocedural pneumothorax. Acad Emerg Med 2010;17:e81–2.
52. Lichtenstein DA, Mezière G, Lascols N, et al. Ultrasound diagnosis of occult pneumothorax. Crit Care Med 2005;33:1231–8.
53. Chan SS. Emergency bedside ultrasound to detect pneumothorax. Acad Emerg Med 2003;10:91–4.
54. Stone MB. Ultrasound diagnosis of traumatic pneumothorax. J Emerg Trauma Shock 2008;1(1):19–20.
55. Liang SJ, Tu CY, Chen HJ, et al. Application of ultrasound-guided pigtail catheter for drainage of pleural effusions in the ICU. Intensive Care Med 2009; 35(2):350–4.
56. Volpicelli G. Sonographic diagnosis of pneumothorax. Intensive Care Med 2011; 37(2):224–32.
57. Givens ML, Ayotte K, Manifold C. Needle thoracostomy: implications of computed tomography chest wall thickness. Acad Emerg Med 2004;11(2):211–3.
58. Gaudio M, Hafner JW. Simple aspiration compared to chest tube insertion in the management of primary spontaneous pneumothorax. Ann Emerg Med 2009;54: 458–60.
59. Zehtabchi S, Rios CL. Management of emergency department patients with primary spontaneous pneumothorax: needle aspiration or tube thoracostomy? Ann Emerg Med 2008;51:91–100.
60. Argall J, Desmond J. Seldinger technique chest drains and complication rate. Emerg Med J 2003;20:169–70.
61. Parry GW, Morgan WE, Salama FD. Management of haemothorax. Ann R Coll Surg Engl 1996;78(4):325–6.
62. Roberts JS, Bratton SL, Brogan TV. Efficacy and complications of percutaneous pigtail catheters for thoracostomy in pediatric patients. Chest 1998;114(4): 1116–21.
63. Kulvatunyou N, Vijayasekaran A, Hansen A, et al. Two-year experience of using pigtail catheters to treat traumatic pneumothorax: a changing trend. J Trauma 2011;71(5):1104–7.
64. Gammie J, Banks MC, Fuhrman CR, et al. The pigtail catheter for pleural drainage: a less invasive alternative to tube thoracostomy. JSLS 1999;3(1): 57–61.
65. Lin YC, Tu CY, Liang SJ, et al. Pigtail catheter for the management of pneumothorax in mechanically ventilated patients. Am J Emerg Med 2010;28(4):466–71.

66. Baker MD. Foreign bodies of the ears and nose in childhood. Pediatr Emerg Care 1987;3(2):67–70.

67. Balbani AP, Sanchez TG, Butugan O, et al. Ear and nose foreign body removal in children. Int J Pediatr Otorhinolaryngol 1998;46(1–2):37–48.

68. Ryan C, Ghosh A, Wilson-Boyd B, et al. Presentation and management of aural foreign bodies in two Australian emergency departments. Emerg Med Australas 2006;18(4):372–8.

69. Marin JR, Trainor JL. Foreign body removal from the external auditory canal in a pediatric emergency department. Pediatr Emerg Care 2006;22(9):630–4.

70. Bressler K, Shelton C. Ear foreign-body removal: a review of 98 consecutive cases. Laryngoscope 1993;103(4 Pt 1):367–70.

71. Timm N, Iyer S. Embedded earrings in children. Pediatr Emerg Care 2008;24(1): 31–3.

72. McRae D, Premachandra DJ, Gatland DJ. Button batteries in the ear, nose and cervical esophagus: a destructive foreign body. J Otolaryngol 1989;18(6):317.

73. Schulze SL, Kerschner J, Beste D. Pediatric external auditory canal foreign bodies: a review of 698 cases. Otolaryngol Head Neck Surg 2002;127(1):73–8.

74. DiMuzio J Jr, Deschler DG. Emergency department management of foreign bodies of the external ear canal in children. Otol Neurotol 2002;23(4):473–5.

75. Ansley JF, Cunningham MJ. Treatment of aural foreign bodies in children. Pediatrics 1998;101(4 Pt 1):638–41.

76. Singh GB, Sidhu TS, Sharma A, et al. Management of aural foreign body: an evaluative study in 738 consecutive cases. Am J Otol 2007;28(2):87–90.

77. Benger JR, Davies PH. A useful form of glue ear. J Accid Emerg Med 2000;17: 149–50.

78. Yasny JS, Stewart S. Nasal foreign body: an unexpected discovery. Anesth Prog 2011;58(3):121–3.

79. Kalan A, Tariq M. Foreign bodies in the nasal cavities: a comprehensive review of the aetiology, diagnostic pointers, and therapeutic measures. Postgrad Med J 2000;76(898):484–7.

80. Hadi U, Ghossaini S, Zaytoun G. Rhinolithiasis: a forgotten entity. Otolaryngol Head Neck Surg 2002;126:48–51.

81. Gomes CC, Sakano E, Lucchezi MC, et al. Button battery as a foreign body in the nasal cavities. Special aspects. Rhinology 1994;32(2):98–100.

82. Cheng CC, Fang TJ, Lee LA, et al. Rhinolith from a plastic object in the nasal cavity for more than 20 years. Pediatr Int 2011;53:135–6.

83. Ezsiás A, Sugar AW. Rhinolith: an unusual case and an update. Ann Otol Rhinol Laryngol 1997;106:135–8.

84. Kumar S, Kumar M, Lesser T, et al. Foreign bodies in the ear: a simple technique for removal analysed in vitro. Emerg Med J 2005;22(4):266–8.

85. Leffler S, Cheney P, Tandberg D. Chemical immobilization and killing of intra-aural roaches: an in vitro comparative study. Ann Emerg Med 1993;22(12):1795–8.

86. Brown L, Denmark TK, Wittlake WA, et al. Procedural sedation use in the ED: management of pediatric ear and nose foreign bodies. Am J Emerg Med 2004;22(4):310–4.

87. Dane S, Smally AJ, Peredy TR. A truly emergent problem: button battery in the nose. Acad Emerg Med 2000;7:204–6.

88. Brown CRS. Intra-nasal button battery causing septal perforation: a case report. J Laryngol Otol 1994;108:589–90.

89. Alvi A, Bereliani A, Zahtz GD. Miniature disc battery in the nose: a dangerous foreign body. Clin Pediatr 1997;36:427–9.

90. Royal SA, Gardner RE. Rhinolithiasis: an unusual pediatric nasal mass. Pediatr Radiol 1998;28:54–5.
91. Kiger JR, Brenkert TE, Losek J. Nasal foreign body removal in children. Pediatr Emerg Care 2008;24(11):785–92.
92. Ryan NJ. Removal of nasal foreign bodies using the fogarty catheter. Emerg Med 1996;8:11–3.
93. Purohit N, Ray S, Wilson T, et al. The 'parent's kiss': an effective way to remove paediatric nasal foreign bodies. Ann R Coll Surg Engl 2008;90(5):420–2.
94. Taylor C, Acheson J, Coats TJ. Nasal foreign bodies in children: kissing it better. Emerg Med J 2010;27:712–3.
95. Botma M, Bader R, Kubba H. 'A parent's kiss': evaluating an unusual method for removing nasal foreign bodies in children. J Laryngol Otol 2000;114(8):598–600.
96. Backlin SA. Positive-pressure technique for nasal foreign body removal in children. Ann Emerg Med 1995;25:554–5.
97. Fox J. Fogarty catheter removal of nasal foreign bodies. Ann Emerg Med 1980; 9:37–8.
98. Sorrels WF. Simple noninvasive effective method for removal of nasal foreign bodies in infants and children. Clin Pediatr (Phila) 2002;41(2):133.
99. Nelson LP, Shusterman S. Emergency management of oral trauma in children. Curr Opin Pediatr 1997;9(3):242–5.
100. Wood GD, Leeming KA. Oral and maxillofacial surgery in accident and emergency departments. J Accid Emerg Med 1995;12(4):270–2.
101. Lamell CW, Fraone G, Casamassimo PS, et al. Presenting characteristics and treatment outcomes for tongue lacerations in children. Pediatr Dent 1999;21:34.
102. Ud-din Z, Aslam M, Gull S. Should minor mucosal tongue lacerations be sutured in children? Emerg Med J 2007;24(2):123–4.
103. Mark DG, Granquist EJ. Are prophylactic oral antibiotics indicated for the treatment of intraoral wounds? Ann Emerg Med 2008;52:368.
104. Maguire S, Hunter B, Hunter L, et al. Diagnosing abuse: a systematic review of torn frenulum and other intra-oral injuries. Arch Dis Child 2007;92(12):1113–7.
105. Schutzman SA, Teach S. Upper-extremity impairment in young children. Ann Emerg Med 1995;26:474–9.
106. Schunk J. Radial head subluxation: epidemiology and treatment of 87 episodes. Ann Emerg Med 1990;19(9):1019–23.
107. Salter RB, Zaltz C. Anatomic investigations of the mechanism of injury and pathologic anatomy of "pulled elbow" in young children. Clin Orthop 1971;77: 134–42.
108. Macias CG. Radial head subluxation. Acad Emerg Med 2000;7:207–8.
109. Macias CG, Bothner J, Wiebe R. A comparison of supination/flexion to hyperpronation in the reduction of radial head subluxations. Pediatrics 1998;102(1):e10.
110. McDonald J, Whitelaw C, Goldsmith LJ. Radial head subluxation: comparing two methods of reduction. Acad Emerg Med 1999;6(7):715–8.
111. Green DA, Linares MY, Garcia Peña BM, et al. Randomized comparison of pain perception during radial head subluxation reduction using supination-flexion or forced pronation. Pediatr Emerg Care 2006;22(4):235–8.
112. Bek D, Yildiz C, Köse O, et al. Pronation versus supination maneuvers for the reduction of 'pulled elbow': a randomized clinical trial. Eur J Emerg Med 2009;16(3):135–8.
113. Toupin P, Osmond MH, Correll R, et al. Radial head subluxation: how long do children wait in the emergency department before reduction? CJEM 2007; 9(5):333–7.

114. Jones J, Cote B. "Irreducible" nursemaid's elbow. Am J Emerg Med 1995;13(4): 491.
115. Corellaa F, Hornaa L, Villab JA, et al. Irreducible 'pulled elbow': report of two cases and review of the literature. J Pediatr Orthop 2010;19:304–6.
116. Bondurant CP, Jimenez DF. Epidemiology of cerebrospinal fluid shunting. Pediatr Neurosurg 1995;23:254–8.
117. Wu Y, Green NL, Wrensch MR, et al. Ventriculoperitoneal shunt complications in California: 1990 to 2000. Neurosurgery 2007;61(3):557–62.
118. McGirt MJ, Leveque JC, Wellons JC 3rd, et al. Cerebrospinal fluid shunt survival and etiology of failures: a seven-year institutional experience. Pediatr Neurosurg 2002;36:248–55.
119. Korinek AM, Fulla-Oller L, Boch AL, et al. Morbidity of ventricular cerebrospinal fluid shunt surgery in adults: an 8-year study. Neurosurgery 2011;68(4):985–94.
120. Key CB, Rothrock SG, Falk JL. Cerebrospinal fluid shunt complications: an emergency medicine perspective. Pediatr Emerg Care 1995;11(5):265–73.
121. Liptak GS, McDonald JV. Ventriculoperitoneal shunts in children: Factors affecting shunt survival. Pediatr Neurosci 1985;12:289–93.
122. McGirt MJ, Zaas A, Fuchs HE, et al. Risk factors for pediatric ventriculoperitoneal shunt infection and predictors of infectious pathogens. Clin Infect Dis 2003;36:858–62.
123. Naradzay JFX, Browne BJ, Rolnick MA, et al. Cerebral ventricular shunts. J Emerg Med 1999;17:311–22.
124. Miller J, Fulop SC, Dashti SR, et al. Rethinking the indications for the ventriculoperitoneal shunt tap. J Neurosurg Pediatr 2008;1:435–8.
125. Pople IK. Hydrocephalus and shunts: what the neurologist should know. J Neurol Neurosurg Psychiatr 2002;73(Suppl 1):i17–22.
126. Lan CC, Wong TT, Chen SJ, et al. Early diagnosis of ventriculoperitoneal shunt infections and malfunctions in children with hydrocephalus. J Microbiol Immunol Infect 2003;36(1):47–50.
127. Noetzel MJ, Baker RP. Shunt fluid examination: risks and benefits in the evaluation of shunt malfunction and infection. J Neurosurg 1984;61:328–32.
128. Maartens NF, Aurorab P, Richards PG. An unusual complication of tapping a ventriculoperitoneal shunt. Europ J Paediatr Neurol 2000;4(3):125–9.
129. Tunkel AR, Hartman BJ, Kaplan SL, et al. Practice guidelines for the management of bacterial meningitis. Clin Infect Dis 2004;39(9):1267–84.
130. Nakagawa K, Smith WS. Evaluation and management of increased intracranial pressure. Continuum (Minneap Minn) 2011;17(5):1077–93.
131. Oliver WJ, Shope TC, Kuhns LR. Fatal lumbar puncture: fact versus fiction—an approach to a clinical dilemma. Pediatrics 2003;112(3 Pt 1):e174–6.
132. López T, Sánchez FJ, Garzón JC, et al. Spinal anesthesia in pediatric patients. Minerva Anestesiol 2012;78(1):78–87.
133. Abo A, Chen L, Johnston P, et al. Positioning for lumbar puncture in children evaluated by bedside ultrasound. Pediatrics 2010;125(5):e1149–53.
134. Rodriques AM, Roy PM. Post-lumbar puncture headache. Rev Prat 2007;57(4): 353–7.
135. Kaur G, Gupta P, Kumar A. A randomized trial of eutectic mixture of local anesthetics during lumbar puncture in newborns. Arch Pediatr Adolesc Med 2003; 157(11):1065–70.
136. Carriaccio C, Feinberg P, Hart LS, et al. Lidocaine for lumbar punctures, a help not a hindrance. Arch Pediatr Adolesc Med 1996;150(10):1044–6.

137. Apiliogullari S, Duman A, Gok F, et al. Spinal needle design and size affect the incidence of postdural puncture headache in children. Paediatr Anaesth 2011; 20(2):177–82.

138. Kokki H, Hendolin H, Turunen M. Postdural puncture headache and transient neurologic symptoms in children after spinal anaesthesia using cutting and pencil point paediatric spinal needles. Acta Anaesthesiol Scand 1998;42(9):1076–82.

139. Friedman JN, Ahmed S, Connolly B, et al. Complications associated with image-guided gastrostomy and gastrojejunostomy tubes in children. Pediatrics 2004; 114(2):458–61.

140. Saavedra H, Losek JD, Shanley L, et al. Gastrostomy tube-related complaints in the pediatric emergency department: identifying opportunities for improvement. Pediatr Emerg Care 2009;25(11):728–32.

141. Wollman B, D'Agostino HB, Walus-Wigle JR, et al. Radiologic, endoscopic, and surgical gastrostomy: an institutional evaluation and meta-analysis of the literature. Radiology 1995;197(3):699–704.

142. Minchff TV. Early dislodgement of percutaneous and endoscopic gastrostomy tube. J S C Med Assoc 2007;103:13–5.

143. Kadakia SC, Cassaday M, Shaffer RT. Prospective evaluation of Foley catheter as a replacement gastrostomy tube. Am J Gastroenterol 1992;87(11):1594–7.

144. Burke DT, El Shami A, Heinle E, et al. Comparison of gastrostomy tube replacement verification using air insufflation versus gastrograffin. Arch Phys Med Rehabil 2006;87(11):1530–3.

145. Ruddy RM. Illustrated techniques of pediatric emergency procedures. In: Fleisher GR, Ludwig S, Henretig FM, editors. Textbook of pediatric emergency medicine. 5th edition. Philadelphia: Lippincott Williams and Wilkins. 1861–955.

146. Kenigsberg K, Levenbrown J. Esophageal perforation secondary to gastrostomy tube replacement. J Pediatr Surg 1986;21(11):946–7.

147. Whiteley S, Liu P, Tellez DW, et al. Esophageal rupture in an infant secondary to esophageal placement of a Foley catheter gastrostomy tube. Pediatr Emerg Care 1989;5(2):113–6.

148. Showalter CD, Kerrey B, Spellman-Kennebeck S, et al. Gastrostomy tube replacement in a pediatric ED: frequency of complications and impact of confirmatory imaging. Am J Emerg Med 2012;30(8):1501–6.

149. Brandt ML. Pediatric hernias. Surg Clin North Am 2008;88(1):27–43, vii–viii.

150. Skinner MA, Grosfield JL. Inguinal and umbilical hernia repair in infants and children. Surg Clin North Am 1993;73(3):439–49.

151. Zamakhshary M, To T, Guan J, et al. Risk of incarceration of inguinal hernia among infants and young children awaiting elective surgery. CMAJ 2008; 179(10):1001–5.

152. Kaya M, Huckstead T, Schier F. Laparascopic approach to incarcerated inguinal hernia in children. J Pediatr Surg 2006;41:567–9.

153. Bradley M, Morgan D, Pentlow B, et al. The groin hernia—an ultrasound diagnosis? Ann R Coll Surg Engl 2003;85(3):178–80.

154. Jamadar DA, Jacobson JA, Morag Y, et al. Sonography of inguinal region hernias. Am J Roentgenol 2006;187(1):185–90.

155. Waseem M, Pinkert H, Devas G. Testicular infarction becoming apparent after hernia reduction. J Emerg Med 2010;38(4):460–2.

156. Zganjer M, Cizmic A, Cigit I, et al. Treatment of rectal prolapse in children with cow milk injection sclerotherapy: 30-year experience. World J Gastroenterol 2008;14(5):737–40.

157. Siafakas C, Vottler TP, Anderson JM. Rectal prolapse in pediatrics. Clin Pediatr 1999;38(2):63.
158. Goldstein SD, Maxwell PJ 4th. Rectal prolapse. Clin Colon Rectal Surg 2011; 24(1):39–45.
159. Ibrahim AI. Prolapsed ileocolic intussusception. Ann Pediatr Surg 2011;7:76–8.
160. Coburn WM, Russell MA, Hofstetter WL. Sucrose as an aid to manual reduction of incarcerated rectal prolapse. Ann Emerg Med 1997;30(3):347.
161. Pollack CV, Pollack ES, Andrew WE. Suprapubic bladder aspiration versus urethral catheterization in ill infants: success, efficacy and complication rates. Ann Emerg Med 1994;23(2):225.

Index

Note: Page numbers of article titles are in **boldface** type.

A

Abdominal trauma, blunt, fluid evaluation in, 311
    focused sonography for examination in, 312–313
Abscess drainage, ultrasound-guided, 140–143
Adenosine, 189
Airway, management of, decision making for, 1–3
  pediatric, anatomic principles of, 336
    difficult, approach to, 338–339
    management of, 336–339
      medications used in, 337
      noninvasive, 336
    rapid sequence intubation of, 336–338
Airway procedures, bridging adjuncts for, 3–5
  in difficult airways, 16–17
  in failed airways, 17–19
Airway skills and procedures, critical, **1–18**
Anesthesia, nasal, 45–46
    field blocks in, 47, 48
Ankle, dislocation of, 282–283
Ankle splint, posterior, 273
Antiarrhythmic medications, 188
Arrhythmias, asystole of PEA arrest, treatment of, 196
  specific therapies in, 185–186, 189
Arterial access and catheterization, 78–83
Arthrocentesis, 261–269
  contraindications to, 265
  indications for, 264
  of elbow joint, 263, 267
  of knee joint, 264, 268
  of shoulder joint, 262, 266–267
  patient preparation for, 265–266
  ultrasound-guided, 129
Auricle, and ear canal, anatomy of, 29, 30
    compression dressing and ear bolster after, 34–35, 36
    field blocks of, 30, 31
    hematoma of, 31–34, 35

B

Bag-valve mask ventilation, technique for, 3, 4
Bartholin abscess, 227–228
Basilic veins, 326

Emerg Med Clin N Am 31 (2013) 377–385
http://dx.doi.org/10.1016/S0733-8627(12)00108-3
0733-8627/13/$ – see front matter © 2013 Elsevier Inc. All rights reserved.

emed.theclinics.com

Bladder aspiration, suprapubic, in pediatric patients, 367–368
Bones, long, anatomy and physiology of, 73
Brachial plexus block, interscalene approach to, 111–113
Breech presentation, 217–219

C

Cardiac pacing, emergent, 157–167
    complications of, 166
    contraindicators to, 160
    indicators for, 159
Cardiac tamponade, symptoms and signs of, 152
Cardiovascular skills and procedures, critical, in emergency department, **151–206**
Cardioversion, and defibrillation, analgesia/sedation for, 192, 195
    in emergency department, 189–195
    steps in, 192, 194
  contraindications to, 191
  electrical, synchronized, indications for, 190, 191
Cardioverter-defibrillator, implantable, chest radiograph of, 174
    complications of, 169–171, 172, 174–176
    discharge of, management of, 177–178, 179
    dysfunction of, symptoms of, 172
    management of, 167–174
    placement of, indicators for, 170
Catheter(s), central venous, placement of, 69–71
     ultrasound for, 69
  pacing, 160, 162
  peripheral venous, placement of, 60–62
  pigtail equipment, 348
Cavernosal aspiration, 246–248
Central nervous system, access to, indications for, and contraindications to, 67–68
    procedure for, 68–69
  procedures in pediatric patients, 359–364
Central venous access, ultrasound-guided, 93
    indications for, 94
Central venous system, anatomy and physiology of, 64–65
Cephalic veins, 326
Cerebrospinal fluid shunt valves, 359, 360
Cesarean section, perimortem, 224–227
Cricothyroidotomy approach, open, 17, 18
Cricothyrotomy, 296–298, 299, 300
  contraindications to, 296
  open, technique of, steps in, 297, 298, 299
  Seldinger technique for, 298–299
Culdocentesis, 232–234

D

Defibrillation, and cardioversion, contraindications to, 192
    in emergency department, 189–195
  indications for, 191
Dorsal slit, 248–250

E

Ear, anesthesia of, 30, 31
  cerumen impaction of, 35–37, 38
  foreign body removal from, 37–40, 350–352
  lacerations of, 30–31, 32, 33
Ear canal, and auricle, anatomy of, 29, 30
    compression dressing and ear bolster after hematoma removal, 34–35, 36
Elbow, anterior recess of, 132
  posterior fossa of, 132, 133
Elbow joint, arthrocentesis of, 263, 267
  dislocation of, 277–278
Elbow splint, 273
Endotracheal intubation, backup devices for, 11–13
  backup procedures in, 14
  equipment for, 6–8, 9
  indications for, 5–6, 296
  postintubation procedures in, 11
  preplanning for, 6
  technique of, 8–11
ENT skills and procedures, critical, in emergency department, **29–58**
Episiotomy, 213–215
Epistaxis, 41–42
  direct pressure in, 42–43
  nasal packing in, 43–45
  silver nitrate cauterization in, 43
Etomidate, for rapid sequence intubation, 15

F

Fasciotomy, for acute limb compartment syndrome, 322–323, 325
Femoral nerve block, indications for, 105
  pitfall of, 107
  survey scan for, 105–106, 107
Femoral vein, anatomy of, 67
  special considerations for, 67
Focused sonography, diagnostic peritoneal lavage versus, for trauma, 307–308
Foreign body removal, from ear, 37–40, 350–352
  from nose, 352–355
  in pediatric patients, 349–355
  ultrasound-guided, 143–145
Fractures, management of, 269–272, 273

G

Gastrointestinal procedures, in pediatric patients, 364–367
Gastrostomy tube replacement, in pediatric patients, 364–365
Genital trauma, 228
Gynecologic procedures, 227–228
  and obstetric procedures, critical, in emergency department, **207–236**

H

Hematoma, of auricle, 31–34, 35
    of nasal septum, 48–50
        incision and drainage of, 49–50
    vulvar, 228
Hemorrhage, postpartum, 219–220
    posttonsillectomy, 53–54
Hip, dislocation of, 278–280
Hypothermia, induced, exclusion criteria for, 198, 199

I

Inguinal hernia, incarcerated, reduction of, in pediatric patients, 365–366
Intraosseous access, 72
    infusions and medications for, 75–77
    procedure for, 73–75

J

Joint dislocations, complications of, 283
        reduction of, 272–283
Jugular vein, internal, anatomy of, 65–66
            and imaging of, 94–95
        imaging of, pitfalls of, 99–100
            techniques for, 95–99
        special considerations for, 66

K

Ketamine, for rapid sequence intubation, 15–16
King laryngeal tube, 13
Knee, effusion of, 129–132
Knee joint, arthrocentesis of, 264, 268
    dislocation of, 280–282

L

Laryngeal mask airway, 12–13
LEMON, 3
Leopold maneuvers, 209, 211
Limb compartment syndrome, acute, 283–288, 313–323, 324
        causes of, 319
        complications of, 321–322
        diagnosis of, 315
        fasciotomy for, 322–323, 325
        needle-manometer technique in, 284, 285, 287, 320–321, 323, 324
        pressure interpretation in, 287–288
        pressure measurements in, 285, 286, 320
        procedure technique in, 317–320
        symptoms and signs of, 319

Lumbar puncture, in children, 362
    complications of, 363–364
    contraindications to, 362–363
    monitoring in, 364
    technique of, 363
  ultrasound-guided, 134–139, 140, 141

M

Mechanical ventilation, 19, 20
  postventilation sedation in, 19, 20
MOANS, 2

N

Nasal septum, hematoma of, 48–50
    incision and drainage of, 49–50
Neck, anatomy and physical examination of, 50–53
Nerve block technique, 105
Nerve blocks, general pitfalls of, 113–114
  ultrasound-guided, 104–105
Nose, 40
  anatomy of, 40–41
  anesthesia of, 45–47, 48
  foreign body removal from, 352–355
  physical examination of, 41
Nursemaid's elbow, reduction of, 357

O

Obstetric procedures, and gynecologic procedures, critical, in emergency department,
  207–236
  breech presentation and, 217–219
  emergent vaginal delivery, 209–215
  labor and, 207–209
  vaginal lacerations, in complicated delivery, 215–216
Oral lacerations, in pediatric patients, 355–357
Orthopedic injuries, common, and splints, 270
Orthopedic procedures, in pediatric patients, 357–358
Orthopedic skills and procedures, critical, **261–290**

P

Pacemaker, implantable, 167, 170
    complications of, approach to patient with, 169–171, 172, 174–177
      chest radiograph of, 174, 175
    dysfunction of, symptoms of, 172
    management of, 167–175
    nomenclature, 167, 171
    placement of, indications for, 167, 169
    sudden cardiac arrest and, 178

Pacing catheter, 160, 162
Pacing generator, 159–160, 161
Paracentesis, ultrasound-guided, 123
        indications for, 123–124
        pitfalls of, 128
        technique of, 126–128
Paralytics, for rapid sequence intubation, 16
Paraphimosis, reduction of, 250–252
Pediatric emergency medicine, critical procedures in, **335–376**
Penile nerve block, dorsal, 244–246
Penis, fractured, 252–253
Pericardiocentesis, blind subxyphoid approach to, 154, 155
    emergent, 151–157
        complications of, 158
        equipment for, 154
    ultrasound-guided, 117–123
        pitfalls of, 121–123
        technique of, 119–120, 121, 122
Pericardium, anatomy of, 118
    normal, 156
Peripheral venous access, ultrasound-guided, 100–104
        anatomy and imaging in, 100–101, 102
        indications for, 100
        pitfalls of, 103–104
        technique of, 101–103
Peritoneal lavage, diagnostic, pitfalls and suggestions for, 313, 314, 315, 316, 317, 318
        procedure for, closed, 310–311
            open, 131, 309–310, 312
            semiopen, 308–309
        versus focused sonography for trauma, 307–308
Peritonsilar abscess, 51–52
    complications of, 54
    drainaage of, 52–53
Phimosis, 248–250
Placenta, delivery of, 213
Pleural cavity, anatomy of, 124–126
Posttonsillectomy hemorrhage, 53–54
Priapism, 246, 247, 248
Pulse generator/defibrillator, portable, 160, 163
Pulsus paradoxus, 152, 153

R

Rapid sequence intubation, 14–16
Rectal prolapse, in pediatric patients, 366–367
Ritgen maneuver, 210, 211

S

Saline, agitated, 157
Sciatic nerve block, distal, at popliteal fossa, 108

survey scan for, 108–110
   technique of, 110–111
Sedation, and analgesia, medications used in, 342, 344–345
   procedural, for children, 339–342
Seldinger cricothyroidotomy approach, 17, 18
Shapenous veins, 328
Shoulder dystocia, management of, 222–223
Shoulder joint, arthrocentesis of, 262, 266–267
   dislocation of, 274–277
Skills annd procedures, critical, in emergency medicine, **59–86**
Spinal tap, in children. See *Lumbar puncture, in children*.
Splinting, complications of, 274
   techniques of, 270–272, 273
Splints, and common orthopedic injuries, 270
Subclavian vein, anatomy of, 66
   special considerations for, 66–67
Sudden cardiac arrest, 178
Suprapubic catheterization, 240–242
Synovial fluid analysis, 268–269

T

Tachyarrhythmias, in children, 185
   management of, in emergency department, 179–185
   vagal maneuvers in, 185, 189
Tachycardia(s), narrow complex, 180–183, 184
   QT interval, drugs known to prolong, 184–185, 187
   ventricular, and ventricular fibrillation, pulseless, treatment of, 197
   wide complex, 184–185, 186, 187
Testicular torsion, 242–243, 244
Thoracentesis, ultrasound-guided, 123–128
    indications for, 123–124
    pitfalls of, 128
    technique of, 126–128
Thoracostomy, chest tube, 299–305
    blunt dissection technique for, 302–303
    chest tube management in, 304–305
    complications of, 302, 305
    equipment for, 301, 302
    guidewire (Seldinger) technique for, 303–304
    preprocedural evaluation for, 300
   in emergency department, 305–307
   needle, in pediatric patients, 343, 346
   procedures in pediatric patients, 342–349
   tube, in pediatric patients, 343–349
Thumb spica splint, 272
Tracheotomies, permanent, in pediatric patients, 339
Transcutaneous pacing, 157, 163
Transvenous pacing, equipment for, 157, 161
   steps in, 163–165
Trauma patients, disposition of, 296

Trauma (*continued*)
    initial evaluation of, 291
    injuries of, physical examination for identification of, 295
    prehospital management of, 292
    primary survey of, 292–294
    secondary survey of, 294–296
Trauma skills and procedures, critical, in emergency department, **291–334**

    U

Ulnar gutter splint, 271
Ultrasound, for placement of central venous catheters, 69
    physics principles of, and instrumentation, 88–89
    procedural, artifacts in, 91–93
        background of, 87–88
        image orientation for, 89–90, 91
        imaging modalities for, 90–91
        probe selection for, 88–89
Ultrasound-guided arthrocentesis, 129
Ultrasound-guided central venous access, 93
    indications for, 94
Ultrasound-guided nerve blocks, 104–105
Ultrasound-guided paracentesis. See *Paracentesis, ultrasound-guided.*
Ultrasound-guided pericardiocentesis, 117–123
Ultrasound-guided peripheral venous access. See *Peripheral venous access, ultrasound-guided.*
Ultrasound-guided procedures, in emergency department, **87–115, 117–149**
Ultrasound-guided thoracentesis. See *Thoracentesis, ultrasound-guided.*
Umbilical cord, entanglement of, 211–212, 224
    prolapse of, 223–224
Umbilical stump, anatomy and physiology of, 77
Umbilical vessel access, 77–78
Urethral catheterization, 217–240
Urinary retention, acute, 237–238
Urologic problems, common, management of, 253–254
Urologic procedures, complications of, 254
    in pediatric patients, 367–368
Urologic skills and procedures, critical, in emergency department, **237–260**
Uterine atomy, 220–221
Uterine inversion, 221–222

    V

Vascular access, in children, 339, 340
Vasopressors, in postresuscitative care, 198
Venous access, peripheral, skills and procedures for, 60–63, 64
Venous cutdown, 325–331
    clinical examples of, 326
    complications of, 328
    equipment for, 327
    peripheral, 62–63, 64

technique of, 325–328, 329–330, 331
Ventricular fibrillation, and ventricular tachycardias, pulseless, treatment of, 197
Ventricular shunt, in children, diagnostic tap of, 361–362
    evaluation of, 359–360
Ventriculoperitoneal shunt system, 359, 360
Volar splint, 272
Vulnar and vaginal laceration, 230–232
Vulvar hematoma, 228–229

EmergencyMed **Advance**

All the latest emergency medicine news and research you need, all in one place

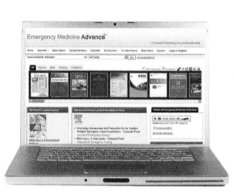

EmergencyMedAdvance.com is a new essential online resource offering valued high-quality content and news for the global community of Emergency Medicine professionals to save time and stay current—from physicians and nurses to EMTs.

Stay current
• Emergency Medicine news

• Upcoming meetings and events

Save time
• Access relevant articles in press from 16 participating journals

• Search across 500+ health sciences journals
• Learn how to submit a manuscript

And more...
• Journals' profiles
• Personalized search results
• Emergency Medicine bookstore

• Sign up for free e-Alerts
• Emergency Medicine jobs

Bookmark us today at
EmergencyMedAdvance.com